ADVANCES IN HOST DEFENSE MECHANISMS
Volume 9

Mucosal Immunology:
Intraepithelial Lymphocytes

ADVANCES IN HOST DEFENSE MECHANISMS

Advances in Host Defense Mechanisms
Volume 9

Mucosal Immunology: Intraepithelial Lymphocytes

Editors

Hiroshi Kiyono, D.D.S., Ph.D.

Jerry R. McGhee, Ph.D.

Immunobiology Vaccine Center

University of Alabama at Birmingham

Birmingham, Alabama

Raven Press New York

Raven Press, Ltd., 1185 Avenue of the Americas, New York, New York 10036

Made in the United States of America

Library of Congress Cataloging-in-Publication Data

Mucosal immunology : intraepithelial lymphocytes (IEL) / editors,
  Hiroshi Kiyono, Jerry R. McGhee.
      p.   cm. —(Advances in host defense mechanism ; v. 9)
    Includes bibiographical references and index.
    ISBN 0-7817-0117-1
    1. T cells.   2. Intestinal mucosa—Immunology.   3. Cytokines.
  4. Immune reponse—Regulation.   I. Kiyono, H. (Hiroshi)
  II. McGhee, Jerry R.   III. Series
      [DNLM: 1. Intestinal Mucosa—immunology.   2. T-Lymphocyte Subsets—
    immunology.   W1 AD636 v.9 1994 / WI 402 M942 1994]
QR185.8.T2M83   1994
616.07′9—dc20
DNLM/DLC
for Library of Congress   93-34356
                                                                                        CIP

ISBN: 0-7817-0117-1

9 8 7 6 5 4 3 2 1

To Momoyo Kiyono,
Erika Kiyono,
Mary-Lou McGhee,
Jerry R. McGhee, Jr., and
Dr. Kimberley K. McGhee

Contents

Contributors

Terrence A. Barrett, M.D.
Assistant Professor
Department of Medicine
Northwestern University Medical School
Chicago, Illinois

Jeffrey A. Bluestone, Ph.D.
Professor
Department of Pathology
University of Chicago
Chicago, Illinois

Marc Bonneville, D.V.M.
CNRS Researcher
Department of Immunology
Institut de Biologie
Nantes, France

Per Brandtzaeg, Ph.D.
Professor and Chairman
Institute of Pathology
Head, Laboratory for
*   Immunohistochemistry and*
*   Immunopathology (LIIPAT)*
The National Hospital
University of Oslo
Oslo, Norway

R. Pat Bucy, M.D., Ph.D.
Associate Professor
Departments of Pathology, Microbiology
*   and Medicine*
University of Alabama at Birmingham
Birmingham, Alabama

Chen-lo H. Chen, Ph.D.
Research Associate Professor
Division of Developmental and Clinical
*   Immunology*
Department of Microbiology
University of Alabama at Birmingham
Birmingham, Alabama

Max D. Cooper, M.D.
Professor of Medicine, Pediatrics and
*   Microbiology*
Director, Division of Developmental and
*   Clinical Immunology*
University of Alabama at Birmingham
Birmingham, Alabama

Kenneth Croitoru, M.D.C.M.
Assistant Professor
Department of Medicine
McMaster University
Hamilton, Ontario, Canada

Christopher Cuff, Ph.D.
Assistant Professor
Department of Microbiology and
*   Immunology*
West Virginia University School of
*   Medicine*
Morgantown, West Virginia

Erastus C. Dudley
Section of Immunobiology and Howard
*   Hughes Medical Institute*
Yale University School of Medicine
New Haven, Connecticut

Ellen C. Ebert, M.D.
Associate Professor of Medicine
Department of Medicine
Division of Gastroenterology
University of Medicine and Dentistry of
*   New Jersey*
Robert Wood Johnson Medical School
New Brunswick, New Jersey

Peter B. Ernst, D.V.M., Ph.D.
Associate Professor
Department of Pediatrics
University of Texas Medical Branch
Children's Hospital
Galveston, Texas

Kohtaro Fujihashi, D.D.S.
Research Instructor
Department of Oral Biology
University of Alabama at Birmingham
Birmingham, Alabama

Thomas W. F. Göbel, D.V.M.
Postdoctoral Fellow
Division of Developmental and Clinical
* Immunology*
University of Alabama at Birmingham
Birmingham, Alabama

Delphine Guy-Grand, M.D.
Directeur de Recherche INSERM
UNITE INSERM U132
Hôpital des Enfants-Malades
Paris, France

Trond S. Halstensen, M.D., Ph.D.
Department of Environmental Medicine
National Institute of Public Health
Oslo, Norway

Adrian C. Hayday, Ph.D.
Associate Professor
Department of Biology
Yale University
New Haven, Connecticut

Stephen D. Hurst, B.A., M.S.
Graduate Student
Departments of Microbiology and
* Immunology*
Northwestern University
Chicago, Illinois

Yoshihito Kasahara, M.D.
Postdoctoral Fellow
Department of Microbiology
University of Alabama at Birmingham
Birmingham, Alabama

Hiroshi Kiyono, D.D.S., Ph.D.
Professor of Dentistry
Co-Director, Immunobiology Vaccine
* Center*
Department of Oral Biology
University of Alabama at Birmingham
Birmingham, Alabama

John R. Klein, Ph.D.
Associate Professor of Immunology
Department of Biological Science
University of Tulsa
Tulsa, Oklahoma

Ann M. Koons, B.S.B.
Lab Technician I
Department of Medicine
Section of Gastroenterology
Northwestern University
Chicago, Illinois

Leo Lefrançois, Ph.D.
Associate Professor
Department of Medicine, Division of
* Rheumatic Diseases*
University of Connecticut Health Center
Farmington, Connecticut

Thomas T. MacDonald, BSc.,
MRCPath.
Professor
Department of Paediatric
* Gastroenterology*
The Medical College of St. Bartholomew's
* Hospital*
London, England

Jerry R. McGhee, Ph.D.
Professor of Microbiology
Director, Immunobiology Vaccine Center
University of Alabama at Birmingham
Birmingham, Alabama

R. Lee Mosley, Ph.D.
Research Fellow
Department of Pathology and
* Experimental Toxicology*
University of Michigan Medical School
Ann Arbor, Michigan

Scott J. Roberts
*Section of Immunobiology and Howard
    Hughes Medical Institute
Yale University School of Medicine
New Haven, Connecticut*

Benedita Rocha, M.D., Ph.D.
*Directeur de Recherche, CNRS
UNITE INSERM
Faculté Necker
Paris, France*

Jo Spencer, Ph.D.
*Professor
Department of Histopathology
University College and Middlesex School
    of Medicine
London, England*

Warren Strober, M.D.
*Deputy Director, Division of Intramural
    Research
Chief, Mucosal Immunity Section
Laboratory of Clinical Investigations
National Institute of Allergy and Infectious
    Diseases
National Institute of Health
Bethesda, Maryland*

Pierre Vassalli, M.D., Ph.D.
*Professor
Département de Pathologie
Centre Médical Universitaire
Geneve, Switzerland*

Masafumi Yamamoto, D.D.S.
*Postdoctoral Fellow
Department of Oral Biology
University of Alabama at Birmingham
Birmingham, Alabama*

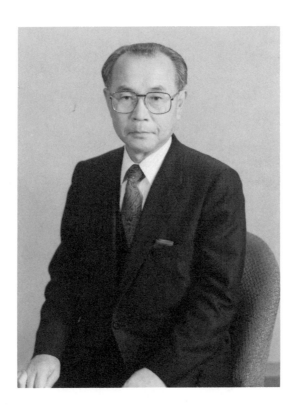

In Memoriam

During the planning and preparation of this book, my father, Dr. Seichi Kiyono, unexpectedly died on June 7, 1992, in Hotaka, Matsumoto, Japan. Since 1951 until his death, he was an anesthesiologist, academician, researcher, and administrator at Shinshyu University, Faculty of Medicine, in Matsumoto, Japan. Although he was a hard-working and dedicated physician, he also knew how to enjoy his life and family. His commitment to clinical science and the academic setting, as well as his personal life style, influenced me to make my career in the basic health sciences in the academic setting. Although we worked in different areas—my father spent his career in anesthesiology while my interest has been in the area of immunology—we had always a common background as health scientists. I will never forget that my father always said, "medicine equals human being": in Japanese, "Hito nakushite i wa nashi." He taught me that we can never forget that our research is for human-kind. I would like to share some of the accomplishments in his life:

1950	M.D.	Matsumoto Medical School
1957	D.M.Sc.	Shinshyu University, Matsumoto College of Medicine
1957–1960	Resident	Department of Anesthesiology, Rhode Island Hospital
1960	Assistant Professor	Shinshyu University, School of Medicine
1963	Associate Professor	Same as above
1967–1992	Professor and Chairman	Department of Anesthesiology, Shinshyu University
1986–1988	Chief of Staff	Shinshyu University Hospital
1988–1990	Dean	Shinshyu University School of Medicine
1990	President	Japanese Society of Anesthesiology
1992	Director	Nagano Cancer Institute
1992	Emperor's Medal (Kun-nitto)	Tokyo, Japan

Although I could not show this book to my father, I dedicate it to him.

Hiroshi Kiyono
At the first anniversary of my father's death.
Matsumoto–Birmingham

Preface

The immune system of the host is continuously exposed to numerous environmental antigens via the mucosa and the skin. The total surface area of the former site is at least 200 times larger than skin, and it is comparable to the surface area of a basketball court. Among these mucosal surface areas, approximately 80 percent is represented by the intestine in humans. Since intraepithelial lymphocytes (IELs) reside in these large epithelial areas, one must realize that large numbers of lymphocytes, especially T cells, occur at the mucosal surface barrier. Thus, it is important to elucidate the origin and immunobiological functions of IELs. Since IELs were discovered in the mid-1800s, a significant number of papers have been published that suggest several possible functions and origins of these lymphocytes residing in the intestinal epithelium. A turning point in IEL research was the discovery in the late 1980s of high numbers of $\gamma\delta$ TCR$^+$ T cells in murine IELs. Since then, the most updated cellular and molecular biological concepts and approaches have been put forth to understand the precise nature of IELs, including their origin, development, and immunological function. This book is the first to devote entire chapters to the most current view of IELs and their role in mucosal immunology. The book will enhance knowledge of IELs and help both basic health and clinical scientists, as well as students, who are interested in the area of mucosal immunology.

The Editors
Summer, 1993
Birmingham, Alabama

Acknowledgments

We thank our expert contributors who have provided a most comprehensive and modern view of IELs. We thank Debra Clisby for her help in collecting and organizing the individual chapters. We would like to express our appreciation to Raven Press who provided us with the opportunity to put together this important book. Finally, I would like to express my appreciation to the co-editor, my former mentor, my long-term collaborator and friend, Dr. Jerry R. McGhee, as well as the individual contributors who allowed me to dedicate this book to my late father, Dr. Seichi Kiyono.

ADVANCES IN HOST DEFENSE MECHANISMS
Volume 9

Mucosal Immunology:
Intraepithelial Lymphocytes

Mucosal Immunology: Intraepithelial Lymphocytes,
edited by H. Kiyono and J. R. McGhee.
Raven Press, Ltd., New York © 1993.

1

T Cell and Cytokine Regulation of Mucosal Antibody Responses with Emphasis on Intraepithelial Lymphocytes Helper Functions

Jerry R. McGhee, Warren Strober*, Kohtaro Fujihashi, and Hiroshi Kiyono

*Departments of Microbiology and Oral Biology, The Mucosal Immunization Research Group, Immunobiology Vaccine Center, University of Alabama at Birmingham, Medical Center, UAB Station, Birmingham, AL and *Mucosal Immunity Section, Laboratory of Clinical Investigation, National Institute of Allergy and Infectious Diseases, NIH, Bethesda, MD.*

We have known for 20 years now that IgA responses are highly T helper (Th) cell dependent, and this knowledge largely stemmed from early studies in athymic, nude mice; neonatally thymectomized mice, rats, or rabbits; or from patients with immunodeficiencies. For example, nude mice have deficient levels of serum IgA as well as IgG subclasses, while IgM levels are normal or even elevated (1,2). Subsequent studies showed that both serum IgA and intestinal IgA plasma cells were deficient in nude mice (3). Furthermore, neonatal thymectomy led to depressed levels of IgA in serum and in external secretions as well as diminished secretory IgA (S-IgA) responses (4,5). Finally, it was shown that patients with ataxia telangiecstasia often showed complex B and T cell abnormalities that resulted in IgA deficiency (6), and some work has shown that T cell abnormalities occur in IgA deficient subjects (7). However, this has not been a universal finding, and a deficiency in Th cells alone does not explain this defect.

It is now generally accepted that the mucosal immune system can be anatomically and functionally divided into two separate but interconnected compartments. Mucosal inductive sites include the gut-associated and nasal-associated lymphoreticular tissues (GALT and NALT), which are strategically placed in the gastrointestinal (GI) tract and the nasopharyngeal area (tonsils), where they encounter environmental antigens. Several studies have now shown that stimulation of Th cells and IgA precursor B cells in GALT, and most especially in the Peyer's patches (PP), with orally administered antigens leads to the dissemination of B and Th cells to mucosal effector tissues, such as the lamina propria (LP) of the GI and upper respiratory tracts (URT), and to secretory glands for subsequent antigen-specific S-IgA antibody responses (reviewed in 8). These mucosal effector tissues share several characteristics: (a) they consist mainly of T cells, and the predominant types are CD4[+] memory/effector T cells; (b) they are also enriched for B cells and plasma cells, mainly of the IgA isotype; and (c) they are covered by epithelial cells, which produce the polymeric Ig (pIg) receptor secretory component (SC) that transports pIgA (and pIgM) into the external secretions as S-IgA. The induction of immune B and Th cells in GALT (or PP) followed by their migration to effector sites for the development of mucosal immune responses is termed the *Common Mucosal Immune System* (CMIS) (8). It remains premature to consider intraepithelial lymphocytes (IELs) as a mucosal effector compartment site until we gain a better understanding of IEL functions; however, we discuss below recent experiments that suggest that certain IEL T cell subsets exhibit helper T cell functions. Approximately one-third (or more) of IEL T cells express the Lyt-2/Lyt-3 (α/β) phenotype of CD8, which suggests thymic development. Further, approximately 40 to 50% of IELs express the α/β form of TCR and are thought to be the progeny of blasts that proliferate and migrate from the thymus to PP and then to the intestinal epithelium (9,10). Thus, certain IEL T cell subsets of thymic origin that are stimulated in PP may migrate to the epithelium and exhibit effector functions in mucosal immunity.

In this chapter, we emphasize the general characteristics of Th cells in GALT and derived cytokines and their function in IgA plasma cell responses in mucosal effector tissues. However, T cells and certain cytokines, e.g., TGF-β have also been shown to induce B cells to switch from IgM to IgA (and to IgG), and this also receives appropriate emphasis here. Finally, we briefly summarize recent studies that suggest that certain IEL T cell subsets produce cytokines and exhibit helper functions and these cells may contribute to mucosal immune responses in underlying LP tissues as well as promote the differentiation of epithelial cells (also see Chapter 7).

GENERAL CHARACTERISTICS OF TH CELLS IN MUCOSAL INDUCTIVE SITES

Activation of Th cells by antigen requires processing of the protein and subsequent re-expression of specific peptide by antigen presenting cells (APCs) in GALT. All major types of APC occur in PP and include dendritic cells (DC), macrophages, and B cells. It is well known that B cell subsets in PP express class II MHC, and more studies of the possible role of PP B cells in antigen presentation should be carried out. The APCs in GALT process antigen in endocytic compartments into peptide epitopes, which become associated with MHC class II molecules. In the PP, Th cells are CD3[+], α/β TCR[+], and most (but not all) are CD4[+], and these CD4[+] subsets respond to peptide epitopes associated with MHC class II in the membrane of the APC (11,12). APC-Th cell contact occurs between the α/β TCR and the presented MHC class II–peptide epitope forming a ternary complex that is reinforced by reaction of the CD4 molecule with a conserved class II determinant (12). Other recognition systems also stabilize the APC–Th cell interaction (13) and contribute to Th cell activation via the CD3 peptides (14).

Activated Th cells and their derived cytokines are sufficient to induce B cells to enter G_1 phase, to complete the cell cycle and divide, and to undergo terminal differentiation into plasma cells. It is interesting that IL-4, IL-5, and IL-6, which are tandem products of Th2 cells, are most adept at inducing these three major steps. Nevertheless, the exact requirements for induction of B cell entry into cell cycle and subsequent division are not known; however, studies (15) have suggested that Th–B cell contact is required, while other work (16) showed that Th cell derived cytokines, e.g., IL-2, IL-4, IL-5, and IL-6, are sufficient to stimulate resting B cells to become plasma cells. It has been difficult to separate the inductive phase of Th–B cell interactions in mucosal immunity from the events that result in B cell terminal differentiation and plasma cell formation. It is tempting to suggest that the initial induction of Th cells by APC occurs in GALT, for example, in the PP; however, memory B cells and Th cells (in G_0) in mucosal effector sites such as the LP of the small intestine may represent the major locale for Th–B cell interactions resulting in the IgA response.

GALT mainly consists of PP, the appendix, and solitary lymphoid nodules, yet most studies, especially in mice, have been done with PP (8). The parafollicular regions of PP are enriched for T cells and are immediately adjacent to the follicles, or B cell zones, containing the germinal centers. These T cell areas possess high endothelial venules (HEVs), which are the entry sites for lymphocytes to continually populate the PP. Furthermore, the T cell zones contain DC, an important type of APC in GALT for induction of Th cells (17,18). In the GALT, approximately 35 to 40% of mononuclear cells are $CD3^+$ T cells with a CD4:CD8 ratio of about 2:1.

The first direct evidence that T cells in PP regulate IgA production came from a seminal comparative study with mitogen-activated T cells from PP and spleen (SP) of mice. Con A-stimulated PP T cells selectively induced IgA synthesis in LPS-triggered PP or SP B cell cultures, while identically treated SP T cells suppressed IgA, IgG, and IgM production in these cultures (19). This work implied that IgA isotype-specific T cells were present in higher frequencies in PP, and helped explain why IgA responses were selectively induced in mucosal tissues. Additional support for this was provided in antigen-specific systems where oral administration of TD antigens, e.g., sheep erythrocytes (SRBC), whole bacteria, and soluble proteins, induced Th cell responses in PP with resultant IgA responses in spleen and mucosal effector regions (20,21).

T Cells Involved in $\mu \rightarrow \alpha$ Switches and for Enhanced IgA Responses

Studies undertaken just over 10 years ago used T cell cloning techniques to isolate and characterize PP T cells. It is interesting that two distinct types of cells were identified and were shown to affect the IgA responses at different stages in B cell development. These two types of T cells should not be confused with the two Th cell subsets, Th1 and Th2, which are described in more detail below. One category

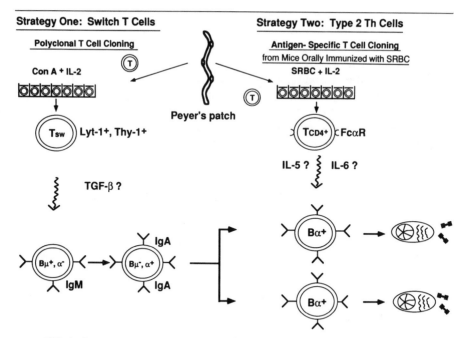

FIG. 1. Generation of two types of Th cell clones which regulate B cell responses.

of T cell clones induced surface IgM positive (sIgM$^+$) B cells to switch to surface IgA (sIgA) expression (22–24), while the second group of Th cells preferentially induced sIgA$^+$ B cells to undergo IgA responses (25–27). The initial studies with T switch (Tsw) cells used T cell clones derived by mitogen stimulation and IL-2 supported outgrowth, and when added to sIgM$^+$, sIgA$^-$ B cell cultures, resulted in marked increases in sIgA$^+$ cells (22) (Fig. 1). PP Tsw cells did not induce IgA secretion, even when incubated with sIgA$^+$ B cell enriched cultures; however, addition of B cell growth and differentiation factors readily induced cultures to secrete IgA (23). Additional work (24) showed that Tsw cells were autoreactive and suggested that continued uptake of gut lumenal antigens into the PP resulted in a unique microenvironment for T–B cell interactions and subsequent IgA responses.

Clones of antigen-specific PP Th cells were shown to support proliferation and differentiation of sIgA$^+$ B cells into IgA-producing plasma cells (25,26) (Fig. 1). These Th cell clones were derived from PP of mice fed sheep erythrocytes (SRBC), and SRBC-specific Th cell clones were generally divisible into two groups. The first type supported IgM, low IgG1, and high IgA anti-SRBC responses, while the second group preferentially supported only IgA anti-SRBC antibody responses (25,26). These PP Th cell clones expressed Fc receptors for IgA (FcαR) (25), and hybridomas derived from them secreted IgA binding factors (27), which could help explain their preferential induction of IgA responses. A recent study (28) has provided interesting new evidence that the expression of FcαR is always associated with Th2-type but not with Th1-type clones (see below for discussion of Th1 and Th2 cells). More recently, others (29) have also isolated Th cell clones specific for keyhole limpet hemocyanin (KLH) from mouse PP, and one of four clones supported KLH-specific IgA responses. Unfortunately, cytokine profiles of Tsw cells or cloned PP Th cells were not done, and thus no conclusions could be drawn as to the role of cytokines for μ→α switches or for preferential help for IgA responses. However, in conjunction with current knowledge of Th1 and Th2 cells as well as their derived cytokines (see below), one could postulate that T cells that are involved in isotype-switching might be TGF-β-producing cells, while Th cells that promote IgA responses may express FcαR and preferentially produce IL-5, IL-6, and IL-10 upon antigen stimulation (Fig. 2). Thus, the latter group of Th cells could be Th2 type cells. On the other hand, Tsw cells could be either Th1 or Th2 type cells, since TGF-β is produced by both types of Th cells as well as by other cell types.

Evidence for Tsw cells in human IgA responses has stemmed from work with malignant T cells from a patient Rac (T_{Rac} cells) who suffered from a mycosis fungoides/Sézary-like syndrome. The T_{Rac} cells induced tonsillar sIgM$^+$ B cells to switch and secrete IgG and IgA (30). Furthermore, T_{Rac} cells, when added to B cell cultures obtained from patients with hyper-IgM immunodeficiency, induced eight of nine cultures to secrete IgG and three of nine to produce IgA (31). T cell clones

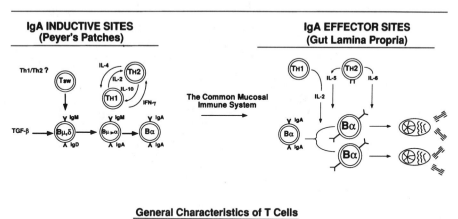

FIG. 2. T cell and cytokine regulation of the IgA response.

have also been obtained from human appendix, and these clones, and their derived culture supernatants, exhibited preferential help for IgA synthesis (32). Direct evidence was provided that CD3[+], CD4[+], CD8[−] T cell clones induced $\mu \rightarrow \alpha$ B cell switches as well as the terminal differentiation of sIgA[+] B cells into IgA producing plasma cells (32). Additional studies are needed to determine the mechanism(s) for the observed class switches and the possible contribution of cytokines to this process.

Role of Th1 and Th2 Cells in the Immune Response and for Immunity to Infection

Murine Th cell clones can be separated into specific subsets on the basis of the overall pattern of cytokines produced. It should be emphasized that some CD4[+] T cell clones do not fit into the Th0, Th1, or Th2 subset categories. Nevertheless, in the original study, a total of 22 different murine Th cell clones were isolated from systemic lymphoid tissue and were examined for IL-2, IFN-γ, and IL-4 production, and approximately one-half of the Th cell clones produced only IL-2 and IFN-γ, while the others preferentially secreted IL-4 (33). The former pattern was designated Th1 type, while IL-4 producers were termed Th2 type. Using additional cytokine-specific bioassays and mRNA analysis, a distinct pattern of cytokine production by murine Th1 and Th2 cells was established (34–37). On the other hand, the Th1 subsets selectively produced IL-2, IFN-γ, and TNF-β (or lymphotoxin; LT), while Th2 cells did not produce these cytokines (Table 1). On the other hand, Th2 cells were shown to preferentially secrete IL-4, IL-5, and IL-6 (and, in later studies, IL-10) upon antigen or mitogen stimulation (Table 1). Thus far, no specific cell surface molecules that differentiate between Th1 and Th2 cells have been identified.

TABLE 1. *Th1 and Th2 cells and derived cytokines with emphasis on IgA responses*

T helper subsets	Cytokines	Effect on IgA responses
Th1 Cells	IL-2	Synergizes with TGF-β for $\mu \rightarrow \alpha$ switches. Augments IgA synthesis in presence of IL-5
	IFN-γ	Down regulates Th2 cells and the effects of IL-4 on B cells
	TNF-β (LT)	Unknown
	TGF-β	Induces $\mu \rightarrow \alpha$ switches
Th2 Cells	IL-4	Enhances $\mu \rightarrow \alpha$ switches and augments IL-5-induced IgA synthesis
	IL-5	Synergizes with TGF-β for $\mu \rightarrow \alpha$ switches. Major cytokine for induction of sIgA[+] B cells to secrete IgA
	IL-6	Major cytokine for induction of sIgA[+] B cells to rapidly differentiate into IgA producing plasma cells
	IL-10	Down regulates Th1 cells via macrophages. Augments TGF-β induced $\mu \rightarrow \alpha$ switches in human sIgD[+] B cell cultures
	TGF-β	Induces $\mu \rightarrow \alpha$ switches

It should be noted that Th1 and Th2 cells communicate regulatory signals via these respective cytokines (35–37). For example, IL-2 and IL-4 produced by Th1 and Th2 cells, respectively, are important for the growth of both types of T cells; whereas IFN-γ, a product of Th1 cells, down regulates Th2 cell function, while IL-10, secreted by Th2 cells, inhibits Th1 cells (36,37).

Both Th1 and Th2 cells can provide helper activity for B cells and subsequent antibody responses; however Th2 cells are more adept at facilitating B cell responses (34,35). These differences in helper activity are largely due to the profile of cytokines secreted by Th1 and Th2 cells. For example, high doses of IFN-γ are immunosuppressive and induce inhibition of B cell responses (35,38). Further, Th1 cells have been shown to kill B cells directly, probably by production of LT and IFN-γ (39). Since these two molecules are powerful cytokines for the elimination of intracellularly infected host cells via activation of MØ and direct cytolytic activity, Th1 cells more efficiently enhance host defense against intracellular parasites (35–37). In addition, it has been shown that Th1 cells are involved in the regulation of a Jones-Mote type DTH reaction, since coinjection of a Th1 clone and antigen into the footpads of virgin mice led to the induction of antigen-specific and MHC-restricted inflammation (40); whereas injection with Th2 cells did not result in the presence of inflammatory lesions.

The cytokines produced by Th2 cells, i.e., IL-4, IL-5, and IL-6, are potent soluble factors for the activation, proliferation, growth, and differentiation of B cells. In this regard, Th2 cell clones have been shown to induce growth and differentiation of the majority of B cells in limiting dilution cultures (41). Th2 cells and their secreted cytokines affect both resting and large (activated) B cell populations. In most cases, resting B cells require direct cell contact with Th cells for their activation, growth, and differentiation (42). However, B cell blasts can proliferate and differentiate in response to culture supernatants from Th2 cells without any physical Th–B cell contact (43).

The unique cytokine patterns of Th1 and Th2 cells have endowed each subset with the ability to support certain B cell isotypes or subclasses. For example, Th1 cells preferentially support IgG2a synthesis in B cell cultures (34,35), and this is due to production of IFN-γ. Since IgG2a antibody–antigen complexes bind C1 and activate the classical C cascade, and possesses a high-affinity FcγR on MØ, this would further support the view that Th1 cells and their secreted cytokines (e.g., IFN-γ) are important in host defense against intracellular pathogens and represent DTH type responses. Th2 cells, in contrast, support IgG1, IgE, and IgA responses when compared with Th1 cells (34,35). Th2 cell-derived IL-4 enhanced IgG1 secretion in LPS triggered B cell cultures by increasing isotype switching of sIgG$^-$ B cells to sIgG1$^+$ B cells (44). However, Th1 cells can also support IgG1 responses (34), and these responses were induced in an IL-4 independent manner. Several lines of evidence, both *in vivo* and *in vitro*, strongly demonstrate that IL-4 produced by Th2 cells is important for the induction of IgE synthesis (41,44,45). Thus, IL-4 acts directly on sIgM$^+$ B cells and induces them to switch to sIgE$^+$ B cells (41,44). It is interesting that anti-IL-4 or anti-IFN-γ treatment inhibits IgE responses both *in vivo* and *in vitro* (45,46). This clearly suggests that Th1 and Th2 cells can cross-regulate each other, and this would be important in isotype-specific responses where IgE synthesis would be Th2 cell and IL-4 dependent, while IFN-γ produced by Th1 cells would attenuate or down regulate IL-4 induced IgE responses. Although Ig genes that encode ε- and α-chains are closely clustered in the 3′ region, IgE responses are rarely seen in normal mucosa. Since relatively high numbers of cytokine producing Th1 and Th2 cells can be isolated from both IgA inductive and effector sites (47,48), the IFN-γ produced by Th1 cells may specifically suppress IL-4 production by Th2 cells, while the production of other Th2 type cytokines (e.g., IL-5 and IL-6), which are essential for IgA synthesis, may be maintained.

Th1 and Th2 Cell Subsets in Regulation of Mucosal IgA Responses

Studies briefly reviewed above have shown that Th cells and certain cytokines, e.g., IL-5 and IL-6, are of particular importance for inducing committed, post-switched sIgA$^+$ B cells to differentiate into IgA producing plasma cells. One logical prediction from this would be that Th2-type cells may be the predominant Th cell type in mucosal effector sites. It was shown that CD4$^+$ T cells from either the LP of the GI tract (47) or salivary glands (48) of mice have more IL-5- (Th2-type) than IFN-γ- (Th1-type) producing T cells. Nevertheless, these studies have involved measurements of total Th2 cell populations, and IL-5 and IL-6 induced IgA responses were done in polyclonal B cell populations (see below). More relevant work should assess the role of Th2 cells and secreted cytokines in antigen-specific systems in response to mucosal vaccination.

In order to focus on antigen-specific Th cell responses, sensitive cytokine-specific ELISPOT assays for IFN-γ and IL-2 (Th1-type), and IL-4, IL-5, and IL-6 (Th2-type) were used for enumeration of increased numbers of Th1 and Th2 type cells present following antigen-specific priming of mucosal inductive sites after oral immunization. It was shown that oral immunization with a T cell dependent antigen, sheep erythrocytes (SRBC), preferentially induced SRBC-specific IL-5-producing T cells in PP, while systemic immunization (intraperitoneal; i.p.) resulted principally in IFN-γ T cell responses in spleen (SP) (49). The results of this study, if generally applicable to mucosal immunization with protein antigens, could have significant implications for design and delivery of mucosal vaccines. For example, orally administered antigens that induce effective levels of mucosal S-IgA antibodies do so by induction of Th2-type cells in GALT. Likewise, antigens that induce significant Th2 cell responses in PP would be expected to supply these continuously for S-IgA responses in mucosal effector tissues, while antigens that preferentially induce Th1 cell responses will not be as effective for provision of help for B cells undergoing IgA responses. However, the Th1 cell response may provide optimal cell-mediated immunity to intracellular pathogens and to toxic environmental antigens that elicit DTH reactions. Therefore, to test these assumptions, more relevant antigens, e.g., cholera toxin (CT), first as an oral immunogen and second as an adjuvant with tetanus toxoid (TT), were used to assess whether oral immunization induced Th2 cells that directly correlate with S-IgA responses in the GI tract of mice (50,51). Controls for these studies have included systemic immunization of mice with CT only or with CT plus TT by the intravenous (i.v.) route.

PP CD4$^+$ Th cells from mice orally immunized with CT and stimulated *in vitro* with CT-B resulted in significant Th2-type responses as manifested by IL-4 and IL-5 producing, spot-forming cells (SFCs). Significantly higher numbers of Th2-type cells occurred in these cultures at all time intervals when compared with Th1-type cells producing IFN-γ and IL-2. Furthermore, SP CD4$^+$ Th cell cultures from mice orally immunized with CT also showed higher frequencies of Th2-type cells. However, SP CD4$^+$ Th cell cultures from mice given CT by the i.v. route exhibited increased numbers of both Th1-type and Th2-type cells. These results suggest that CT, unlike other antigens such as SRBC, induces both Th2-type and Th1-type responses when given by the i.v. route and may explain why significant IgG anti-CT responses occur following i.v. injection of a single dose of this antigen (51).

It was of importance to determine whether the mucosal adjuvant CT could enhance Th2-type responses to other protein antigens when given by the oral route. Dose-response studies (51) showed that 250 μg of TT coadministered with CT induced maximum IgA antibody responses in the GI tract. When PP CD4$^+$ Th cell subsets from these mice were assessed for frequencies of TT-specific Th1- and Th2-type cell responses, higher numbers of TT-specific IL-5 SFC were induced in PP CD4$^+$ Th cell cultures in comparison to IFN-γSFC (51). These findings have shown that both CT and TT, when given orally to mice, preferentially induce Th2 cell responses (Table 2).

The studies summarized above showed that oral immunization resulted in enhanced Th2-type cell responses in IgA inductive sites, e.g., PP. Furthermore, this immunization regimen also resulted in significant IgA anti-CT and anti-TT SFC responses in the LP of the GI tract, a major IgA effector site (Table 2). The re-

TABLE 2. *Oral immunization preferentially induces Th2 cells that mediate IgA responses*

Antigen and mode of delivery	Th cell subsets		B cell responses (isotype)	
	GALT	Spleen	Lamina propria	Spleen/serum
Oral				
SRBC	Th2>>Th1	Th2>Th1	ND	ND
CT	Th2>>Th1	Th2>Th1	High IgA anti-CT	IgG and IgA anti-CT
CT + TT	Th2>>Th1	Th2>Th1	High IgA anti-CT	IgG and IgA anti-CT
			IgA anti-TT	IgG and IgA anti-TT
Systemic				
SRBC	0	Th1>>Th2	ND	ND
CT	0	Th1 = Th2	0	IgM/IgG anti-CT
CT + TT	0	Th1 = Th2	0	IgM/IgG anti-CT and anti-TT

CT, cholera toxin; ND, not done; SRBC, sheep erythrocytes; TT, tetanus toxoid.

sponses in LP lymphocytes (LPLs) were entirely of the IgA isotype, while splenic SFC responses to CT and TT were largely of IgG and IgA isotypes (Table 2). These studies provide the first clear evidence that oral immunization preferentially induces Th2-type responses that directly correlate with antigen-specific IgA responses in mucosal effector sites. It is tempting to suggest that activated, antigen-specific Th cells leave the PP and home to IgA effector sites via the CMIS. It is likely that Th2-type producing IL-5 and IL-6 direct antigen-specific sIgA$^+$ B cells to become IgA producing plasma cells. Nevertheless, additional studies will be required to establish that IgA responses to T cell dependent antigens depend on Th2-type derived help. In summary, these studies show that several antigens, e.g., SRBC (49), CT, and TT (50,51), induce antigen-specific Th2-type cell responses in PP. A direct correlation exists between antigen-specific Th2-type cells in PP, in higher frequencies of polyclonal Th2-type cells in mucosal effector tissues, and antigen-specific IgA and total IgA SFC in these sites, respectively.

CYTOKINES THAT REGULATE IgA RESPONSES

Cytokines of most relevance to IgA responses and thus to mucosal immunity, as with T cells described above, can for simplicity be divided into two broad classes. The first are cytokines that influence the isotype switch to IgA as well as cytokines that facilitate or enhance this switch process. The second class of cytokines are those that effectively induce memory, sIgA$^+$ B cells to divide and to differentiate into plasma cells that secrete high levels of IgA. A complication to the above classification involves cytokines that regulate IgA responses in mice versus humans. Generally, some cytokines have similar effects in both species, e.g., TGF-β and IL-6, while others such as IL-5 do not.

TGF-β is a 25 Kda cytokine with a wide array of inflammatory and immunologic effects; however, we focus only on studies with TGF-β for induction of μ→α switches. Convincing evidence has now been presented to establish that TGF-β induces sIgM$^+$ B cells to undergo switches to IgA. This cytokine specifically enhanced IgA synthesis in LPS-stimulated mouse splenic B cell cultures (52), and this effect was significantly augmented by either IL-2 (53) or IL-5 (54). In these instances, IL-2 and IL-5 enhance the TGF-β induced switching to α, since these cytokines alone (or in combination) did not induce switching. Recent studies (55) have shown that transcription of the germline Cα gene precedes the TGF-β induced switch to IgA. Furthermore, TGF-β also induced B cell switches to IgA in either pokeweed mitogen (PWM) (56) or bacterial mitogen (57,58) stimulated SP cells. Again, TGF-β induced sterile-α transcripts and in the case of human B cells for both α1 and α2 in mitogen- and TGF-β treated cultures (58). In the human system, IL-10 may serve as a switch cofactor since it was shown (59) that activation of sIgD$^+$ tonsillar B cells with anti-CD40 and coaddition of TGF-β and IL-10 resulted in significant IgA synthesis.

At present, all Th2 cell-derived cytokines, e.g., IL-4, IL-5, IL-6, and IL-10, have been shown to support or to enhance IgA responses in either mouse or human systems. The first studies in this area (60–65) showed that murine IL-5 selectively enhances IgA synthesis. For example, it was shown (61) that an autoreactive T-cell line derived from mouse PP, incubated with splenic LPS-induced B-cell blasts, resulted in enhanced synthesis of both IgG1 and IgA. Furthermore, supernatants from the original cell line, and from one of two daughter cell lines, yielded IL-4 and IL-5 and enhanced both IgG1 and IgA production. When added to LPS-driven B-cell cultures, highly purified IL-5 enhanced IgA production, and this effect was further increased by IL-4 (61). Other studies (62) have shown that supernatants from Th2 cell clones enhanced IgA synthesis in LPS-triggered splenic B-cell cultures. This IgA-enhancing factor (IgA-EF) was purified from culture supernatants of a Th2 cell clone and a resulting 21-amino-acid sequence was found to correspond to that predicted from a cDNA clone of murine IL-5, confirming that the IgA-EF produced by the various T-cell lines was indeed IL-5 (62,63).

The mechanisms of IL-5 regulation of IgA synthesis have been studied in more detail (60,64,65), and the results obtained in these studies clearly indicate that IL-5 induces IgA-committed B cells to secrete IgA. Since the PP possess a high frequency of B cells that are committed to IgA and that express sIgA, PP B-cell subsets have been used to study IL-5-induced effects. In this regard, it was shown (64) that IL-5 induced IgA synthesis in LPS-stimulated sIgA$^+$ but not in sIgA$^-$ B cells. IL-5 also induced increased numbers of IgA-secreting cells, but did not enhance cell division in culture, suggesting that IL-5 induces terminal differentiation of IgA-committed B cells to secrete IgA.

Studies have also been carried out on the target PP B-cell population affected by IL-5 in a system that did not require LPS stimulation. It is now established that GALT cells are naturally exposed to environmental microbial stimulants and that approximately 30 to 40% (or more) of PP B cells are in cell cycle (60,66). It was thus feasible to separate PP B cells into large blasts and small, resting lymphocytes using Percoll gradients. The addition of recombinant IL-5 (rIL-5) to PP B-cell cultures resulted in increased synthesis of IgA, with little or no effect on the production of IgM or IgG isotypes (60). The IL-5-induced increase in IgA synthesis was restricted to large blast, sIgA$^+$ cells and the rIL-5-enhanced IgA synthesis occurred in a dose-dependent fashion (62). These studies suggest that IL-5 induces activated sIgA$^+$ B cells to differentiate into cells secreting IgA, and that LPS alone may induce B-cell switching to IgA and the increased expression of receptors for IL-5 (IL-5R). The presence of IL-5, therefore, would be sufficient to direct the IgA-committed, IL-5R$^+$ B cells to become IgA-secreting cells.

IL-6 is a well characterized cytokine that induces terminal differentiation of mitogen or antigen activated B cells, including PP B cells, to become IgA producing cells (67). In these studies, when rIL-5 or rIL-6 was added to PP B cell cultures, rIL-6 appeared to be two to three times more potent than rIL-5. Furthermore, both rIL-5 and rIL-6 induced significant increases in IgA levels in the large blast B-cell population. On the other hand, when PP B cells were separated into sIgA$^+$ and sIgA$^-$ B-cell subsets by flow cytometry, removal of sIgA$^+$ B cells abolished the effect of both rIL-5 and rIL-6 for IgA synthesis. However, subsets enriched for sIgA$^+$ cells and incubated with rIL-5 or rIL-6 increased IgA synthesis in a dose-dependent manner, with rIL-6 appearing to be two to four times more potent than rIL-5. Thus, both IL-5 and IL-6 induce sIgA$^+$ blast B-cell subsets to differentiate into IgA-secreting cells. Since IL-6 induced increased numbers of B cells secreting IgA at higher levels of total IgA synthesis, it is more effective for terminal differentiation than IL-5 (67). In order to induce appropriate IgA responses at mucosal surfaces, it may be most efficacious to induce antigen-specific CD4$^+$ Th cells, which can provide the appropriate cytokines such as IL-5 and IL-6 (e.g., Th2 type cells) to antigen-specific sIgA$^+$ B cells to support their differentiation into IgA-producing plasma cells. Furthermore, it is feasible to consider that the delivery of these cytokines, together with specific antigens, to mucosal effector sites could allow the maximum production of antigen-specific IgA responses.

POSSIBLE ROLES FOR TH CELLS AND CYTOKINES IN THE IEL COMPARTMENT

The IELs in the GI tract represent a numerically large lymphocyte population with a frequency of one IEL for every six epithelial cells (68). The IELs collectively possess several unique properties, and this has generated considerable interest in their potential functions in host defense. Epithelial cells and IELs are continually exposed to a myriad of environmental antigens, toxicants, and pathogens and must serve in various capacities as a first line of mucosal defense. The epithelium and component cells may thus be considered a mucosal effector site, perhaps in the same sense as the underlying LP regions. Other chapters in this book place emphasis on the class I restricted, as well as general cytotoxic, functions of IELs and their role in host immunity (see Chapters 2,3,6,9,10,11, and 14). In this section, we briefly discuss the potential role for IEL T cell subsets that express the α/β TCR (about 40 to 45% of all mouse IELs) (47,69) and that, in some instances, produce cytokines and provide help for B cell responses.

Generally, 80 to 90% of lymphocytes from the mouse small intestinal epithelium express the CD3-TCR complex, and about 75% of these are CD4$^-$, CD8$^+$ (70,71). Other subsets in somewhat equal, albeit smaller, numbers are CD4$^+$, CD8$^-$, or CD4$^+$, CD8$^+$ (double positives; DPs) or CD4$^-$, CD8$^-$ (double negatives; DNs). Of interest, on the one hand, approximately two-thirds of CD8$^+$ IELs express the γ/δ TCR, while all DNs are γ/δ TCR$^+$ (47). On the other hand, about one-third of CD8$^+$ IELs are α/β TCR$^+$, and all CD4$^+$, CD8$^-$ as well as DPs use this form of TCR (47). Thus, as a composite, the γ/δ TCR$^+$ IELs are the most dominant in mice and represent approximately 45 to 65% of the entire population (47, 69–71).Nevertheless, α/β TCR$^+$ IELs are also numerically important and in some situations can represent the major cell fraction among IELs; and, as recent studies indicate, the murine large intestine also contains IELs, the majority of which are of a α/β TCR$^+$, CD4$^+$, CD8$^-$ phenotype (Beagley et al., manuscript submitted for publication).

The first clue that IELs may contain Th cell subsets came from the observation that CD3$^+$ TCR$^+$ IELs produce IFN-γ and IL-5 (47). This earlier work showed that both γ/δ TCR$^+$ and α/β TCR$^+$ IELs, including the CD8$^+$ subset, produce both IFN-γ and IL-5, and this could suggest their involvement in regulatory or inflammatory responses. In this regard, it was recently shown (72) that both α/β TCR$^+$ and γ/δ TCR$^+$ IELs synthesize a large array of cytokines including IFN-γ, IL-2, IL-3, IL-6, TNF-α, and TGF-β, which would indeed support their roles in immune regulation and in inflammation.

The first direct evidence for the presence of Th cells among IELs came from our studies of regulatory IEL T cell subsets that, when adoptively transferred to mice made orally tolerant to SRBC, could in fact "redirect" these mice to undergo anti-SRBC antibody responses (73,74) (Chapter 7). Our evidence pointed to γ/δ TCR$^+$ T cells as the "contrasuppressors" that could abrogate oral tolerance to SRBC, and we showed (73,74) that both CD8$^+$ γ/δ TCR$^+$ and DN γ/δ TCR$^+$ IELs had this unique property. One could, however, raise the point that, in fact, the γ/δ TCR$^+$ "contrasuppressors" were perhaps a super helper family of T cells that, through production of cytokines, could simply overcome antigen-specific tolerance. This was not the case, however, since our studies (73,74) showed that γ/δ TCR$^+$ IELs exhibited no helper functions in either antigen-specific or in polyclonal B cell systems although they were capable of producing regulatory cytokines. We noticed that α/β TCR$^+$ IELs in these same experiments were effective helpers for B cell responses (Table 3).

In more recent experiments (75), we have focused on the subsets of α/β TCR$^+$ IELs that exhibit helper functions. We first purified the α/β TCR$^+$ IEL subset and then determined the relative frequency of CD4$^-$, CD8$^+$ or CD4$^+$, CD8$^+$ or CD4$^+$, CD8$^-$ T cells present; this distribution was 65%, 20%, and 15%, respectively. Again, even among α/β TCR$^+$ IELs, the CD8$^+$ phenotype predominates. We then analyzed these subsets for cytokines by assay for production at the single-cell level,

TABLE 3. *Evidence for helper T cell subsets in the α/β TCR$^+$ fraction of IELs*

IEL T cells tested	Helper cell function for	
	Antigen-specific B cell responses (SRBC)	Polyclonal B cell responses
α/β TCR	+ + +	+ + +
γ/δ TCR	—	—

Subsets of α/β TCR T cells tested	Th1-type and Th2-type cytokine synthesis					
	Th1		Th2			Helper function for B cells
	IFN-γ	IL-2	IL-4	IL-5	IL-6	
CD4$^+$, CD8$^-$	+ + +	—	+ +	+ + +	+	Yes
CD4$^+$, CD8$^+$ (DP)	+ +	—	±	+ + +	+	Yes
CD4$^-$, CD8$^+$	+ + +	—	—	+ +	+	No

as well as by mRNA analysis, and finally, for their ability to support PP B cell Ig synthesis of all three major isotypes.

The mRNA was extracted from these three subsets of freshly isolated IEL T cells and examined for IFN-γ, IL-2, IL-4, IL-5, and IL-6 messages by cytokine-specific reverse transcription-polymerase chain reaction (RT-PCR). After 35 cycles of amplification, CD4$^+$, CD8$^-$ T cells expressed strong messages for the Th2 cell type, e.g., IL-4, IL-5, and IL-6 (Table 3). Furthermore, mRNA for Th1 cytokine such as IFN-γ was seen; however, no IL-2 mRNA was detected. Thus, the profile of cytokine mRNA for CD4$^+$, CD8$^-$, α/β TCR$^+$ was IL-4, IL-5, IL-6, and IFN-γ, but not IL-2 (Table 3). In the case of mRNA from DP T cells, a similar pattern of cytokine message was noted; however, in this case neither IL-2 nor IL-4 mRNA was found (Table 3). When mRNA isolated from CD4$^-$, CD8$^+$ T cells was examined, a pattern quite similar to that of DP T cells was seen, e.g., message for IL-4, IL-5, and IL-6 and IFN-γ. However, mRNA for IL-2 was not detected in either CD4$^-$, CD8$^+$ T cells or DP T cells, and the latter IEL T cell subset lacked IL-4 mRNA as well (Table 3).

We then confirmed this pattern of cytokine production by the CD4$^+$, CD8$^-$ and DP T cells using IFN-γ, IL-2, IL-4, IL-5, and IL-6 single-cell ELISPOT assays. When freshly isolated CD4$^+$, CD8$^-$ T cells, DP T cells, or CD4$^-$, CD8$^+$ T cells were examined, the CD4$^+$, CD8$^-$ T cell subset always contained higher numbers of IL-4, IL-5, and IL-6 SFC when compared with DP T cells. Among Th2-type cytokine producing cells, IL-5 secreting cells were present in highest numbers. In terms of Th1-type cytokine production, IFN-γ SFC were noted; however, no IL-2 producing cells were detected. In studies with DP T cells, although this subset contained IL-4, IL-5, and IL-6 SFC, the frequency of IL-4 and IL-6 secreting cells was low. As with CD4$^+$, CD8$^-$ T cells, IFN-γ producing cells were seen in the DP T cell population, but again no IL-2 SFC were detected. Consequently, the major profile for cytokine production by CD4$^+$, CD8$^-$ T cells and DP T cells freshly isolated from IELs confirmed the mRNA analysis (Table 3).

We next assessed these three subsets of α/β TCR$^+$ IELs for provision of help for B cells since CD4$^+$, CD8$^-$ T cells and CD4$^-$, CD8$^+$ T cells in IELs contained Th1- and Th2-type cytokine producing cells (Table 3). To do this, each of the three T cell subsets was tested for its ability to induce B cell differentiation to Ig producing cells by using PP B cells cultured *in vitro*. When individual T cell subsets (1×10^6 cells/well) were added to PP B cell cultures (5×10^6 cells/well), CD4$^+$, CD8$^-$ T cells provided helper function (Table 3). DP T cells also enhanced IgM, IgG, and IgA SFC responses, for which 1.5 to 3.0-fold increases of isotype-specific SFC were noted when compared with control B cell cultures containing PP B cells only, whereas CD4$^-$, CD8$^+$ T cells did not provide any helper function for B cells.

The predominant CD8$^+$ IELs have been extensively studied for their immunological functions, and it has been suggested (76) that CD8 bearing IELs are central players for the immune surveillance of the mucosal epithelial cell barrier. Thus, IELs have been shown to harbor various cytolytic activities including those of antigen-specific and MHC class I restricted CTLs (76,77), ADCC (78), alloreactive

CTL (79,80), NK cell type cytotoxicity (81–83), and spontaneous cytotoxic activity (78,84) (see Chapters 2,3,6,9,10, and 14). In contrast to these past experiments on CD8$^+$ IELs, the studies summarized here were the first to address the immuno-biological function of α/β TCR$^+$ IELs, with emphasis on the CD4$^+$, CD8$^-$ and DP T cell subsets in IELs, and they have provided new information concerning the ability of these CD4$^+$ IELs to produce Th1 and Th2 cell type cytokines and to provide helper function to support B cell responses.

These studies have provided new evidence that both α/β TCR bearing CD4$^+$, CD8$^-$ T cells and DP T cells are capable of producing Th1- (IFN-γ and IL-2) and Th2- (IL-4, IL-5, and IL-6) type cytokines (75). Therefore, this array of cytokine production has suggested that IEL T cells are an important population of effector cells which could be involved in all aspects of cell-to-cell interactions for the induction and regulation of mucosal immune responses.

It is, of course, intriguing that IELs contain subsets of T cells, namely CD4$^+$, CD8$^-$ T cells and DP T cells, which are capable of providing helper function for B cell responses. Since it is generally accepted that there are essentially no B cell populations in IELs, it is difficult to envision that CD4 bearing IELs will direct B cell responses in the epithelium. Instead, CD4$^+$, CD8$^-$ T cells and DP T cells in IELs may communicate with B cells as well as with antigen presenting cells that reside in the LP region. In this regard, some IELs were seen to be situated on the basement membrane side of the epithelial cell layer when serial longitudinal sections of villi were examined. Furthermore, it was suggested that most IELs situated in or along the basement membrane leave the epithelium and re-enter the LP region of the small intestine (85). Alternatively, since intestinal epithelium has been shown to provide an environment for the development of T cells without thymic influence (86), it is also possible that some CD4$^+$ T cells in the LP might originate from IELs. Current work in our group is focused on these relevant issues of IEL T cell regulation for mucosal immunity.

SUMMARY

The mucosal immune system is composed of IgA inductive and effector sites, which are represented by gut-associated lymphoid tissues (GALT) and epithelial and LP regions in the GI tract. For the regulation of IgA immune responses, CD4$^+$ Th cells, especially those of the IL-5 and IL-6 producing Th2 type, have been shown to be important. In this regard, orally administered protein antigen induced antigen-specific Th2-type cells in GALT. It is suggested that following antigen encounter, antigen-specific sIgA$^+$ B cells and CD4$^+$ Th2-type cells leave GALT and migrate to IgA effector tissues via the common mucosal immune system. Antigen-specific cognate interactions between CD4$^+$ Th cells and sIgA$^+$ B cells in the LP region of the GI tract leads to cell-to-cell communication via regulatory cytokines such as IL-5 and IL-6. These cell interactions result in the induction of IgA plasma cells in mucosal effector tissues.

In the mucosal effector tissues of the GI tract, lymphocytes frequently reside in the gut epithelium, where they are commonly termed intraepithelial lymphocytes (IELs) and, as such, may be considered to be part of a regulatory T cell network for IgA responses. Although CD4$^-$, CD8$^+$ T lymphocytes are a dominant T cell fraction in IELs, a substantial number of IELs are CD4$^+$ T cells that express the α/β heterodimer chains of TCR. Thus, CD4$^+$, CD8$^-$ T cells and CD4$^+$, CD8$^+$ (DP) T cells represent approximately 7.5% and 10% of CD3$^+$ T cell in IELs, respectively. Both CD4$^+$, CD8$^-$ and DP T cell subsets from freshly isolated IELs possess cytokine-specific mRNA for Th1- (IFN-γ) and Th2- (IL-4, IL-5, and IL-6) type cells. These two subsets of IEL T cells are also capable of producing Th1- and Th2-type cytokines. Further, CD4$^+$, CD8$^-$ T cells and DP T cells can provide helper functions, since addition of these two subsets of T cells to GALT-derived B cell cultures resulted in the induction of Ig synthesis including that of the IgA isotype. Thus, in addition to GALT derived CD4$^+$ Th2-type cells, CD4$^+$ T cells, including both CD4$^+$, CD8$^-$ and DP T cells, in IELs are also able to provide helper function for mucosal IgA responses.

ACKNOWLEDGMENTS

The results summarized in this chapter were supported in part by U.S. Public Health Service Contract AI 15128 and grants DK 44240, AI 30366, DE 09837, AI 18958, DE 04217, and DE 08228. Dr. H. Kiyono is the recipient of an NIH Research Career Development Award DE 00237. We thank Ms. Sheila Weatherspoon for preparation and Drs. Dennis W. McGee and Katherine W. Merrill for their critical review of the material covered in this chapter.

REFERENCES

1. Crewther P, Warner NL. Serum immunoglobulins and antibodies in congenitally athymic (nude) mice. *Aust J Exp Biol Med Sci* 1972;50:625–635.
2. Pritchard H, Riddaway J, Micklem HS. Immune responses in congenitally thymusless mice. II: Quantitative studies of serum immunoglobulins, the antibody response to sheep erythrocytes, and the effect of thymus allografting. *Clin Exp Immunol* 1973;13:125–138.
3. Guy-Grand D, Griscelli C, Vassalli P. Peyer's patches, gut IgA plasma cells and thymic function: study in nude mice bearing thymic grafts. *J Immunol* 1975;115:361–364.
4. Clough JD, Mims LH, Strober W. Deficient IgA antibody responses to arsanilic acid bovine serum albumin (BSA) in neonatally thymectomized rabbits. *J Immunol* 1971;106:1624–1629.
5. Ebersole JL, Taubman MA, Smith DJ. The effect of neonatal thymectomy on the level of salivary and serum immunoglobulins in rats. *Immunology* 1979;36:649–657.
6. Waldmann TA, Broder S, Goldman CK, Frost K, Korsmeyer SJ, Medici MA. Disorders of B cells and helper T cells in the pathogenesis of the immunoglobulin deficiency of patients with ataxia teleangiectasia. *J Clin Invest* 1983;71:282–295.
7. Waldmann TA, Broder S, Krakauer R, Durm M, Meade B, Goldman C. Defects in IgA secretion and in IgA specific suppressor cells in patients with selective IgA deficiency. *Trans Assoc Am Physicians* 1976;89:215–223.
8. McGhee JR, Mestecky J, Elson CO, Kiyono H. Regulation of IgA synthesis and immune response by T cells and interleukins. *J Clin Immunol* 1989;9:175–199.

9. Guy-Grand D, Cerf-Bensussan N, Malissen B, Malassis-Seris M, Briottet C, Vassalli P. Two gut intraepithelial CD8[+] lymphocyte populations with different T cell receptors: a role for the gut epithelium in T cell differentiation. *J Exp Med* 1991;173:471–481.
10. Guy-Grand D, Griscelli C, Vassalli P. The mouse gut T lymphocyte, a novel type of T cell: nature, origin, and traffic in mice in normal and graft-versus-host conditions. *J Exp Med* 1978;148:1661–1677.
11. Marrack P, Kappler J. The antigen-specific, major histocompatibility complex-restricted receptor on T cells. *Adv Immunol* 1986;38:1–30.
12. Bierer BE, Sleckman BP, Ratnofsky SE, Burakoff SJ. The biologic roles of CD2, CD4 and CD8 in T-cell activation. *Annu Rev Immunol* 1989;7:579–599.
13. Kupfer A, Singer SJ. Cell biology of cytotoxic and helper T-cell functions: immunofluorescence microscopic studies of single cells and cell couples. *Annu Rev Immunol* 1989;7:309–337.
14. Clevers H, Alarcon B, Wileman T, Terhorst C. The T cell receptor/CD3 complex: a dynamic protein ensemble. *Annu Rev Immunol* 1988;6:629–662.
15. Owens T. A noncognate interaction with anti-receptor antibody-activated helper T cells induces small resting murine B cells to proliferate and to secrete antibody. *Eur J Immunol* 1988;18:395–401.
16. Leclercq L, Cambier JC, Mishel Z, Julius MH, Theze J. Supernatant from a cloned helper T cell stimulates most small resting B cells to undergo increased I-A expression, blastogenesis and progression through cell cycle. *J Immunol* 1986;136:539–545.
17. Spalding DM, Koopman WJ, Eldridge JH, McGhee JR, Steinman RM. Accessory cells in murine Peyer's patch. I: Identification and enrichment of functional dendritic cells. *J Exp Med* 1983; 157:1646–1959.
18. Spalding DM, Williamson SI, Koopman WJ, McGhee JR. Preferential induction of polyclonal IgA secretion by murine Peyer's patch dendritic cell–T cell mixtures. *J Exp Med* 1984;160:941–946.
19. Elson CO, Heck JA, Strober W. T-cell regulation of murine IgA synthesis. *J Exp Med* 1979; 149:632–643.
20. Richman LK, Graeff AS, Yarchoan R, Strober W. Simultaneous induction of antigen-specific IgA helper T cells and IgG suppressor T cells in the murine Peyer's patch after protein feeding. *J Immunol* 1981;126:2079–2083.
21. Kiyono H, Mosteller LM, Eldridge JH, Michalek SM, McGhee JR. IgA responses in *xid* mice: oral antigen primes Peyer's patch cells for *in vitro* immune responses and secretory antibody production. *J Immunol* 1983;131:2616–2622.
22. Kawanishi H, Saltzman L, Strober W. Mechanisms regulating IgA class-specific immunoglobulin production in murine gut-associated lymphoid tissues. I: T cells derived from Peyer's patches that switch sIgM B cells to sIgA B cells *in vitro*. *J Exp Med* 1983;157:433–450.
23. Kawanishi H, Saltzman L, Strober W. Mechanisms regulating IgA class-specific immunoglobulin production in murine gut-associated lymphoid tissues. II: Terminal differentiation of postswitch sIgA-bearing Peyer's patch B cells. *J Exp Med* 1983;158:649–669.
24. Kawanishi H, Ozato K, Strober W. The proliferative response of cloned Peyer's patch switch T-cells to syngeneic and allogeneic stimuli. *J Immunol* 1985;134:3586–3591.
25. Kiyono H, McGhee JR, Mosteller LM, et al. Murine Peyer's patch T-cell clones: characterization of antigen-specific helper T cells for immunoglobulin A responses. *J Exp Med* 1982;156:1115–1130.
26. Kiyono H, Cooper MD, Kearney JF, et al. Isotype-specificity of helper T cell clones: Peyer's patch Th cells preferentially collaborate with mature IgA B cells for IgA responses. *J Exp Med* 1984; 159:798–811.
27. Kiyono H, Mosteller-Barnum LM, Pitts AM, Williamson SI, Michalek SM, McGhee JR. Isotype-specific immunoregulation: IgA binding factors produced by Fcα receptor[+] T cell hybridomas regulate IgA responses. *J Exp Med* 1985;161:731–747.
28. Sandor M, Gajewski T, Thorson J, Kemp, JD, Fitch FW, Hoover G. CD4[+] murine T cell clones that express high levels of immunoglobulin binding belong to the interleukin 4-producing T helper cell type 2 subset. *J Exp Med* 1990;171:2171–2176.
29. Maghazachi A, Phillips-Quagliata JM. Keyhole limpet hemocyanin-propagated Peyer's patch T cell clones that help IgA responses. *J Immunol* 1988;140:3380–3388.
30. Mayer L, Postnett DN, Kunkel HG. Human-malignant T-cells capable of inducing an immunoglobulin class switch. *J Exp Med* 1985;161:134–144.
31. Mayer L, Kwan SP, Thompson C, et. al. Evidence for a defect in "switch" T cells in patients with immunodeficiency and hyperimmunoglobulin M. *New Engl J Med* 1986;314:409–413.

32. Benson EB, Strober W. Regulation of IgA secretion by T cell clones derived from the human gastrointestinal tract. *J Immunol* 1988;140:1874–1882.
33. Mosmann TR, Cherwinski H, Bond MW, Giedlin MA, Coffman RL. Two types of murine helper T cell clone. I: Definition according to profiles of lymphokine activities and secreted proteins. *J Immunol* 1986;136:2348–2357.
34. Coffman RL, Seymour BW, Lebman DA, et al. The role of helper T cell products in mouse B cell differentiation and isotype regulation. *Immunol Rev* 1988;102:5–28.
35. Mosmann TR, Coffman RL. Th1 and Th2 cells: different patterns of lymphokine secretion lead to different functional properties. *Annu Rev Immunol* 1989;7:145–173.
36. Street NE, Mosmann TR. Functional diversity of T lymphocytes due to secretion of different cytokine patterns. *FASEBJ* 1991;5:171–177.
37. Mosmann TR, Moore KW. The role of IL-10 in cross regulation of Th1 and Th2 responses. *Immunol Today* 1991;12:A49–A53.
38. Reynolds DS, Boom WH, Abbas AK. Inhibition of B lymphocyte activation of interferon-γ. *J Immunol* 1987;139:767–773.
39. Janeway CA Jr, Carding S, Jones B, et al. CD4$^+$ T cells: specificity and function. *Immunol Rev* 1988;101:39–80.
40. Cher DJ, Mosmann TR. Two types of murine helper T cell clone II: delayed-type hypersensitivity is mediated by T_h1 clones. *J Immunol* 1987;138:3688–3694.
41. Lebman DA, Coffman RL. Interleukin 4 causes isotype switching to IgE in T cell-stimulated clonal B cell cultures. *J Exp Med* 1988;168:853–862.
42. Rasmussen R, Takatsu K, Harada N, Takahashi T, Bottomly K. T cell-dependent hapten-specific and polyclonal B cell responses require release of interleukin 5. *J Immunol* 1988;140:705–712.
43. Herron LR, Coffman RL, Bond MW, Kotzin BL. Increase autoantibody production by NZB/NZW B cells in response to interleukin 5. *J Immunol* 1988;141:842–848.
44. Paul WE. Interleukin 4/B cell stimulatory factor 1: one lymphokine, many functions. *FASEBJ* 1987; 1:456–461.
45. Finkelman FD, Holmes J, Katona IM, et al. Lymphokine control of *in vivo* immunoglobulin isotype selection. *Annu Rev Immunol* 1990;8:303–333.
46. Coffman RL, Carty J. A T cell activity that enhances polyclonal IgE production and its inhibition by interferon-γ. *J Immunol* 1986;136:949–954.
47. Taguchi T, McGhee JR, Coffman RL, et al. Analysis of Th1 and Th2 cells in murine gut-associated tissues: frequency of CD4$^+$ and CD8$^+$ T cells which secrete IFN-γ and IL-5. *J Immunol* 1990; 145:68–77.
48. Mega J, McGhee JR, Kiyono H. Cytokine and Ig producing cells in mucosal effector tissues: analysis of IL-5 and IFN-γ producing T cells, TCR expression and IgA plasma cells from mouse salivary gland associated tissues. *J Immunol* 1992;148:2030–2039.
49. Xu-Amano J, Aicher W.K, Taguchi T, Kiyono H, McGhee JR. Selective induction of Th2 cells in murine Peyer's patches by oral immunization. *Intern Immunol* 1992;4:433–445.
50. Xu-Amano J, Jackson RJ, Fujihashi K, Kiyono H, Elson CO, McGhee JR. Helper Th1 amd Th2 cell responses following mucosal or systemic immunization with cholera toxin. 1993; *submitted for publication.*
51. Xu-Amano J, Kiyono, H, Jackson R, et al. Helper T cell subsets for immunoglobulin A responses: Oral immunization with tetanus toxoid and cholera toxin as adjuvant selectively induces Th2 cells in mucosa-associated tissues. *J Exp Med* 1993 (*in press*).
52. Coffman RL, Lebman DA, Shrader B. Transforming growth factor β specifically enhances IgA production by lipopolysaccharide-stimulated murine B lymphocytes. *J Exp Med* 1989;170:1039–1044.
53. Lebman DA, Lee FD, Coffman RL. Mechanism for transforming growth factor β and IL-2 enhancement of IgA expression in lipopolysaccharide-stimulated B cell cultures. *J Immunol* 1990;144:952–959.
54. Sonoda E, Matsumoto R, Hitoshi Y, et al. Transforming growth factor β induces IgA production and acts additively with interleukin 5 for IgA production. *J Exp Med* 1989;170:1415–1420.
55. Lebman DA, Nomura DY, Coffman RL, Lee FD. Molecular characterization of germline immunoglobulin A transcripts produced during transforming growth factor type β-induced isotype switching. *Proc Natl Acad Sci USA* 1990;87:3962–3966.
56. Van Vlasselaer, P Punnonen J, De Vries JE. Transforming growth factor-β directs IgA switching in human B cells. *J Immunol* 1992;148:2062–2067.

57. Islam KB, Nilsson L, Sideras P, Hammarström L, Smith CIE. TGF-β1 induces germline transcripts of both IgA subclasses in human B lymphocytes. *Intern Immunol* 1991;3:1099–1106.

58. Nilsson L, Islam KB, Olafsson O, et al. Structure of TGF-β1-induced human immunoglobulin Cα1 and Cα2 germ-line transcripts. *Intern Immunol* 1991;3:1107–1115.

59. Defrance T, Vandervliet B, Briére F, Durand I, Rousset F, Banchereau J. Interleukin 10 and transforming growth factor β cooperate to induce anti-CD40-activiated naive human B cells to secrete immunoglobulin A. *J Exp Med* 1992;175:671–682.

60. Beagley KW, Eldridge JH, Kiyono H, et al. Recombinant murine IL-5 induced high rate IgA synthesis in cycling IgA-positive Peyer's patch B cells. *J Immunol* 1988;141:2035–2041.

61. Murray PD, McKenzie DT, Swain SL, Kagnoff MF. Interleukin 5 and interleukin 4 produced by Peyer's patch T-cells selectively enhance immunoglobulin A expression. *J Immunol* 1987;139: 2669–2674.

62. Coffman RL, Shrader B, Carty J, Mosmann TR, Bond MW. A mouse T cell product that preferentially enhances IgA production. I: Biologic characterization. *J Immunol* 1987;139:3685–3690.

63. Bond MW, Shrader B, Mosmann TR, Coffman RL. A mouse T cell product that preferentially enhances IgA production. II: Physicochemical characterization. *J Immunol* 1987;139:3691–3696.

64. Harriman GR, Kunimoto DY, Elliott JF, Paetkau V, Strober W. The role of IL-5 in IgA B cell differentiation. *J Immunol* 1988;140:3033–3039.

65. Lebman DA, Coffman RL. The effects of IL-4 and IL-5 on the IgA response by murine Peyer's patch B cell subpopulations. *J Immunol* 1988;141:2050–2056.

66. Lebman DA, Griffin, PM, Cebra JJ. Relationship between expression of IgA by Peyer's patch cells and functional IgA memory cells. *J Exp Med* 1977;166:1405–1418.

67. Beagley KW, Eldridge JH, Lee F, et al. Interleukins and IgA synthesis: human and murine IL-6 induce high rate IgA secretion in IgA-committed B cells. *J Exp Med* 1989;169:2133–2148.

68. Brandtzaeg P. Overview of the mucosal immune system. *Curr Top Microbiol Immunol* 1989;146: 13–25.

69. Bonneville M, Itohara S, Krecko EG, et al. Transgenic mice demonstrate that epithelial homing of γ/δ T cells is determined by cell lineages independent of T cell receptor specificity. *J Exp Med* 1990;171:1015–1026.

70. Goodman T, Lefrançois L. Expression of the γ-δ T cell receptor on intestinal CD8[+] intraepithelial lymphocytes. *Nature* 1988;333:855–858.

71. Bonneville M, Janeway CA Jr, Ito K, et al. Intestinal intraepithelial lymphocytes are a distinct set of gamma delta T cells. *Nature* 1988;333:479–481.

72. Barret TA, Gajewski TF, Danielpour D, Chang EB, Beagley KW, Bluestone JA. Differential function of intestinal intraepithelial lymphocyte subsets. *J Immunol* 1992;149:1124–1130.

73. Fujihashi K, Taguchi T, McGhee JR, et al. Regulation function for the murine intraepithial lymphocytes: two subsets of CD3[+] T cell receptor-[1+] intraepithelial lymphocyte T cells abrogate oral tolerance. *J Immunol* 1990;145:2010–2019.

74. Fujihashi K, Taguchi T, Aicher WK, et al. Immunoregulatory functions for murine intraepithelial lymphocytes: γ/δ T cell receptor-positive (TCR[+]) T cells abrogate oral tolerance while α/β TCR[+] T cells provide B cell help. *J Exp Med* 1992;175:695–707.

75. Fujihashi K, Yamamoto M, McGhee JR, Beagley KW, Kiyono H. Function of α/β TCR bearing intraepithelial lymphocytes: Th1 and Th2 type cytokine production by CD4[+] CD8[−] and CD4[+] CD8[+] T cells possess helper activity. *Intern Immunol* 1993; in press.

76. Janeway CA Jr, Jones B, Hayday A. Specificity and function of T cells bearing γδ receptors. *Immunol Today* 1988;9:73–76.

77. Klein JR, Kagnoff MF. Nonspecific recruitment of cytotoxic effector cells in the intestinal mucosa of antigen-primed mice. *J Exp Med* 1984;160:1931–1936.

78. Offit PA, Cunningham SL, Dudzik KI. Memory and distribution of virus-specific cytotoxic T lymphocytes (CTLs) and CTL precursors after rotavirus infection. *J Virol* 1991;65:1318–1324.

79. Guy-Grand D, Malassis-Seris M, Briottet C, Vassalli P. Cytotoxic differentiation of mouse gut thymodependent and independent intraepithelial T lymphocytes is induced locally: correlation between functional assays presence of perforin and granzyme transcripts and cytoplasmic granules. *J Exp Med* 1991;173:1549–1552.

80. Arnaud-Battandier F, Bundy BM, O'Neill M, Bienenstock J, Nelson DL. Cytotoxic activities of gut mucosal lymphoid cells in guinea pigs. *J Immunol* 1978;121:1059–1065.

81. London SD, Cebra JJ, Rubin DH. Intraepithelial lymphocytes contain virus-specific MHC-restricted

cytotoxic cell precursors after gut mucosal immunization with reovirus serotype 1/Lang. *Reg Immunol* 1989;2:98–102.

82. Tagliabue A, Befus AD, Clark DA, Bienenstock J. Characteristics of natural killer cells in the murine intestinal epithelium and lamina propria. *J Exp Med* 1982;155:1785–1796.

83. Ernst PB, Clark DA, Rosenthal KL, Befus AD, Bienenstock J. Detection and characterization of cytotoxic T lymphocytes precursors in the murine intestinal intraepithelial leukocyte population. *J Immunol* 1986;136:2121–2126.

84. Klein JR. Ontogeny of the Thy-1$^-$ Lyt-2$^+$ murine intestinal intraepithelial lymphocytes: characterization of a unique population of thymus-independent cytotoxic effector cells in the intestinal mucosa. *J Exp Med* 1986;164:309–314.

85. Marsh MN. Studies of intestinal lymphoid tissue. II: Aspects of proliferation and migration of epithelial lymphocytes in the small intestine of mice. *Gut* 1975;16:674–682.

86. Poussier P, Edouard P, Lee C, Binnie M, Julius M. Thymus-independent development and negative selection of T cells expressing T cell receptor α/β in the intestinal epithelium: evidence for distinct circulation patterns of gut- and thymus-derived T lymphocytes. *J Exp Med* 1992;176:187–199.

Mucosal Immunology: Intraepithelial Lymphocytes,
edited by H. Kiyono and J. R. McGhee.
Raven Press, Ltd., New York © 1993.

2

Origin and Development of Gut Intraepithelial Lymphocytes

Delphine Guy-Grand*, Benedita Rocha†, and Pierre Vassalli‡

*INSERM U 132, Hôpital des Enfants-Malades, 149, rue de Sèvres, 75743 Paris, France.
†INSERM U 345, Faculté Necker, 156, rue de Vaugirard, 75015 Paris, France.
‡Département de Pathologie, Centre Médical Universitaire,
CH-1211 Geneve 4, Switzerland.

The gut wall of normal adult mice contains both B lymphocytes (mainly IgA plasma cells) and CD3$^+$ T lymphocytes. IgA plasma cells are located in the lamina propria, while T cells are found in both the lamina propria and between the epithelial cells of the villi (intraepithelial lymphocytes; IEL). Gut T lymphocytes are very numerous: it has been calculated that the IEL lodged in the small bowel are more than half as numerous as all the T lymphocytes in the peripheral lymphoid organs (1); further-more, the number of T lymphocytes located in the lamina propria appears to be similar to that of IEL.

Fichtelius (2) (1968) thought that IEL evolved in mammals as a "bursa equiva-lent." In 1974 (3), they were identified as T cells by the use of anti-Thy-1 anti-bodies. In 1988, the observation by Goodman and Lefrançois (4) and Bonneville et al. (5) that an unusually high percentage of gut IEL bear the T cell receptor γδ TCR led immunologists, who had previously paid little attention to mucosal immunol-ogy, to take a fresh look at these lymphocytes. Now, mAbs against the two chains of the CD8 molecule have been used to identify T cell populations more or less specific to the gut epithelium, and to show the dual lineage of IEL (6).

PHENOTYPE OF GUT WALL T LYMPHOCYTES

The gut wall contains CD4$^-$CD8$^-$, CD4$^+$, CD8$^+$ and small numbers of CD4$^+$ CD8$^+$ cells. The majority of these cells are CD3$^+$. With regard to their pheno-type and TCR expression, some of these cells resemble the bulk of mature T cells found in the spleen and lymph nodes, as they consist of CD4$^+$ T lymphocytes that predominate in the lamina propria and are rare in the epithelium, and CD8$^+$ T lymphocytes (6), which, like peripheral CD8$^+$ T cells, coexpress CD8 molecules made of α and β chains. Both these cell populations express Thy-1, and bear αβ

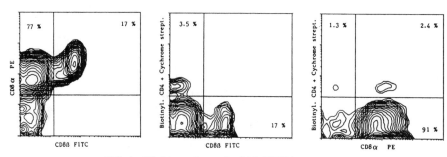

FIG. 1. IEL from a 3-month-old C₃H/DBA₂ mouse.

TCR. These lymphocytes are referred to as the CD4⁺/CD8αβ⁺ subset. The phenotypes of the other T cell populations, which largely predominate in the epithelium, are very peculiar to the gut, at least by their frequency. Some cells are CD4⁻CD8⁻, but the majority are CD8⁺. The CD8 molecules expressed are, however, made of a homodimeric chain (Fig. 1), and these cells contain no CD8 β chain transcripts (6). Whatever their phenotype (6), these populations bear similar amounts of αβ TCR and γδ TCR, and the majority lack Thy-1. They are referred to as CD4⁻CD8β⁻ IEL.

The gut also contains rare populations of CD4⁺CD8⁺ (double positive; DP) αβ TCR⁺ lymphocytes, which differ from immature DP thymocytes. While all DP thymocytes coexpress CD4 and CD8αβ, DP IEL bear CD8 made of homodimeric α chains (Fig. 1). CD4⁺CD8αβ⁺ IEL are as rare in the gut as in peripheral lymphoid organs. DP IEL are thought to be a mature CD4⁺ population that acquires CD8α chains in the gut wall.

THE CD4⁻CD8αβ⁻ SUBSET IS THYMUS-INDEPENDENT (TID) AND THE CD4⁺/CD8αβ⁺ SUBSET IS THYMUS-DEPENDENT (TD)

In nude mice, IEL can be isolated in small numbers (one-eighth of value in normal mice), but CD4⁺ and CD8αβ⁺ IEL are not found. Only the CD4⁻CD8β⁻ subset differentiates. Indeed, about 85% of IEL bear CD8αα chains, but only 40% of these cells are CD3⁺; the majority express γδ TCR. The percentage of CD3⁺ cells within nude IEL increases with age, and some αβ TCR⁺ IEL emerge.

In contrast, when Thy 1.2⁺ nude mice are injected with lymph node T cells (CD8αβ⁺, αβ TCR or CD4⁺, αβ TCR⁺ TD population) from syngeneic Thy 1.1⁺ donors, CD4⁺ and CD8αβ⁺ populations, all of donor origin, appear in the gut mucosa. These cells coexist with the normal CD4⁻CD8β⁻ subset in nude mice (7).

In normal mice, the CD4⁻ CD8β⁻ subset can differentiate in the absence of a thymus. This was shown in thymectomized lethally irradiated mice (T × BM), reconstituted with T-depleted bone marrow from beige mice (6). IEL of donor origin are recognizable because of their giant granules and show a phenotype identical to that in nude mice, i.e., CD4⁻CD8β⁻. CD4⁺ and CD8αβ⁺ cells were also found in the IEL of these mice, but all were of recipient origin, containing characteristic small granules. We found that a large fraction of gut lymphocytes were strikingly radioresistant. After lethal irradiation, when no T lymphocytes were found in the thymus or the peripheral pool, the yield of IEL was only reduced by half (unpublished observations). $\gamma\delta$ TCR$^+$ IEL are also found in TxBM mice reconstituted with CD3$^-$ fetal liver precursors, identified by a Thy-1 allotype marker (8).

It has recently been reported (9,10) that in thymectomized semiallogeneic mice, injection of bone marrow or fetal liver cells reconstitutes both CD4$^-$CD8β^- and CD4$^+$/CD8$\alpha\beta^+$ IEL subsets. In these experiments, the identification of CD4$^+$ and CD8$\alpha\beta^+$ IEL as being of donor origin and thymoindependent was based on the use of an anti-H2 mAb to detect the parental donor antigen in the semiallogeneic combination. The conclusion that CD4$^+$ and CD8$\alpha\beta^+$ IEL are thymus-independent is, however, in conflict with a number of observations, mainly the absence of IEL with this phenotype in nude mice and the above evidence that most Thy-1$^+$ IEL were the progeny of T blasts circulating in the thoracic duct. Another type of transfer experiment with another marker to recognize donor and recipient cells led to the conclusion that CD4$^+$ and CD8$\alpha\beta^+$ IEL originated, in contrast to IEL with other phenotypes, from thymus-derived donor cells. As a result, several types of transfer experiments with several types of markers are required to avoid erroneous interpretations.

THE CD4$^+$/CD8$\alpha\beta^+$ SUBSET AND THE CD4$^-$CD8$^-$ SUBSET ARE OF DIFFERENT ORIGINS, SHOW DIFFERENT CIRCUITS, AND EMERGE UNDER DIFFERENT CONDITIONS

Since the work by Gowans and Knight (1964) (11), it is clear that some lymphoid cells located in the gut mucosa derive from dividing precursors circulating in the mesenteric lymph nodes and the thoracic duct lymph into the blood and then selectively returning to the gut wall. These precursors represent 1% of total circulating lymphocytes and are either IgA-bearing blasts or Thy-1$^+$ blast cells (3,12–15). In contrast, blasts of other origins, blasts obtained by culture, and small lymphocytes show minimal migration into the gut wall (15). T blasts circulating in the thoracic duct lymph bear $\alpha\beta$ TCR and either CD4 or CD8$\alpha\beta$ coreceptors (6) and migrate into both the lamina propria and the epithelium. In separate transfer experiments, purified CD8$^+$ blasts from the thoracic duct or mesenteric lymph nodes (16) migrated better into the epithelium than CD4$^+$ blasts, possibly explaining the relative distribution of the two populations within the gut in normal mice (Fig. 2).

Activated cells recirculating in mesenteric lymph nodes or the thoracic duct originate in Peyer's patches (PP) (15). Topical (^{3}H)TdR labeling of the PP leads, 48 hours later, to the appearance of labeled lymphocytes in the thoracic duct lymph and in the entire epithelium and lamina propria. Furthermore, selective and continuous (5-day) irradiation of the PP (with ^{32}P-labeled polyvinylchloride strips) drastically decreases the number of Thy-1$^+$ gut lymphocytes, as well as the number of IgA plasma cells in the lamina propria (15). Similar observations were made in acute

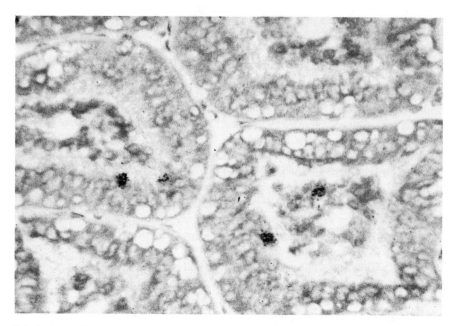

FIG. 2. Autoradiography of the gut wall 24 hours after transfer into a syngeneic normal mouse of CD8αβ$^+$ T blasts from the thoracic duct lymph and labeled with [^{3}H] TdR *in vitro* (16). The labeled cells are found within the lamina propria and between epithelial cells.

GVHR in lethally irradiated animals. This condition leads to massive and exclusive proliferation of allogeneic donor CD4$^+$ and CD8αβ$^+$, αβ TCR$^+$ cells that invade the gut wall. Irradiation of the PP leads to the disappearance of these cells from the gut epithelium and the lamina propria (15) without modifying the course of GVHR in the peripheral lymph nodes or spleen. Moreover, canulation of the thoracic duct in these animals also prevents infiltration of the gut by activated allogeneic T cells (15).

As soon as PP T lymphocytes proliferate they leave the patches. In conditions of strong immunization [GVHR (16) and nematode infestation (17)], the PP are small and the lymph contains numerous blasts. During this cycle, which allows the dissemination of the immune response to the whole gut (and to the body), T cells [and precursors of IgA plasma cells (3)] differentiate and mature. Only in the gut wall do they acquire the granules characteristic of terminal differentiation. Blasts can proliferate in the PP as the result of both allogeneic stimulation (GVHR) and exogenous antigenic stimulation in normal mice. In germ-free mice and suckling mice, gut lymphocytes are found in small numbers, and the proportion of CD4$^+$ and CD8αβ$^+$ IEL does not exceed 15%. The size of this thymus-dependent population increases proportionally to the intensity of the foreign antigenic stimulation (6).

Cells with the CD8αα phenotype are not found in the thoracic duct lymph of normal, nude, or suckling mice. The CD8αα$^+$ IEL population does not originate from circulating CD8αβ$^+$ blasts: after treatment *in vivo* with an anti-CD8β mAb,

CD8$\alpha\beta^+$ IEL disappear, together with peripheral CD8$^+$ T cells, while CD8$\alpha\alpha^+$ IEL persist with an unchanged percentage of $\alpha\beta$ TCR$^+$ and $\gamma\delta$ TCR$^+$ lymphocytes. It thus appears that precursors of the TID IEL population home directly from the bone marrow to the gut.

The ontogeny of TID IEL and TD IEL differs, as does their susceptibility to exogenous antigenic stimulation. Like TD IEL, TID IEL are not found at birth, but $\gamma\delta$ TCR$^+$ IEL are detectable at around day 16 in mice (8). TID IEL are the dominant population in the gut of germ-free mice, although their numbers are reduced relative to normal mice. The TD $\gamma\delta$ TCR$^+$ IEL/$\alpha\beta$ TCR$^+$ IEL ratio in germ-free mice depends on the strain.

TID IEL may be influenced by the appearance of TD IEL through the release of lymphokines or an acceleration of epithelium renewal kinetics (16): the influx of TD IEL into the gut results in an increase in the TID pool, as well as in modifications of the $\gamma\delta$ TCR$^+$/$\alpha\beta$ TCR$^+$ IEL ratio, with an increasing percentage of TID IEL bearing $\alpha\beta$ TCR.

THE CD4$^+$/CD8$\alpha\beta^+$ SUBSET AND THE CD4$^-$CD8$^-$ SUBSET ACQUIRE THE CD3-TCR COMPLEX IN DIFFERENT ENDODERM DERIVATIVES: THE THYMUS AND THE GUT, RESPECTIVELY.

CD4$^+$, $\alpha\beta$ TCR$^+$ or CD8$\alpha\beta^+$, $\alpha\beta$ TCR$^+$ lymphocytes are the progeny of cells that differentiate in the thymus. They migrate early in life to the PP and are part of the continuously recirculating pool of mature small lymphocytes. When stimulated, they migrate as blast cells to the gut. Double-negative and double-positive thymocytes do not migrate to the gut wall (unpublished data).

In contrast, gut CD4$^-$ CD8β^- IEL differentiate in the gut microenvironment. In young athymic nude mice, mature CD3/TCR$^+$ lymphocytes are virtually absent outside of the gut. By Northern blot analysis of the IEL δ TCR, mature transcripts that migrate as a 2-kD band are detectable, as are a few immature transcripts (1.7-kD band); in contrast, only the immature forms are detectable in bone marrow cells enriched with lymphoid precursors. The ability of precursors to differentiate fully in the gut wall is also striking in nude mice bearing a transgene against the HY antigen (18). These mice are the result of the back-crossing of H2b transgenic euthymic mice with H2b nude mice. Cells bearing the $\alpha\beta$ transgene are not detectable in the peripheral lymphoid organs or bone marrow (19). In contrast, numerous CD8$\alpha\alpha^+$ IEL bearing the transgene are found in male mice (Fig. 3).

Thus it appears that the gut epithelial microenvironment is able to induce in TID cells $\alpha\beta$ TCR/CD3 and $\gamma\delta$ TCR/CD3 complexes, the hallmarks of T cells. Indeed, the enzymatic machinery required for TCR rearrangement is not detectable in the thymocyte progeny but is found in IEL (6). *In situ* hybridization has shown that RAG-1 protein transcripts are detectable in the small population of TCR$^-$ IEL (20).

The pathway of TCR rearrangement appears to be different in TID IEL when compared with thymocytes. First, in the thymus, RAG-1 transcripts are detectable

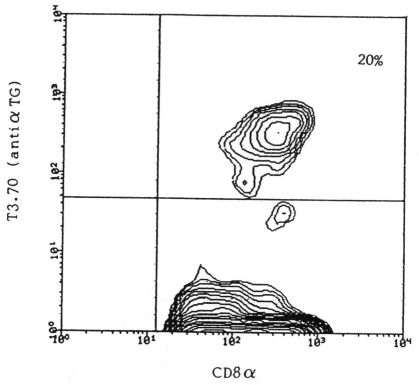

FIG. 3. CD8α$^+$ IEL from a transgenic male nude mouse (a kind gift from H. Von Boehmer). T3.70 mab recognizes the α chain of the anti-HY αβ transgene.

in both TCR$^-$ CD4$^-$CD8$^-$ and in TCR$^+$ CD4$^+$CD8αβ$^+$ thymocytes, as α TCR rearrangements continue to occur during the expansion of double positive thymocytes. In contrast, RAG-1 transcripts in IEL appear to be restricted to the TCR$^-$ population (20). This suggests that, in contrast to the progeny of double positive thymocytes, IEL undergo limited TCR rearrangements giving rise locally to TCR$^+$ cells without prior extensive local expansion and selection. Second, no thymocytes coexpress αβ and γδ TCRs. By contrast, cells bearing the β TCR chain as well as the γδ TCR chains are present among IEL, representing about 15 to 40% of all γδ TCR$^+$ IEL (21). It is likely that these IEL express both types of TCR, since their β TCR chains do not associate with δ TCR chains in cocapping experiments; however, these experiments do not rule out the possibility that the β chains are present in the form of ββ homodimers (22), since a monoclonal antibody against the framework of α chains was not available. However in mice bearing anti-HY αβ TCR transgenes (18 and below), the specific chains of which can be recognized by monoclonal antibodies, coexpression of αβ and γδ TCR chains on IELs has been demonstrated (21). Thus, the mechanisms that control the expression of TCRs may differ between TD and TID cells.

The gut microenvironment also induces the appearance of CD8αα molecules. This coreceptor, found on TID TCR$^+$ IEL, also appears on TCR$^-$ IEL, which are numerous in nude mice (6) and which are the only population in mice with the SCID mutation (6,23). CD8α molecules are also induced on TD CD4$^+$ cells (Fig. 1) and possibly on TD CD8αβ$^+$ IEL.

GUT TD CD4$^+$CD8αβ$^+$ LYMPHOCYTES AND TID CD4$^-$CD8β$^-$ LYMPHOCYTES SHOW DIFFERENT RULES OF SELECTION

The progeny of double-positive thymocytes show a deletion of Vβ6$^+$, Vβ8.1$^+$ and Vβ11$^+$ lymphocytes in Mls − 1^a IE$^+$ mice (24,25). When TD and TID αβ TCR$^+$ gut IEL are separated and studied for expression of these Vβ chains, TD IEL show the same deletions as peripheral T cells, while TID IEL do not. On the contrary, these Vβ families are frequently overrepresented in the TID lineage.

Studies of mice bearing a transgenic αβ TCR specific for the male antigen (HY) clearly demonstrated that the negative and positive selection processes that shape the repertoire of TD αβ TCR$^+$ lymphocytes do not take place in TID IEL. In these mice, recognition of HY is MHC class I-restricted and requires the expression of the αβ TCR transgenic receptor and high levels of CD8 coreceptors at the cell surface (26). In female mice, CD8αβ$^+$ transgene-expressing HY-specific cells are positively selected in the thymus by MHC class I in the absence of specific peptide; they migrate in the lymphoid organs as CD8αβ^{bright} lymphocytes, and some are found among TD gut IEL (unpublished data). In contrast, lymphocytes with the transgenic TCR are very rare among TID IEL, and are exclusively of the CD4$^-$ CD8$^-$ phenotype (21). In male transgenic mice, HY-specific thymocytes are deleted and CD8αβ^{bright} transgene-positive lymphocytes are absent from the TD lymphocyte population. Among TD IEL, however, transgenic CD8αα^{bright} cells are numerous and have not thus undergone negative selection. Rather than causing deletion, recognition of HY appears to lead to the differentiation of male-specific TID IEL. Among transgenic TCR$^+$ IEL, only those that are CD8αα^{bright} (not those that are double-negative), display intracytoplasmic granules (21), the hallmark of gut IEL differentiation. Thus, CD8αα chains (induced by the gut epithelium, probably at random) act in transgenic mice as αβ TCR coreceptors in a recognition process that has an effect opposite to that observed in the thymus: not only does it not result in deletion but it also leads to increased differentiation (8,21).

As for TID γδ TCR$^+$ IEL, their rules of selection are a matter of some controversy, even in the thymus. While they appear to be deleted in the thymus, they seem to be progressively anergized in the gut wall (27). Since the representation of Vγ and Vδ gene families is similar in nude and euthymic mice (28), it is probable that the γδ TCR IEL repertoire develops largely independently of thymic selection, probably under antigenic influence. CD8α molecules are not necessarily required for the differentiation process since the proportion of γδ TCR$^+$ lymphocytes containing granules is similar among CD8αα$^+$ and CD8αα$^-$ lymphocytes (21).

TD CD4$^+$/CD8αβ$^+$ IEL AND TID CD4$^-$CD8$^-$ IEL ARE BOTH MATURE CELLS WITH CYTOTOXIC PROPERTIES

It is difficult to induce proliferation of gut IEL *in vitro* (29 and unpublished data). Recently, Poussier et al. (10) reported that, in contrast to the CD8β$^-$ subset, the CD4$^+$/CD8αβ$^+$ subset proliferates. They concluded that the CD8β$^-$ subset is immature. In contrast to this view, it is likely that this subset is fully differentiated, since it contains a higher percentage (65 to 85%) of cells with intracytoplasmic granules than the CD4$^+$/CD8αβ$^+$ subset. IEL granules contain perforin and granzyme, two cytotoxic proteins (30). In addition, TD IEL and TID IEL (bearing αβ or γδ TCR) became cytotoxic on cross-linkage of their TCRs by mAbs in directed cytotoxicity assays (30–32). Strikingly, and in contrast to agranular peripheral T cells, both TD and TID IEL are cytotoxic against class II$^+$ targets coated with enterotoxin superantigens (Fig. 4). αβ TCR$^+$ TID IEL, a subset not deleted by self-

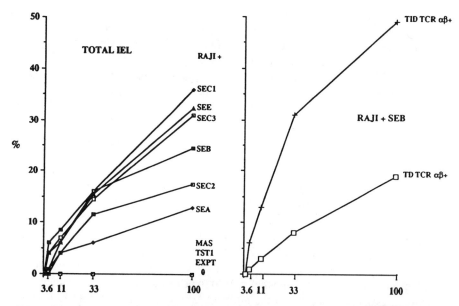

FIG. 4. Cytotoxic activity of IEL against Raji tumor cells coated with enterotoxins (1 μg/ml), at various ratios, after 3 hours' incubation. For isolation of TD and TID TCRαβ$^+$ IEL, IEL were labeled with biotinylated anti-δ mab (GL3) + PE and with FITC-labeled anti-CD4 and anti-CD8β mab (6). Subsets were sorted with a FACStar® flow cytometer.

superantigens, can be highly cytotoxic, probably reflecting the abundance of cells bearing Vβ chains reactive against enterotoxins.

SUMMARY

The long-ignored T lymphocytes of the gut epithelium are a peculiar population of special interest. They comprise two subsets: TD lymphocytes were probably added to the ancestral TID system during the evolution, while gut IgA plasma cells originating from PP probably reinforce the system of precursors originating from the omentum (33).

The TD population must be sensitized in the PP to the antigens they will reencounter in the gut. The TID population is selected and induced to differentiate by antigens present on the surface of the villous epithelium, and they may play a major role as a first line of defense. Both populations are cytotoxic and are probably able to destroy epithelial cells. The mechanisms of antigen presentation by epithelial cells are not fully understood. Epithelial cells appear able to present peptides and superantigens, since they express not only class I but also class II molecules [in large amounts under IFN-γ stimulation (16)], as well as the class Ib molecules Tla and CD1 (34–36).

When epithelial cells are destroyed, crypt cells show accelerated proliferation via an adaptive process known to occur in other epithelial stem cells (37). Gut damage occurs when this restorative process is insufficient. Finally, it appears unlikely that the gut epithelium and lamina propria are closed compartments. The ratio of TD to TID lymphocytes in the lamina propria is unknown. The lamina propria is probably a reservoir of TD and TID lymphocytes. The life spans of IEL subsets remain to be accurately determined.

REFERENCES

1. Rocha B, Vassalli P, Guy-Grand D. The Vβ repertoire of mouse gut homodimeric CD8[+] intraepithelial αβ TCR[+] lymphocytes reveals a major extrathymic pathway of T cell differentiation. *J Exp Med* 1991;173:483–486.
2. Fichtelius KE. The gut epithelium: a first level lymphoid organ? *Exp Cell Res* 1968;49:87–104.
3. Guy-Grand D, Griscelli C, Vassalli P. The gut-associated lymphoid system: nature and properties of the large dividing cells. *Eur J Immunol* 1974;4:435–443.
4. Goodman T, Lefrançois L. Expression of the γδ T-cell receptor on intestinal CD8[+] intraepithelial lymphocytes. *Nature* 1988;333:855–858.
5. Bonneville M, Janeway CA Jr, Ito K, Haser W, Ishida I, Nakanishi N, Tonegawa S. Intestinal intraepithelial lymphocytes are a distinct set of γδ T-cells. *Nature* 1988;336:479–481.
6. Guy-Grand D, Cerf-Bensussan N, Malissen B, Malassis-Seris M, Briottet C, Vassalli P. Two gut intraepithelial CD8[+] lymphocyte populations with different T cell receptors: a role for the gut epithelium in T cell differentiation. *J Exp Med* 1991;173:471–481.
7. Rocha B, Vassalli P, Guy-Grand D. The extrathymic T cell development pathway. *Immunol Today* 1992;13:449–454.
8. Bandeira A, Itohara S, Bonneville M, Burlen-Defranoux O, Mota-Santos T, Coutinho A, Tonegawa S. Extrathymic origin of intestinal intraepithelial lymphocytes bearing T-cell antigen receptor γδ. *Proc Natl Acad Sci USA* 1991;88:43–47.

9. Mosley RL, Styre D, Klein JR. Differentiation and functional maturation of bone marrow derived intestinal epithelial T cells expressing membrane T cell receptor in athymic radiation chimeras. *J Immunol* 1990;145:1369–1375.

10. Poussier P, Edouard P, Lee C, Binnie M, Julius M. Thymus-independent development and negative selection of T cells expressing T cell receptor $\alpha\beta$ in the intestinal epithelium: evidence for distinct circulation patterns of gut- and thymus-derived T lymphocytes. *J Exp Med* 1992;176:187–199.

11. Gowans JL, Knight EJ. The route of re-circulation of lymphocytes in the rat. *Proc R Soc Lond* 1964;139:257–282.

12. Husband AJ, Gowans JL. The origin and antigen-dependent distribution of IgA-containing cells in the intestine. *J Exp Med* 1978;48:1146–1160.

13. McWilliams M, Phillips-Quagliata JM, Lamm ME. Mesenteric lymph node B lymphoblasts which home to the small intestine are precommitted to IgA synthesis. *J Exp Med* 1977;145:866–875.

14. Sprent J. Fate of H2-activated T lymphocytes in syngeneic hosts. *Cell Immunol* 1976;21:278–302.

15. Guy-Grand D, Griscelli C, Vassalli P. The mouse gut T lymphocyte, a novel type of T cell: nature, origin and traffic in mice in normal and graft-versus-host conditions. *J Exp Med* 1978;148:1661–1677.

16. Guy-Grand D, Vassalli P. Gut injury in mouse graft-versus-host reaction: study of its occurrence and mechanisms. *J Clin Invest* 1986;77:1584–1595.

17. Guy-Grand D, Dy M, Luffau G, Vassalli P. Gut mucosal mast cells: origin, traffic and differentiation. *J Exp Med* 1984;160:12–28.

18. Von Boehmer H. Developmental biology of T cells in T cell-receptor transgenic mice. *Annu Rev Immunol* 1990;8:531–556.

19. Von Boehmer H, Kirberg J, Rocha B. An unusual lineage of $\alpha\beta$ T cells that contains autoreactive cells. *J Exp Med* 1991;174:1001–1008.

20. Guy-Grand D, Vanden Broecke C, Briottet C, Malassis-Seris M, Selz F, Vassalli P. Different expression of the recombination activity gene RAG-1 in various populations of thymocytes, peripheral T cells and gut thymus-independent intraepithelial lymphocytes suggests two pathways of T cell receptor rearrangement. *Eur J Immunol* 1992;22:505–510.

21. Rocha B, Von Boehmer H, Guy-Grand D. Selection of intraepithelial lymphocytes with CD8$\alpha\alpha$ coreceptors by self-antigen in the murine gut. *Proc Natl Acad Sci USA* 1992;89:5336–5340.

22. Von Boehmer H. Thymic selection: a matter of life and death. *Immunol Today* 1992;13:454–458.

23. Croitoru K, Stead RH, Bienenstock J, Fulop G, Harnish DG, Shultz LD, Jeffery PK, Ernst PB. Presence of intestinal intraepithelial lymphocytes in mice with severe combined immunodeficiency disease. *Eur J Immunol* 1990;29:645–651.

24. MacDonald HR, Schneider R, Lees RK, et al. T-cell receptor Vβ use predicts reactivity and tolerance to Mlsa-encoded antigens. *Nature (Lond.)* 1988;332:40.

25. Bill J, Kanagawa O, Woodland DL, Palmer E. The MHC molecule I-E is necessary but not sufficient for the clonal deletion of Vβ11-bearing T cells. *J Exp Med* 1989;169:1405.

26. Huesmann M, Scott B, Kisielow P, Von Boehmer H. Kinetics and efficacy of positive selection in the thymus of normal and T cell receptor transgenic mice. *Cell* 1991;66:533–540.

27. Barrett TA, Delvy ML, Kennedy DM, et al. Mechanism of self-tolerance of $\gamma\delta$ T cells in epithelial tissue. *J Exp Med* 1992;175:65–70.

28. Ota Y, Kobata T, Seki M, et al. Extrathymic origin of Vγ1/Vδ6 T cells in the skin. *Eur J Immunol* 1992;22:595–598.

29. Mosley RL, Whetsell M, Klein JR. Proliferative properties of murine intestinal intraepithelial lymphocytes (IEL): IEL expressing TCR$\alpha\beta$ or TCR$\gamma\delta$ are largely unresponsive to proliferative signals mediated via conventional stimulation of the CD3-TCR complex. *Int Immunol* 1991;3:563–569.

30. Guy-Grand D, Malassis-Seris M, Briottet C, Vassalli P. Cytotoxic differentiation of mouse gut thymodependent and independent intraepithelial T lymphocytes is induced locally: correlation between functional assays, presence of perforin and granzyme transcripts, and cytoplasmic granules. *J Exp Med* 1991;173:1549–1552.

31. Goodman T. Lefrancois L. Intraepithelial lymphocytes: anatomical site, not T cell receptor form, dictates phenotype and function. *J Exp Med* 1989;170:1569–1581.

32. Viney JL, Kilshaw PJ, MacDonald TT. Cytotoxic $\alpha\beta^+$ and $\gamma\delta^+$ T cells in murine intestinal epithelium. *Eur J Immunol* 1990;20:1623–1626.

33. Solvason N, Lehuen A, Kearney JF. An embryonic source of Ly1 but not conventional B cells. *Intern Immunol* 1991;3:543–550.

34. Hershberg R, Eghtesady P, Sydora B, Brorson K, Cheroutre H, Modlin R, Kronenberg M. Expres-

sion of the thymus leukemia antigen in mouse intestinal epithelium. *Proc Natl Acad Sci USA* 1990; 87:9727–9731.

35. Wu M, Van Kaer L, Itohara S, Tonegawa S. Highly restricted expression of the thymus leukemia antigens on intestinal epithelial cells. *J Exp Med* 1991;174:213–218.

36. Bleicher PA, Balk SP, Hagen SJ, Blumberg RS, Flotte TJ, Terhorst C. Expression of murine CD1 on gastrointestinal epithelium. *Science* 1990;250:679–681.

37. Cotsarelis G, Cheng SZ, Dong G, Sun TT, Lavker RM. Existence of slow-cycling limbal epithelial basal cells that can be preferentially stimulated to proliferate: implications on epithelial stem cells. *Cell* 1989;57:201–209.

Mucosal Immunology: Intraepithelial Lymphocytes,
edited by H. Kiyono and J. R. McGhee.
Raven Press, Ltd., New York © 1993.

3

Phenotypic and Cytotoxic Characteristics of Intraepithelial Lymphocytes

John R. Klein[*] and R. Lee Mosley[†]

*Department of Biological Science, University of Tulsa, 600 S. College Avenue, Tulsa, OK.
†Department of Pathology and Experimental Toxicology, University of Michigan
Medical School, 2800 Plymouth Road, Ann Arbor, MI.*

Intestinal intraepithelial lymphocytes (IEL) comprise part of the gut-associated lymphoid tissues (GALT). Prior to methodologies for characterizing lymphocyte subsets either functionally or phenotypically, little attention had been paid to the IEL. However, beginning in the 1960s and continuing to the present, there has been increased interest in the IEL, both as a component of the mammalian immune system, and with regard to the role of the IEL in protection from and/or induction of disease states within the gastrointestinal tract. This chapter discusses phenotypic and cytotoxic properties of the intestinal IEL, particularly in the context of studies done in mice and rats. Although IEL also are present in extraintestinal mucosal tissues (e.g., skin, reproductive tract, lung, etc.), the present review focuses on IEL of the intestinal tract. In understanding a dynamic and changing area of biology such as the IEL, it is important to bear in mind that until the clear and complete picture emerges, contradictions in experimental findings will exist. Many factors undoubtedly account for those differences, including variations in experimental approaches used among laboratories, differences in the immunophysiologic and pathophysiologic status of laboratory animals, and perhaps most importantly, differences imparted onto data when viewed as a portion of the whole due to an incomplete understanding of the overall biology. Even so, the surge in interest in the intestinal IEL has provided a surprisingly rapid and accurate characterization of several key aspects of intestinal T cell biology that were not appreciated but a few years ago.

MORPHOLOGICAL CHARACTERISTICS OF THE IEL

The murine intestinal mucosa can be compartmentalized anatomically according to lamina propria and epithelial regions demarcated by a basement membrane. Prior to the availability of monoclonal antibodies (mAb) and the widespread use of flow cytometric (FCM) analyses using the flourescent-activated cell sorter, much had been learned about the IEL based on properties of physical and morphological criteria, as discussed in earlier review articles (1–4). Those reports provide interesting insights into the general nature of the IEL and demonstrate that in nearly every aspect of IEL biology, similarities and differences exist when compared to lymphocytes in other peripheral immune compartments. By morphologic and phenotypic criteria, lymphoid cells in the small intestine of rats and mice are nearly all lymphocytes. Polymorphonuclear leukocytes and mast cells are rarely present in the gut epithelium (4–6), although increases in those cells may occur during parasitic infections (7–10) and may be regulated by lymphokine secretion locally (6). Exact numbers of IEL present in the small intestine epithelium of mice are difficult to determine due in part to variations in cell recoveries in epithelium-extracted cell preparations. However, *in situ* there are between 50 and 100×10^6 IEL per small intestine (4,11,12,17), making the IEL compartment equivalent in size to the murine spleen. In purified IEL preparations, about 5 to 10×10^6 purified IEL are obtained per mouse or rat small intestine (11–18), depending on the extraction procedure used (11,12,17,19,21). Consequently, even with the best procedures, the number of IEL recovered in epithelium-extracted preparations rarely exceeds 50% of the total lymphocytes present in the gut epithelium (11,12,17,21).

Intracytoplasmic Granules

One of the earliest morphological characteristics that distinguished murine IEL from other lymphocyte populations was the presence of intracytoplasmic granules similar in some respects to those found in natural killer (NK) cells (4). Intracytoplasmic granules are readily evident in Giemsa-stained tissue sections of mouse (5,6,12,20,22–24), rat (15,25–27), rabbit (28), and human (28,29) IEL. Cytoplasmic granules do not contain histamine, nor do IEL bear Fcε receptors (4,5). In mice and rats, the proportion of granulated lymphocytes may range from 30 to 80% of the total IEL (5,6,11,12,20,22,25–27) and may vary according to size of granules (4,6) and as to the proportion of granulated IEL in animal strains within a species (22). Functionally, it is likely that granules are involved in target cell destruction by cytotoxic IEL, as inferred from findings of perforin and granzymes in granulated IEL (30). Yet, granulation is not a hallmark of cytotoxic activity of IEL given that lytic activity also is present among nongranulated IEL (4,5,27), and considering the extensive variation noted in the distribution and morphology of IEL granules (4,22).

Properties of Cell Size and Density

When physical characteristics of IEL are studied by FCM analyses, the majority of IEL in adult mice are indistinguishable from other murine lymphocytes. By criteria of cell size and granularity, murine IEL consist of small-to-medium-sized lymphocytes. That property can be seen in Fig. 1, which compares lymphocytes from adult thymus (A), spleen (B), lymph nodes (C), and the intestinal epithelium (IEL) (D). Using the leukocyte common antigen (CD45) to track hematopoietic cells

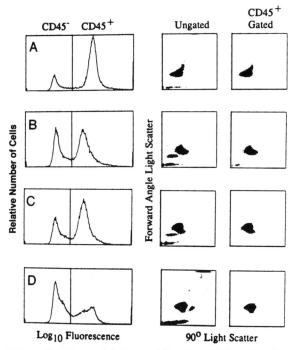

FIG. 1. Cells from adult thymus (*A*), spleen (*B*), lymph nodes (*C*), and intestine epithelium (*D*) were stained with mAb to the leukocyte common antigen, CD45, to identify total lymphoid cells. The distribution of unstained and CD45$^+$ cells from each tissue is shown in the center and right panels according to cell size (forward-angle light scatter) and cell granularity (90° light scatter) in each population, indicating a high degree of similarity between IEL and other lymphocyte populations according to those parameters. (RL Mosley and JR Klein, unpublished.)

(31,32), and by comparing each population according to similar parameters of cell size (forward scatter) and cell granularity (90° scatter), the distribution of the total cell population (ungated) and the CD45$^+$ cell population (CD45$^+$ gated) is evident. Only minor differences are noted in the size of IEL, and in the degree of granularity of those cells, compared to lymphocytes of the thymus, spleen, and lymph nodes, demonstrating that most IEL are indistinguishable from lymphocytes in other immune compartments. However, IEL also contain a minor subset of slightly larger, more heavily granulated lymphoid cells (32–36). Those IEL comprise about 10 to 15% of the total IEL and correlate with the percentage of asialo GM$_1$$^+$ IEL (32–35).

By other criteria, the IEL exhibit a high degree of cellular heterogeneity that is most evident in properties of cell density. Studies in which discontinuous Percoll gradients are used to purify murine IEL indicate that viable lymphocytes are present at several levels between 30% (1.048 g/ml) and 70% (1.095 g/ml) Percoll (5,6,

11,12). Although most IEL migrate through 40% (1.062 g/ml) Percoll but not into 55% (1.075 g/ml) Percoll, some IEL consistently penetrate 55% Percoll (5,6,11, 12). IEL isolated in high-density Percoll gradients (>45 to 50% Percoll) frequently result in substantial loss of total IEL (11,12) and may cause deletions of potentially important subsets. In experiments using 40/50/55% discontinuous Percoll gradients to separate IEL in our laboratory, approximately 60% of the IEL migrate to the 40/50% Percoll interface; 20% migrate to the 50/55% Percoll interface; and 20% migrate below 55% Percoll (36a). In similar studies using splenic lymphocytes, a reverse pattern of cell migration occurs such that only 3% of nucleated spleen cells migrate to the 40/50% Percoll interface; 14% migrate to the 50/55% Percoll interface; and the bulk of splenic lymphocytes, 83%, migrate below 55% Percoll. Thus, a major difference exists between lymphocytes of the gut epithelium and the spleen with regard to cell density. The IEL that migrate to the 40/50% Percoll interface are most characteristic of murine IEL with regard to phenotypic properties; however, several important functional properties of IEL are specifically associated with certain subsets. It has been shown, for example, that most cytotoxic activities mediated by IEL NK cells migrate above 55% Percoll (5), whereas CD3- or T cell receptor (TCR)-induced proliferation of IEL is greatest in the IEL population that migrates at the 50/55% Percoll interface (36a). Those differences demonstrate that cell density can be an extremely useful criterion for studying functionally distinct IEL groups, and point to the need to carefully select methods of extraction and purification for studies of IEL in order to avoid skewing or deletion of component IEL subsets. IEL extraction techniques that provide high viability and purity with maximum overall cell recovery are especially important for studies aimed at understanding the total IEL, such as for analyses of the TCR repertoire, or for phenotypic studies of the IEL.

GENERAL PHENOTYPIC PROPERTIES OF THE IEL

Early phenotypic studies of intestinal IEL revealed that most lymphocytes within the gut epithelium are T cells, as determined by a lack of immunoglobulin (Ig)[+] cells in histologic sections stained by immunocytochemical techniques and/or by expression of broadly distributed T cells markers such as Thy-1 and CD8 (22,37–39). Those phenotypic properties have been confirmed in many studies using freshly extracted IEL and by immunochemical staining in situ. However, more detailed studies (4–6,11,12,14,16,18,21,31,33–35,41–55), of the IEL have revealed that as much as half of the CD8[+] IEL lack Thy-1 expression, thereby defining a large and rather unusual subset of Thy-1[−], CD8[+] peripheral T cells (Fig. 2). Although that IEL phenotype now is a well-documented component of the gut epithelium, considerable variation may occur in the proportion of Thy-1[+] IEL.

With regard to other lymphocyte markers, essentially all IEL express the leukocyte common antigen (CD45), a marker that can be used to discriminate IEL from enterocytes (32,56). IEL in humans (57–58) but not in rats (59,60) express CD2.

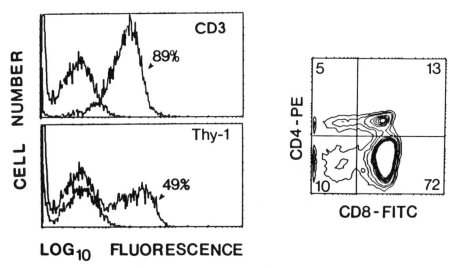

FIG. 2. General phenotypic profile of murine IEL demonstrating that most cells are CD3[+], CD8[+], CD4[−] T cells of which about half express Thy-1. Also present among IEL are CD4[+] CD8[+] T cells and a CD4[−]CD8[−] subset. (RL Mosley and JR Klein, unpublished.)

About 30 to 50% of IEL in mice and rats express CD5 (Lyt-1) (6,33,34,52,61) and/ or the lymphocyte-function associated antigen, LFA-1 (CD11a) (31,35). Surface antigens such as NK1.2 or asialo GM_1 are expressed on a minor proportion of the IEL (12,33–35). In rats virtually all IEL express Thy-1 and CD8 (59,60) as well as CD43 (59). The majority of IEL in mice are B220[−] (61). The heat-stable antigen (HSA) generally is not expressed on murine IEL, although a minor subset of IEL, which are T cells and not B cells, occasionally expresses HSA (40,51); that subset is highly variable and may be a transient IEL population (D Stickney and JR Klein, unpublished). Other lymphocyte markers of IEL are discussed in the context of specific IEL functional properties.

CD4[−]CD8[+] and CD4[+]CD8[−] Single-Positive IEL Subsets

Overall, about 80 to 90% of the CD3[+] IEL in mice and rats are CD8[+]CD4[−] T cells (Fig. 2). The remaining CD3[+] IEL can be accounted for by two CD4[+] subsets: one is a CD4[+]CD8[−] subset; the other is an unusual CD4[+]CD8[+] phenotype (discussed below), each of which usually comprises less than 15% of the total IEL (14,15,17,18,32,40–42,46,49,50–54,62–66). CD4[+]CD8[−] IEL are primarily Thy-1[+] T cells that express the αβ TCR (62,63) are not contaminants from the lamina propria or the Peyer's patches, but appear to be true components of the gut epithelium. The specific functional role of the CD4[+]CD8[−] IEL subset is not yet evident.

Understanding the CD8[+] IEL is further complicated by the fact that the CD8 molecular complex can be expressed in one of two mutually exclusively forms on IEL (66), consisting of either a CD8αβ heterodimer or a CD8αα homodimer (67–69). In mice the proportion of CD8αα IEL usually exceeds that of CD8αβ IEL (30,43,52,53,61,62), a finding also true for IEL in wild mice (70). Most γδTCR$^+$ IEL are CD8αα T cells, whereas αβTCR$^+$ IEL can be either CD8αβ or CD8αα T cells (43,50,52,53,61,62). The CD8αβ subset is primarily Thy-1$^+$ (18,43,60). In mice lethally irradiated with 950 rads, CD8αβ cells are quickly lost from the gut epithelium, whereas CD8αα are retained (54), implying that CD8αβ IEL are radiosensitive cells with a rapid turnover rate. There is an increase in CD8αβ on αβTCR$^+$ IEL following *in vitro* exposure to staphylococcal enterotoxin A (SEA) (53) and also in mice with age (62), suggesting that the presence of CD8αβ IEL subset within the gut epithelium is influenced by environmental factors. Although in congenitally athymic nude mice the overall proportion of αβTCR$^+$ IEL also increases with age, there is no concomitant increase in CD8β expression in those animals (53).

CD4$^+$CD8$^+$ Double-Positive and CD4$^-$CD8$^-$ Double-Negative IEL Subsets

In both mice and rats a peripheral CD4$^+$CD8$^+$ double-positive (DP) T cell subset is present among the IEL (49,52,63,64). In mice, most DP IEL are CD3$^+$ and Thy-1$^+$ (18,49,52), are αβTCR$^+$ (52,63), and also are present in athymic mice (18,51,71). Most DP IEL are CD8α$^+$ T cells (18,52). In rats the number of DP IEL increases with age, accounting for 20 to 40% of the total CD4$^+$/CD8$^+$ IEL by six months of age in normal rats, although not in aged germ-free or nude rats (65), suggesting that expression of the DP phenotype may be influenced in some fashion by thymus-dependent factors in conjunction with intestinal microflora. Some strains of mice (e.g., C57BR/cd) have high levels of DP IEL (52), although the effect of age on DP IEL in those mice has not been determined. DP IEL do not appear to be precursors of single-positive IEL, as determined from studies using radiation chimeras, but may arise from the CD4$^+$CD8$^-$ subset (55). The latter possibility is further supported by studies of human lymphocytes demonstrating that mature CD4$^+$ CD8$^-$ T cells acquire CD8 expression upon *in vitro* culture with the T cell-derived cytokine interleukin (IL)-4 (68,72). CD8 expression induced on CD4$^+$ T cell consists principally of the CD8αβ heterodimer and is reversible upon removal of IL-4, indicating a cytokine-dependent effect (68). Conversely, CD4$^-$, CD8αβ$^+$ T cells do not acquire CD4 expression upon culture with IL-4 (68), implying that development of cytokine-induced DP T cells occurs in a precise and apparently regulated manner. DP IEL in rats lack CD45RB, suggesting that those IEL are memory cells (59).

Also present among the IEL is a subset of CD4$^-$CD8$^-$ lymphocytes that are not B cells as shown by expression of TCR (14,18,49,51,62,63,73). Those cells constitute between 5 and 25% of the total IEL and primarily express the γδ TCR (63). Like the DP IEL, the functional role of CD4$^-$CD8$^-$ IEL is largely unknown; however, they may have an immunoregulatory role within the gut (79).

T Cell Receptor Phenotypes of the IEL

With the availability of mAbs that precisely define the TCR and associated molecules (CD3 complex), accurate analyses of IEL T cell subsets within the gut epithelium has been possible. Although the intestinal IEL were initially described as $\gamma\delta$ TCR$^+$ T cells (41,74), phenotypic analyses of IEL using flow cytometry now demonstrate that both $\alpha\beta$ TCR$^+$ and $\gamma\delta$ TCR$^+$ T cells are routinely present within the small intestine epithelium of mice, usually in about equivalent proportions. In fact, of studies done to date, 43.4% of murine IEL were $\alpha\beta$ TCR$^+$ and 46.4% were $\gamma\delta$ TCR$^+$ collectively (14,18,30,42,43,48,55,61–64,75–80). Those findings, however, should not be taken to mean that the distribution of TCR-bearing IEL are always evenly distributed. Indeed, extensive variations exist with regard to expression of TCR class. The reasons for such variations are not clear, however, factors such as age, intestinal flora, or other local microenvironmental events may be important. In wild mice there is a 3:1 ratio of $\gamma\delta$ TCR$^+$ to $\alpha\beta$ TCR$^+$ IEL (70); however, the effect of age cannot be measured in those animals. Thy-1 is expressed on some $\alpha\beta$ TCR$^+$ and $\gamma\delta$ TCR$^+$ IEL in inbred mice (14,16,17,52–54,62), whereas nearly all IEL in wild mice do not express Thy-1 (70). Both $\alpha\beta$ TCR$^+$ and $\gamma\delta$ TCR$^+$ IEL are present among the single-positive IEL subsets (CD4$^-$8$^+$ and CD4$^+$8$^-$) (63), most DP IEL are $\alpha\beta$ TCR$^+$ T cells, and most DN IEL are $\gamma\delta$ TCR$^+$ T cells (63). Unlike in mice, in which a high proportion of IEL are $\gamma\delta$ TCR$^+$ T cells, in rats (15,59) and humans (81), only about 15% of IEL express the $\gamma\delta$ TCR.

T Cell Receptor Phenotypes and the IEL Repertoire

Phenotypic and molecular studies of IEL TCR genes and gene expression indicate that the overall repertoire of both $\alpha\beta$ TCR$^+$ and $\gamma\delta$ TCR$^+$ IEL is probably large. In addition to reactivity of IEL with pan-$\alpha\beta$ and pan-$\gamma\delta$ TCR antibodies, IEL have been shown to contain $\alpha\beta$ TCR$^+$ subsets defined by antibodies to Vβ3 (53), Vβ6 (18,82), Vβ8 (21,82), and Vβ11 (18,21,82). Moreover, compared to $\gamma\delta$ TCR$^+$ cells in anatomical sites such as the skin epidermis or the reproductive tract, intestinal IEL exhibit a high degree of diversity of the $\gamma\delta$ TCR at both the gene and protein level. In mice, rearrangements have been reported for at least four of the six functional γ genes (71,83–85), with preference for Vγ5 (71,77,83–86). Rearrangements of all seven δ genes have been reported for IEL, although Vδ4, Vδ5, Vδ6, and Vδ7 appear to be most frequently used by IEL (83–85, 87). Events of junctional diversity involving gene rearrangements substantially increase IEL TCR diversity at the gene level and also in the γ and δ chain proteins (71,84,87). In addition, diversity of the $\gamma\delta$ TCR at the cell surface can be further inferred from studies of FCM analyses of IEL using mAbs specific for γ (76,78,88) or δ chain molecules (76,78,88). Mice with severe combined immune deficiency (SCID) have CD8$^+$CD4$^-$ IEL, which lack TCR expression (24). In wild mice, $\gamma\delta$ TCR$^+$ T cells use Vγ1.2, Vγ2, and/or Vγ5 genes and Vδ4, Vδ5, and Vδ6 genes, demonstrating a high degree of similarity in γ and δ gene repertoires of laboratory and wild mice.

PHENOTYPIC MARKERS OF IEL LINEAGE AND DEVELOPMENT

Issues of IEL ontogeny and development, particularly as they relate to the thymus-dependency of intestinal T cells, are of considerable interest. Over a quarter of a century ago immunologists recognized that murine IEL are probably not thymus-dependent lymphocytes as determined from studies using neonatally thymectomized mice or radiation chimeras (25,26,89,90). Those early observations now have been firmly established in experiments that demonstrate the presence of phenotypically defined T cell populations among IEL in nude mice or athymic radiation chimeras (18,21,30,40,42,46,50,51,71,82,91). Expression of the recombinase-activating gene in cells from murine small intestine suggests local development of IEL T cells within the gut epithelium (30). While those studies demonstrate that CD3[+], CD8[+] IEL are routinely present in the gut epithelium of athymic mice, they provide little insight into IEL lineage and/or development pathways. Moreover, because Thy-1 is expressed on IEL in athymic chimeras (18,51), that marker is not useful for defining thymus-dependent versus thymus-independent subsets. Thus, identification of IEL markers that accurately discriminate thymus-independent and thymus-dependent IEL lineages is of importance for tracing specific developmental pathways of IEL T cells.

T Cell Receptor as a Phenotypic Marker of IEL Lineage

Both $\gamma\delta$ TCR[+] and $\alpha\beta$ TCR[+] IEL are present in athymic mice, although differences exist in the proportions of TCR-bearing IEL. Studies using nude mice demonstrate a preponderance of $\gamma\delta$ TCR[+] over $\alpha\beta$ TCR[+] IEL (21,30,42,46,48,82). In contrast, IEL that have developed in athymic radiation chimeras consist of both $\alpha\beta$ TCR[+] and $\gamma\delta$ TCR[+] T cells (18,50,51,71,87), frequently with a higher overall proportion of $\alpha\beta$ TCR[+] IEL than $\gamma\delta$ TCR[+] IEL (50,71,87). Given that few mature T cells are found in extraintestinal peripheral tissues of radiation chimeras, and because IEL in those mice are not host-derived T cells (18,50,71,87), $\alpha\beta$ TCR[+] IEL in athymic chimeras appear to be extrathymic in nature. Further evidence of extrathymic IEL development is drawn from studies of radiation chimeras with intact thymus epithelium in which $\alpha\beta$ TCR[+] and $\gamma\delta$ TCR[+] T cells are seeded into the gut epithelium within one week of BM transfer, and 1 to 2 weeks prior to the appearance of T cells in the thymus or the spleen (55), thus demonstrating that both types $\alpha\beta$ TCR[+] and $\gamma\delta$ TCR[+] IEL can develop directly from BM stem cells. The thymopoietic nature of the murine small intestine is further underscored in studies of athymic chimeras engrafted with fetal intestine under the kidney capsule or the shoulder, which leads to seeding of functionally mature T cells into peripheral immune compartments (92). In those mice both $\alpha\beta$ TCR[+] and $\gamma\delta$ TCR[+] T cells are present within intestine grafts, yet nearly all T cells exported to the periphery are CD3[+], $\alpha\beta$ TCR[+] cells that consist of both CD4[+]CD8[−] and CD4[−]CD8[+] subsets

(92). Other studies demonstrate that all phenotypically defined IEL are present in athymic chimeras, and that there is a lack of cross-circulation between the IEL and lymphocytes of other major lymphoid tissues (spleen and Peyer's patches), suggesting minimal interaction between the IEL and peripheral immune compartments (18).

IEL γ and δ gene rearrangements, and the extent of gene diversity, are similar for Vγ and Vδ genes in IEL that have developed in the absence or presence of a thymus (71,85,87). Analyses of gene rearrangements in athymic mice demonstrates gene diversity and protein heterogeneity for both γ and δ gene rearrangements in athymic mice, with the greatest potential for diversity in the δ molecule (71,84,87). In nude mice most, though not all, CD8$^+$ IEL lack Thy-1 expression (21,42,46,48), whereas Thy-1$^+$ IEL are common in athymic chimeras (21,51). That distinction is well drawn in a study (21) of IEL in nude mice and athymic chimeras in which the kinetic development of Thy-1 expression in athymic chimeras was similar to what occurred in thymus-bearing control mice. The reasons for differences between nude mice and athymic chimeras are not evident.

CD8α (Lyt-2) and CD8β (Lyt-3) Phenotypes and IEL Lineage

It has been proposed that CD8$\alpha\beta$ IEL are thymus-dependent T cells, and that CD8$\alpha\alpha$ IEL are thymus-independent cells (30). That conclusion is drawn from studies (5) in nude mice in which most IEL were $\gamma\delta$ TCR$^+$ T cells that expressed CD8$\alpha\alpha$ and lacked $\alpha\beta$ TCR$^+$ IEL. However, as delineated above, those phenotypic characteristics do not hold true for IEL in all types of athymic mice. In athymic chimeras, for example, $\alpha\beta$ TCR$^+$ IEL are present in proportions equaling or exceeding that of $\gamma\delta$ TCR IEL (18,50,51,71,87), and some $\alpha\beta$ TCR$^+$ IEL in athymic chimeras express the CD8$\alpha\beta$ phenotype (18). In a series of over 20 athymic chimeras in our laboratory, no difference has been observed in the overall distribution of CD8$\alpha\alpha$ versus CD8$\alpha\beta$ IEL between athymic chimeras and mice with intact thymus. In mice with intact thymus, 81% of total CD8$^+$ T cells were CD8$\alpha\alpha$ and 19% were CD8$\alpha\beta$; in athymic chimeras 82% were CD8$\alpha\alpha$ and 18% were CD8$\alpha\beta$ (R L Mosley and J R Klein, unpublished), indicating that both CD8$\alpha\alpha$ and CD8$\alpha\beta$ IEL can develop extrathymically. Likewise, in studies of BM reconstitution of mice with intact thymus epithelium, both CD8$\alpha\alpha$ and CD8$\alpha\beta$ T cells repopulate the gut prior to T cell repopulation of the thymus or spleen (R L Mosley and J R Klein, unpublished). Moreover, it has now been established that CD8$\alpha\alpha$, $\gamma\delta$ TCR$^+$ T cells can be derived from intrathymic precursors following activation with mitogen (93), and that CD4$^+$, CD8$\alpha\alpha$ cells can be generated from thymocytes following in vitro culture with T cell derived cytokines (68), thereby providing direct evidence that CD8$\alpha\alpha$ T cells can arise from thymus-derived T cells.

If not developmental, what might account for differences in CD8$\alpha\alpha$ and CD8$\alpha\beta$ expression on IEL? Insights into that can be gained from studies of CD8 expression on T cells outside the gut. It is possible that differences in CD8 phenotype are not determined by lineage but that they reflect either the state of T cell activation, mode of antigen recognition, or the type of IEL-mediated cytotoxicity, i.e., MHC-restricted or unrestricted lysis. In mice, it has been shown that CD8 is necessary for antigen recognition by cytotoxic T lymphocytes (CTL) (67,94), and that both CD8$\alpha\alpha$ and CD8$\alpha\beta$ molecules bear discrete functional domains involved either in enhancement of binding to target cells, or in transmembrane signalling to CTL (67,95,96). On human lymphocytes, correlations exist between CD8 phenotypes and cytotoxic activity such that MHC-restricted cytotoxicity is most common among T cells bearing the classical CTL phenotype CD3$^+$, CD8$\alpha\beta^+$, CD56$^-$; NK cytotoxic activity resides primarily among CD3$^-$, CD8$^-$ (or CD8^{low}), CD56$^+$ cells; and unrestricted cytotoxicity is mediated by CD3$^+$, CD8$\alpha\alpha^+$, CD56$^+$ cells (97). For IEL, the possibility that differences in CD8 phenotype represent functional rather than developmental distinctions is further reinforced by findings that the number of CD8$\alpha\alpha^+$, $\alpha\beta$ TCR$^+$ IEL increases with age in normal (62) but not nude (53) mice, and that expression of the CD8$\alpha\alpha$ homodimer on T cells can be altered by microenvironmental changes, e.g., exposure to lymphokines (68). Thus, until it has been thoroughly established that CD8 expression definitively correlates with lineage development, caution is needed in assigning lineage status to IEL based on CD8$\alpha\alpha$/CD8$\alpha\beta$ phenotypes.

Other Phenotypic Markers and Lineage Development

With regard to other potential markers of IEL lineage, it has been suggested that CD5$^+$ IEL are thymus-dependent T cells based on the lack of CD5 expression in nude mice (98). Further experimental work will be needed to precisely determine the role of CD5 in IEL development. The presence of Thy-1 on IEL in athymic chimeras (18,51) indicates that Thy-1 is not an accurate marker of thymus dependency. At face value, the CD4$^+$CD8$^+$ IEL subset might be mistaken for an early developmental cell lineage. However, evidence now suggests that those IEL are not a precursor population of other IEL subsets. Studies (55) examining the kinetic repopulation of lymphoid tissues after BM reconstitution of irradiated mice demonstrate that DP IEL appear late, rather than early, in IEL repopulation. Moreover, evidence suggests that the DP IEL may be generated from CD4$^+$CD8$^-$ subset (55,65).

Finally, although the lymphocyte markers and/or phenotypic subsets described above may yet provide clues regarding developmental lineages of the IEL, other approaches to understanding IEL development also may be productive. At present virtually nothing is known about the expression on IEL of BM-linked markers such as the stem-cell antigens, Sca-1 and Sca-2 (99), antigens of the Ly-6 family (100–102), or the markers of the Joro series (103), among others. Detailed studies of those markers on IEL in the context of BM or fetal liver repopulation of the IEL should permit early lineage-specific phenotypic subsets to be tracked.

PHENOTYPIC MARKERS OF IEL ACTIVATION, MEMORY, AND HOMING

Based on the presence of cytotoxic activity (16,44,45,51,55,74) and endogenous secretion of some lymphokines (13) in freshly extracted IEL, murine IEL contain T cells activated *in situ*. Exactly which IEL are in a state of activation at any given time has yet to be determined. When classical markers of T cell activation, such as CD25 (IL-2 receptor), are studied for IEL, few freshly extracted IEL in mice express CD25 (16,31), implying that IEL are not activated in the classical sense. Similarly, in rats nearly all IEL express at high density the RT6 antigen (59), which is present on resting T cells but not on activated T cells, implying that few IEL in rats are activated in a conventional manner. However, caution is warranted in interpreting those findings to mean that the IEL are not activated, since it has yet to be established that cell proliferation is a requisite event in the IEL activation pathway, or exactly what proportion of the IEL are responsive to signals of proliferation. In fact, studies of IEL proliferation demonstrate a lower frequency of cells responsive to mitogen stimulation when compared to splenic lymphocytes (104,105) or upon CD3/TCR stimulation (16). Even in studies in which vigorous IEL proliferation occurs, that event is restricted to a subset of the total IEL (e.g., $\alpha\beta$ TCR$^+$ IEL and/ or Thy-1$^+$ subset) (61,36a). Human IEL, by comparison, express CD25, although the proportion of CD25$^+$ IEL can vary widely (81) and may be influenced by disease status (106).

CD28 Expression on IEL

On both human and murine T cells, CD28 is important in immunoregulation as a costimulatory molecule of activation in conjunction with the CD3/TCR complex (107). The functional role of CD28 is consistent with a two-signal activation hypothesis in that stimulation of T cells via CD28 enhances CD3/TCR activation but does not lead to activation independent of CD3/TCR stimulation (107). Because CD28 costimulation occurs most efficiently when CD3/TCR stimulation is at suboptimal levels, activation of T cells via CD28 is probably most important during the early stages of induction. Signal transmission conveyed via CD28 also may be important for preventing anergy of already activated T cells (107), and may be involved in some fashion in the cytolytic process on activated CTL (108–110). Moreover, stimulation of human and murine T cells via CD28 has been shown to overcome the immunosuppressive effects of cyclosporin A (111).

Two mAbs, 37.51 (112) and R2/60 (113), have been isolated that react with the murine CD28 molecule. Both antibodies show similar patterns of tissue staining and costimulatory properties for T cells. Studies of IEL in our laboratory using mAb R2/60 indicate that nearly all CD3$^+$ IEL express CD28 and that CD28 is expressed on both $\alpha\beta$ TCR$^+$ and $\gamma\delta$ TCR$^+$ subsets (Fig. 3). Moreover, stimulation of IEL via CD28 enhances CD3-induced proliferation but does not induce proliferation of IEL by itself (M Hamad and J R Klein, unpublished), implying that requirements

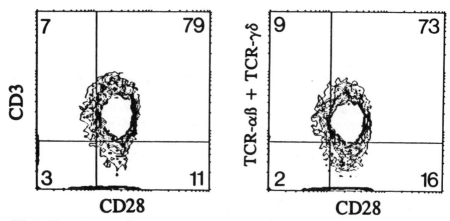

FIG. 3. CD28 on murine IEL is expressed on most CD3$^+$ T cells including both αβ TCR$^+$ and γδ TCR$^+$ IEL. (D Stickney and JR Klein, unpublished.)

for costimulation of IEL are probably similar to those of other peripheral T cells. It is interesting that antibody to CD28 mediates lysis of target cells in a redirected cytotoxic assay (Fig. 4 and discussed below), indicating functional involvement of CD28 on already-activated IEL in mice. For human T cells the natural ligand for CD28 is the B7/BB1 activation molecule expressed on accessory cells and B cells (114); a similar structure now has been identified in mice (115), although involvement of that molecule with murine CD28 remains to be determined. Moreover, it is unclear what types of intercellular relationships exist between CD28 on IEL and other cells in the gut epithelium. It is possible that the ligand for CD28 is expressed on intestinal epithelial cells, perhaps in a manner regulated as a consequence of infection, tissue damage, or exposure to luminal antigens. That possibility is feasible given the rather large number of lymphocyte antigens already described for intestinal epithelia in mice.

In both humans and mice the CTLA-4 molecule is closely related to CD28 at the gene level (116) and may have arisen during evolution as a duplication event from the CD28 gene (117). Unlike CD28, which is expressed on about 80% of human T cells, the CTLA-4 antigen appears to be a true activation molecule that is acquired on resting T cells upon induction with antigen or other stimuli (116,117). At present nothing is known about expression of CTLA-4 on murine IEL, however, that marker may ultimately be highly useful for understanding states of IEL activation.

CD45 and IEL Activation

The CT antigens (CT1 and CT2) are oligosaccharide moieties of the CD45 leukocyte common antigen in mice that are expressed on activated CD8$^+$ T cells *in vitro*, but are not expressed on most resting T cells *in vivo* (118). The CT1 determinant also is expressed on CD4$^-$CD8$^-$ fetal thymocytes (119). Within the gut epithelium, about 50 to 80% of IEL express CT antigens, whereas those markers are not

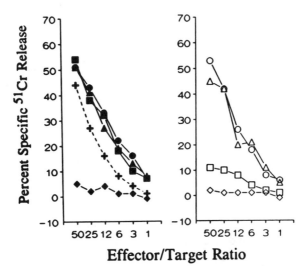

FIG. 4. *Left*: Cytotoxic activity of freshly extracted IEL in the RC assay using mAb to CD3 (*circle*), αβ TCR (*square*), γδ TCR (*triangle*), CD28 (*cross*), and no antibody (*diamond*) demonstrates the presence of activated CTL in IEL isolates. *Right*: Treatment of IEL with anti-Thy-1 mAb plus complement reduces but does not eliminate cytotoxic activity in RC assay (*square*), compared to treatment of IEL with complement in the absence of antibody (*circle*), and to IEL cultured with target cells without RC (*diamond*); RC activity is unaffected following treatment of IEL with anti-CT1 plus complement (*triangle*). (RL Mosley and JR Klein, unpublished.)

expressed on lamina propria or Peyer's patch lymphocytes (31). Interestingly, the CT antigens are differentially expressed on intestine epithelial cells in mice (31). Among the IEL there is some discrepancy as to which subset(s) expresses CT antigens. In one study (31) CT1 expression was associated primarily with Thy-1[+] IEL; another study (47) found CT expression to be exclusively associated with a Thy-1[−] subset.

Recently, a second IEL-associated antigen (M371) has been identified that, like CT, is a carbohydrate determinant of CD45 in mice (43). M371 is present on about one-third of BALB/c IEL and is principally affiliated with a CD3[+], Thy-1[−], CD8αα[+] subset and is not present on lamina propria lymphocytes, other peripheral T cells, or intestinal enterocytes (43). About half of the αβ TCR[+] IEL express M371 based on Vβ8 expression, and by inference a fairly high proportion of γδ TCR[+] IEL probably express M371 (43). Unlike the CT antigens, M371 does not react with the human Tamm-Horsfall glycoprotein or with *in vitro*-derived CTL lines. Moreover, M371 is expressed on a different CD45 molecular isoform than CT (43). The functional and/or developmental roles of the CT and M371 antigens are unknown. Both CT1 (40,31,51) and M371 (43) are present on IEL in normal and nude mice, and thus they are not markers of thymus-dependency.

Additional insights into IEL states of activation (and possible lineage development) in mice as defined by phenotypic markers may be gained from studies of CD45 isoforms. Extensive heterogeneity of CD45 molecular forms has been reported for murine IEL (47), pointing to a high degree of variability in the pattern CD45 glycosylation within the gut epithelium. In mice and rats, most CD8$^+$ IEL are CD45RB$^+$, whereas CD4$^+$ IEL are CD45RB$^-$ (62), implying that the bulk of CD8$^+$ IEL are naive T cells and that some CD4$^+$ IEL are memory T cells (62,59). On human IEL, increases in CD45RO expression have been reported for IEL from patients with coeliac disease, suggesting an accumulation of memory T cells concomitant with that disorder (120).

With regard to other activation markers, it has recently been shown that CD11b (Mac-1) is expressed on virus-specific CTL and memory T cells (121). Whether that antigen will serve as a marker of IEL activation remains to be determined. Likewise, the CD44 molecule on mature T cells in mice has been linked to a population of memory T cells (122). To date, expression of CD44 has received little attention for murine IEL. One study (123) reported that nearly all CD4$^+$ IEL and that about half of the CD8$^+$ IEL express high levels of CD44. Examination of IEL in our laboratory indicates that CD44 is usually not expressed on murine IEL, although CD44 is present on a substantial proportion of lamina propria T cells (D Stickney and J R Klein, unpublished). More detailed experiments are needed to address the role of CD44 on IEL, particularly in the context of antigen-priming or local infection. The MEL-14 lymphocyte selectin molecule, which operates in the migration of lymphocytes through lymph node endothelial cells, is rarely espressed on murine IEL (31). That distinction for IEL is intriguing considering that MEL-14 is expressed on most resting cells but is absent on activated T cells (124).

Markers of IEL Migration and Homing

The migration of lymphocytes into the gut epithelium, and the origin of those cells either as IEL precursors or as mature T cells, is a topic of considerable interest. Lymphocyte markers known to participate in trafficking and/or cell migration include molecules of the integrin group such as the lymphocyte function-associated antigen (LFA-1) (CD11a/CD18) as well as the α and β integrin molecules (β2, α4 class, α4β1, α4βp, α4β7, among others); the selectins molecules such as MEL-14, LAM, ELAM; the antigens of the proteoglycan group (CD44); and/or the cell adhesion molecules (CAM) (e.g., CD2/LFA-3) (reviewed in refs. 125,126). IEL in mice have been shown to bind selectively to intestine-associated high endothelial venules (HEV) but not to peripheral HEV (127), implying an active lymphocyte selection process within the gut epithelium.

It is interesting that most murine IEL (59) do not express CD2 even though that marker is expressed on human IEL (57). Moreover, not all murine CD8$^+$ IEL express LFA-1 (31,35) even though both LFA-1 and CD2 are present on most CTL in the periphery (125,126). On IEL, the LFA-1 molecule has been shown to be functionally important based on the ability of anti-LFA-1 antibody to abrogate lytic activity of IEL-derived CTL (35). Currently, no information is available as to whether LFA-3, the ligand for CD2, or ICAM-1 and ICAM-2, the ligands for LFA-1 (125), are expressed within the gut epithelium of mice. Such information would be valuable given that expression of ICAM-1 is modulated on nonhematopoietic tissues during inflammation or immunologic activation (128). In mice the integrin β1, β2, β3, and β7 molecules are expressed on both peripheral lymphocytes and the IEL (129,130).

In humans (81,131), rats (132), and mice (129,130) a family of molecules related in size and tissue distribution have been termed the mucosal lymphocyte antigens (MLA). Those molecules appear to be involved in migration of lymphocytes into selected tissues (125). In mice, a series of mAbs have been isolated that react with a 135-kDa α-chain integrin molecule (M290, M294, M295), or with a 100-kDa β-chain (possibly β7) integrin molecule (M291, M293, M298, M300, M301) (130). M290 expression is primarily restricted to the IEL in that little or no reactivity is seen for other peripheral lymphocytes, including the lamina propria, Peyer's patches, and the thymus, although expression of the M290 antigen is increased on lymph node lymphocytes following exposure to TGFβ_1 (129,130). The M290 antigen bears a high degree of identity to murine β7 integrin at the gene level (130,133). Paradoxically, studies of the distribution of murine β7 in lymphoid populations as determined by Northern blot analyses indicate an abundance of β7 transcripts in thymocytes, spleen cells, and to a lesser extent in IEL (133,134), raising questions as to the exact relationship of the M290 antigen to murine β7. Of interest, the M290 antigen also is endogenously expressed on some bone marrow T cells.

PHENOTYPIC MARKERS OF INTESTINE EPITHELIA

Because the IEL reside between and among nonhematopoietic epithelial cells of the intestinal mucosa, an understanding of the IEL must ultimately take into account the relationship of the IEL to epithelial cells. Detailed phenotypic and biochemical studies of epithelial cells may provide insights into that relationship. Even though few classical accessory-like cells are found in the gut epithelium, it has been demonstrated that MHC class II molecules are expressed on some intestinal enterocytes and that such cells can function in antigen presentation to T cells (135–137). In mice, intestinal epithelia have been shown to express asialo GM$_1$ (32), the CT determinants (31), thymus-leukemia (TI) antigens (75,138), and CD1 (139), suggesting a potentially complex network of communication between IEL and nonhematopoietic components of intestinal epithelia.

CYTOTOXIC PROPERTIES OF IEL

Although the veritable function of IEL has yet to be elucidated, it is probably safe to assume that the primary purpose of the IEL is similar to that of T cells in other peripheral lymphoid tissues, i.e., the recognition and elimination of host cells bearing foreign and/or nonself antigens. Moreover, given the morphology, granularity, and phenotype of the IEL, it is likely that cytotoxic cells within the intestinal epithelium have a fundamentally important role in host immune protection locally. Both antigen-specific and antigen-nonspecific cytotoxic responses have been described for murine IEL. Those include MHC-restricted and alloreactive cytotoxic activities, spontaneous cytotoxicity (SC), antibody-dependent cell-mediated cytotoxicity (ADCC), and cytotoxicity detected in the redirected cytotoxicity (RC) assay.

Evidence for *In Vivo* Activation of Cytotoxic IEL

Unlike T cells in most other peripheral compartments, a fairly high proportion of IEL are activated CTL. That property is readily evident in the RC assay using IEL without *in vitro* activation (16,44,45,51,55,74,140). Because the RC assay requires effector cells that express TCR or CD3ϵ in conjunction with Fc-receptor (FcR)-bearing, non-NK-susceptible target cells, the RC assay specifically identifies cytotoxic activity mediated by CTL, and not by classical NK or other spontaneous cyctotoxic effector cells. Although cytotoxic IEL are routinely detectable in the RC assay, specific IEL subset(s) that mediate lytic activity, and the factors that influence activation *in vivo*, remain largely undefined. For murine IEL both $\alpha\beta$ TCR$^+$ and $\gamma\delta$ TCR$^+$ IEL can mediate RC (16,44,45,51,55,74,140).

It has been suggested that activation of cytotoxic IEL as measured by the RC assay may be influenced by the presence of intestinal microflora and may be linked to expression of Thy-1 (44). That interpretation is based on the lack of Thy-1 expression and the lack of CD3-mediated RC in IEL from germ-free mice, and by the re-expression of Thy-1 and the return of RC cytotoxic activity in IEL upon removal of mice from germ-free conditions (44). Similarly, depletion of Thy-1$^+$ IEL in normal mice has been shown to abrogate CD3-mediated RC (44). Yet those findings are contrasted to studies that show cytotoxic activity in IEL depleted of Thy-1-bearing cells which had levels of CD3/TCR-mediated RC that were slightly lower (45) or no different (140) than unfractionated IEL. IEL enriched for Thy-1$^+$ T cells have greater CD3- and $\alpha\beta$ TCR-mediated RC activity (45). Likewise, IEL from germ-free mice had normal levels of CD3- and $\gamma\delta$ TCR-mediated RC but substantially lower levels of $\alpha\beta$ TCR-mediated RC (140), a pattern that correlates with the overall distribution of TCR-bearing IEL in germ-free mice (73). Experiments in our laboratory indicate that CD3-mediated RC is substantially reduced but not eliminated in IEL depleted of Thy-1$^+$ cells (Fig. 4), and that depletion of CT1$^+$ IEL does not alter CD3-mediated RC (Fig. 4).

In addition to cytotoxic activity mediated by antibodies directed to the TCR and CD3ϵ, a type of RC has been shown for the CD28 molecule on activated murine CTL as well as freshly extracted IEL (113) (Fig. 4). That phenomenon also has been demonstrated for human peripheral blood CTL by use of a bifunctional CD3/CD28 monoclonal antibody (108–110). Although the mechanisms by which CD28 mediates target cell lysis have yet to be determined, transmembrane signaling via CD28 may involve pathways that are at least partially distinct from those directed through the CD3/TCR complex (discussed in ref. 107).

Developmental Kinetics of IEL Cytotoxic Activity

Activation of cytotoxic IEL does not require a functional thymus, as demonstrated by RC responses in IEL from athymic radiation chimeras (51) and nude mice (45). IEL from athymic chimeras have nearly normal CD3/TCR-mediated RC responses (51). In nude mice, by contrast, CD3-mediated RC responses tend to be lower than those of euthymic littermates (45). The reasons for differences in lytic responses in nude mice and athymic chimeras are not fully evident. A simple explanation might be that there are fewer CD3$^+$ IEL in nude mice (42,46) or that there is an overall reduction of IEL that express functionally important T cell markers (42,46). However, it also must be considered that there is a fundamental impairment of T cell development in nude mice that extends beyond the thymus lineage pathway. That possibility is supported by experiments (141) in which nude mice engrafted with thymus tissues failed to reject third-party tissue grafts, whereas reintroduction of thymus into athymic chimeras leads to rejection of third-party grafts.

In radiation chimeras with intact thymus epithelium, activation of cytotoxic IEL occurs rapidly after BM transplantation as measured by the RC assay (55). In fact, during repopulation of IEL in radiation chimeras with intact thymus epithelium, γδ TCR-mediated RC is detectable as soon as day 7 post-BM-reconstitution; αβ TCR-mediated RC also appears rapidly after BM reconstitution but remains at subnormal levels until after day 21 postreconstitution (55). Likewise, in mice exposed to sublethal irradiation (600 rad) in which lymphoid cell repopulation is derived from radioresistant precursors within the animal, normal levels of cytotoxic CD3$^+$ IEL are present by day 10 postirradiation, even though normal numbers of CD3$^+$ T cells are not evident in mesenteric lymph nodes or Peyer's patches until day 40 (54). Taken together, those findings indicate that there is a rapid development of cytotoxic IEL following seeding of the gut epithelium with T cell precursors, and further confirm that the thymus is not essential for development of cytotoxic IEL.

Antigen-Specific and MHC-Restricted Cytotoxic IEL

Given that most IEL are CD3$^+$, CD8$^+$, TCR$^+$ T cells, it is likely that antigen-specific CTL are an integral part of the intestinal defense repertoire. Antigen-specific CTL can be generated from IEL after antigen priming *in vitro* or *in vivo* (34,66,142–148). There appears to be a fundamental difference in the nature of the CTL response within individual compartments of the GALT as a function of route of priming. This can be seen in experiments in which antigen-specific CTL are generated in all GALT tissues (the IEL, the lamina propria, and Peyer's patches) after intraperitoneal or oral immunization with antigen, whereas subcutaneous immunization leads to generation of antigen-specific CTL in all compartments *except* the IEL (66,147,148).

Antigen-specific, MHC-restricted CTL are present in IEL from rotavirus- and reovirus-infected mice (146–148). Rotavirus-specific MHC-restricted CTL are present in IEL and spleen 6 days after oral or parenteral inoculation with infectious virus (147,148). Rotavirus-specific CTL from IEL and spleen express Thy-1 and are $\alpha\beta$ TCR$^+$ as demonstrated by loss of CTL activity following treatment of cells with antibody plus complement (147,148). In one study (147), rotavirus-specific pCTL were present among lymphocytes from Peyer's patch, mesenteric lymph nodes, and spleen, but *not* IEL, 4 weeks after oral or parenteral inoculation with virus, suggesting a short retention span for virus-specific CTL in the gut epithelium. That interpretation is reinforced by the finding that rotavirus-specific pCTL were present in freshly isolated IEL 1 week postinfection (147).

Preliminary reports suggest some $\gamma\delta$ TCR$^+$ IEL recognize peptides from heat stress proteins in the context of TL antigen (149). IEL responses measured by degranulation of serine esterase-containing granules are specific of recognition of small intestine epithelial cells and do not occur for epithelial cells from other tissues including the colon (149). Moreover, heat-shock treatment of small intestine epithelial cells from germ-free mice augments degranulation of the effectors (149), suggesting that some IEL recognize heat-shock protein epitopes independent of microflora. Antibodies directed against TCR-Vγ5 or TL antigens inhibit the response (149), implying that TCR-Vγ5$^+$ IEL recognizes antigen presented in the context of TL (149).

Alloreactive Cytotoxic IEL

Based on estimates of alloreactive CTL precursors (pCTL) in IEL isolates, there are roughly 2- to 5-fold fewer pCTL in IEL than in spleen, and 3- to 4-fold less pCTL than in the lamina propria (34). The majority of alloreactive pCTL express Thy-1 and CD8 (34), and upon fractionation of IEL by density gradient centrifugation most pCTL migrate above 55% Percoll, although some pCTL are present at the 55/70% Percoll interface (34). IEL alloreactive pCTL also can be distinguished from NK cells by unit gravity sedimentation in that the former sediment faster (3 to 5 mm/hr) than the latter (5 to 8 mm/hr) (34). Alloreactive IEL have been cloned from IEL generated in *in vitro* MLR (34) or following *in vivo* priming (66,143,145). To the present virtually all alloreactive IEL propagated *in vitro* express Thy-1 and CD8 (34,145) and are $\alpha\beta$ TCR$^+$ (R L Mosley and J R Klein, unpublished). Alloreactive CTL generated in bulk IEL cultures express CD5 (34). Expression of CT1 and asialo GM$_1$ is variable on CTL clones and may be dependent on culture conditions such as concentration of growth factors and/or length of time in culture (145). CTL clones from IEL grown over long periods of time have been shown to lose lytic activity for antigen-bearing target cells and to acquire NK-like cytotoxicity even though retaining antigen-specificity for proliferation (145). Those effects are most evident when IEL clones are grown in high concentrations of T cell-derived cytokines (144,145). Similarly, some alloreactive CTL from IEL immunized *in vivo* lyse NK-resistant target cells (34,143), suggesting that antigen recognition by intestinal cells may differ in some ways from that of splenic CTL, or possibly that the IEL pCTL repertoire is different.

Antibody Dependent Cell-Mediated Cytotoxicity (ADCC)

ADCC activity is detected in a 4- to 18-hour *in vitro* culture assay in which anti-target cell antibody (rat anti-P815 or rabbit anti-Chang liver cell) bridges join effector and target cells via the FcR of the effector (150,151). ADCC has been shown for IEL from guinea pigs (150) and rats (151). Although ADCC cytotoxic levels in IEL are 5- to 10-fold greater than that of lymphocytes from mesenteric lymph nodes and Peyer's patches, ADCC by IEL effectors is slightly less efficient than that of splenic effectors (150,151). It is unclear whether those differences are due to numbers of responding cells or to lytic potential (150,151). No information is available as to the phenotype of the IEL ADCC cell; however, it should be noted that cells that mediate NK activity also can mediate ADCC (152), and that NK activity has been demonstrated for IEL (see below). In fact, concomitant NK and ADCC activities have been reported for IEL (151), making it difficult to know whether those activities represent the same or mutually exclusive effector populations.

Natural Killer Cell-Mediated Cytotoxicity

Over the years numerous studies have described NK cytotoxic activities in IEL isolates of mice (5,6,11,12,40,66,153–155), rats (151,156,157), and guinea pigs (150). Both similarities and differences exist between NK responses of the gut and those of other peripheral tissues. In general, IEL NK cells lyse NK-sensitive but not NK-resistant target cells (11,12,66) as can be seen in the RC assay in which little or no lytic activity occurs upon culture with NK-resistant target cells in the absence of antibody (16,45,55,74). As with splenic NK cells, IEL NK activity varies with strains of mice (33,66), is reduced in mice older than 16 weeks compared to mice less than 8 weeks of age (11), and can be enhanced by treatment of cells with interferon (11,151). Developmental studies of rat IEL and lamina propria lymphocytes demonstrates that NK activity is undetectable in fetal rats (18 to 21 days of gestation), is slightly higher in neonates (3 to 5 days post-birth), attains peak activity upon weaning (21 days of age), and is substantially lower than peak activity in adult rats (10 to 12 weeks of age) (157). In short-term assays (4 to 6 hours), IEL from nude mice exhibit slightly enhanced NK activity compared to those from euthymic mice (66). In 18-hour NK cytotoxicity assays, IEL and spleen cells from nude mice and euthymic mice have higher levels of NK activity than are found among spleen cells from euthymic mice (66). NK activity is low for IEL, spleen, and lamina propria lymphocytes from mice expressing the bg/bg mutation (12,66,154). NK activity of the IEL but not the spleen can be augmented by treatment with substance P, a neurotransmitter present in abundance in intestine tissues (153). In germ-free mice, little or no NK activity is detectable in IEL or in lymphocytes from the lamina propria, Peyer's patches, mesenteric lymph nodes, or the spleen (33). In contrast, IEL from germ-free mice effectively lyse targets infected with the enterotropic coronavirus but not targets infected with the nonenterotropic Pichinde virus (33), suggesting that IEL NK effectors may recognize additional target antigens not seen by most peripheral NK cells.

Within both the IEL and the spleen, NK cells comprise a minority of the total lymphoid cells. It is estimated that 5 to 25% of the IEL have NK activity, whereas 5 to 15% of splenic cells are NK cells (6,11,12,33). IEL and splenic NK cells have buoyant densities of less than 1.075 g/ml (33). Like splenic NK cells, IEL that mediate NK activity do not express CD4, CD5, or CD8, as demonstrated in enrichment and depletion experiments (33). Although peripheral NK cells are defined as large granular lymphocytes (LGL) that do not express CD3 or TCR, it has yet to be determined whether IEL NK cells meet that criterion fully. Differences have been noted between IEL and splenic NK effector cells, as demonstrated by selective depletion of specific cell populations using antibodies to Thy-1, asialo GM_1, and NK-1.2 cell surface markers. For example, although NK activities of the IEL and spleen are reduced after depletion of cells bearing Thy-1 (11,12,33), asialo GM_1 (11,12,33), and NK-1.2 (12), that reduction is quantitatively different for IEL and splenic NK cells (12). Depletion of Thy-1$^+$ cells reduced IEL NK activity by 75% compared to only 38% reduction in NK activity mediated by spleen cells (12). In addition, depletion of NK-1.2$^+$ or asialo $GM_1$$^+$ effectors reduced splenic NK activity by 83%, whereas IEL NK activity was reduced by only 34% and 31%, respectively (12). Thus, IEL NK cells appear to express more Thy-1 and less NK-1.2 and asialo GM_1 than splenic NK cells. Conversely, IEL that mediate NK activity toward coronavirus-infected targets cells express lower levels of Thy-1 and higher levels of asialo GM_1, suggesting that there are discrete types of NK effector subsets within the gut (33).

Some NK activity of IEL may be mediated by antigen-specific CTL, as indicated by the gradual loss of antigen-specific cytotoxic activity and concomitant acquisition of NK-like activity upon long-term culture of alloreactive or MHC-restricted IEL-derived clones, implying different mechanisms of antigen recognition by NK cells and CTL (145). Splenic T cell clones maintained under similar culture conditions retain cytotoxic and proliferative specificities (145).

Spontaneous Cytotoxic (SC) Cell-Mediated Cytotoxicity

Also present in freshly extracted IEL are cells that mediate spontaneous cytotoxic (SC) activity (40,150), which is broadly defined by the ability spontaneously to lyse

NK-resistant, and also possibly NK-sensitive, target cells. SC activity of the IEL requires a higher effector:target ratio than NK cells (31,40), suggesting that SC cells constitute a very minor population of the total IEL (32). Moreover, cells that mediate SC activity in the gut are larger and more granular cells than most IEL (40), likewise suggesting a very minor IEL subset. SC activity of IEL can be abrogated by treatment with antibody plus complement to CT1 or HSA (40); however, on the basis of the low frequency of SC cells in the gut epithelium, it is clear that all IEL bearing those markers are *not* SC cells. As with NK cells, the significance of SC cells to IEL immunity remains uncertain.

SUMMARY

The studies cited above demonstrate the heterogeneity, complexity, and dynamic nature of murine IEL. In addition to the many similarities that exist between IEL and T cells in other peripheral compartments, there are important differences between those populations, such as the nature of development, and possibly also differences in mode of activation and/or antigen recognition by IEL. Unlike T cells in other compartments, the environment of the gut epithelium is perpetually changing due to continual exposure to intestinal flora, luminal antigens, and other external environmental factors. Overlaid onto those variables are age-related changes in the IEL population as noted in many IEL studies cited herein. Whether such changes are the consequence of environmental factors or whether they are dictated by physiologic or genetic events independent of external influences is difficult to determine. It is also interesting that notable age-dependent changes occur in the spatial organization of intestine epithelial tissues in mice, as delineated in transgenic studies of intestine epithelium (158,159). Similarly, age-related changes in GALT lymphocyte populations in mice occur in a temporal fashion that is different from that of lymphocytes in other peripheral compartments (160). Those findings coupled with information regarding IEL development, phenotypic properties, and the functional involvement of IEL in host immune protection, emphasize the need to view the IEL as a dynamic cell population across time.

ACKNOWLEDGMENT

This work was supported by NIH grant DK35566.

REFERENCES

1. Otto HF. The intraepithelial lymphocytes of the intestine: morphological observations and immunologic aspects of intestinal enteropathy. *Curr Top Pathol* 1973;57:81–121.
2. Ferguson A. Intraepithelial lymphocytes of the small intestine. *Gut* 1977;18:921–937.
3. Bienenstock J, Befus AD. Mucosal immunology. *Immunology* 1980;41:249–270.
4. Ernst PB, Befus AD, Bienenstock J. Leukocytes in the intestinal epithelium: an unusual immunologic compartment. *Immunol Today* 1985;6:50–55.

5. Petit A, Ernst PB, Befus AD, Clark DA, Rosenthal KL, Ishizaka T, Bienenstock J. Murine intestinal intraepithelial lymphocytes. I: Relationship of a novel Thy-1-, Lyt-1-, Lyt-2+, granulated subpopulation to natural killer cells and mast cells. *Eur J Immunol* 1985;15:211–215.

6. Ernst PB, Petit A, Befus AD, Clark DA, Rosenthal KL, Ishizaka T, Bienenstock J. Murine intestinal intraepithelial lymphocytes. II: Comparison of freshly isolated and cultured intraepithelial lymphocytes. *Eur J Immunol* 1985;15:216–221.

7. Despommier D, Weisbroth S, Fass C. Circulating eosinophils and trichinosis in the rat: the parasitic stage responsible for induction during infection. *J Parasitol* 1974;60:280–287.

8. Haig DM, McKee TA, Jarrett EE, Woodbury RG, Miller HRP. Generation of mucosal mast cells is stimulated in vitro by factors derived from T cells of helminth-infected rats. *Nature* 1982;300:188–191.

9. Dillon SB, MacDonald TT. Limit dilution analyses of mast cell precursor frequency in the gut epithelium of normal and *Trichinella spiralis* infected mice. *Parasite Immunol* 1986;8:503–508.

10. Wang CH, Korenaga M, Greenwood A, Bell RG. T-helper subset function in the gut of rats: differential stimulation of eosinophils, mucosal mast cells and antibody-forming cells by OX8⁻ OX22⁻ and OX8⁻ OX22⁺ cells. *Immunology* 1990;71:166–175.

11. Tagliabue A, Luini W, Soldateschi D, Boraschi D. Natural killer activity of gut mucosal lymphoid cells in mice. *Eur J Immunol* 1981;11:919–922.

12. Tagliabue A, Befus AD, Clark DA, Bienenstock J. Characteristics of natural killer cells in the murine intestinal epithelium and lamina propria. *J Exp Med* 1982;155:1785–1796.

13. Taguchi T, McGhee JR, Coffman RL, Beagley KW, Eldridge JH, Takatsu K, Kiyono H. Analysis of Th1 and Th2 cells in murine gut-associated tissues: frequencies of CD4+ and CD8+ T cells that secrete IFN-γ and IL-5. *J Immunol* 1990;145:68–77.

14. Fujihashi K, Tagushi T, McGhee JR, et al. Regulatory function for murine intraepithelial lymphocytes: two subsets of CD3+ T cells receptor-1+ intraepithelial lymphocyte T cells abrogate oral tolerance. *J Immunol* 1990;145:2010–2019.

15. Torgils Vaage J, Dissen E, Ager A, Roberts I, Fossum S, Bent R. T cell receptor-bearing cells among rat intestinal intraepithelial lymphocytes are mainly α/β+ and are thymus dependent. *Eur J Immunol* 1990;20:1193–1196.

16. Mosley RL, Whetsell M, Klein JR. Proliferative properties of murine intestinal intraepithelial lymphocytes (IEL): IEL expressing TCRαβ or TCRγδ are largely unresponsive to proliferative signals mediated via conventional stimulation of the CD3-TCR complex. *Int Immunol* 1991;3:563–569.

17. Mosley RL, Klein JR. A rapid method for isolating murine intestine intraepithelial lymphocytes with high yield and purity. *J Immunol Meth*; 1992;156:19–26.

18. Pousier P, Edouard P, Lee C, Binnie M, Julius M. Thymus-independent development and negative selection of T cells expressing T cell receptor α/β in the intestinal epithelium: evidence for distinct circulation patterns of gut- and thymus-derived T lymphocytes. *J Exp Med* 1992;176:187–199.

19. Leventon GS, Sulabha SK, Meinstrich ML, Newland JR, Zander AR. Isolation of murine small bowel intraepithelial lymphocytes. *J Immunol Meth* 1983;63:35–44.

20. Davies MDJ, Parrott DMV. Preparation and purification of lymphocytes from the epithelium and lamina propria of murine small intestine. *Gut* 1981;22:481–488.

21. Bandeira A, Itohara S, Bonneville M, Burlen-Defanoux O, Mota-Santos T, Coutinho A, Tonegawa S. Extrathymic origin of intestinal intraepithelial lymphocytes bearing T-cell antigen receptor γδ. *Proc Natl Acad Sci USA* 1991;88:43–47.

22. Guy-Grand D, Griscelli C, Vassalli P. The mouse gut T lymphocyte, a novel type of T cell: nature, origin, and traffic in mice in normal and graft-versus-host conditions. *J Exp Med* 1978;148:1661–1677.

23. Schrader JW, Scollay R, Battye F. Intramucosal lymphocytes of the gut: Lyt-2 and Thy-1 phenotypes of the granulated cells and evidence for presence of both T cells and mast cell precursors. *J Immunol* 1983;130:558–564.

24. Croitoru K, Stead RH, Bienenstock J, et al. Presence of intestinal intraepithelial lymphocytes in mice with severe combined immunodeficiency disease. *Eur J Immunol* 1990;20:645–651.

25. Mayrhofer G, Whately RJ. Granular intraepithelial lymphocytes of the rat small intestine. I: Isolation, presence in T lymphocyte-deficient rats and bone marrow origin. *Int Arch Allerg Appl Immunol* 1983;71:317–327.

26. Mayrhofer G. Thymus-dependent and thymus-independent subpopulations of intestinal intraepithelial lymphocytes: a granulated subpopulation of probable bone marrow origin. *Blood* 1980;55:532–535.

27. Flexman JP, Shellman GR, Mayrhofer G. Natural cytotoxicity, responsiveness to interferon and morphology of intra-epithelial lymphocytes from the small intestine of the rat. *Immunology* 1983;48:733–741.
28. Rudzik O, Bienenstock J. Isolation and characterization of mucosal lymphocytes. *Lab Invest* 1974;30:260–265.
29. Cerf-Bensussan N, Schneeberger EE, Bhan AK. Immunohistologic and immunoelectron microscopic characteristics of the mucosal lymphocytes in human small intestine by the use of monoclonal antibodies. *J Immunol* 1983;130:2615–2622.
30. Guy-Grand D, Cerf-Bensussan N, Malissen B, Malassis-Seris M, Briottet C, Vassalli P. Two gut intraepithelial CD8 $^+$ lymphocyte populations with different receptors: a role for the gut epithelium in T cell differentiation. *J Exp Med* 1991;173:471–481.
31. Lefrancois L. Carbohydrate differentiation antigens on murine T cells: expression on intestinal lymphocytes and intestinal epithelium. *J Immunol* 1987;138:3375–3384.
32. Klein JR, Mosley RL, Kaiserlian D. Expression of the asialo GM_1 determinant on murine intestinal epithelia. *Proc Soc Exp Biol Med* 1990;195:329–334.
33. Carman P, Ernst PB, Rosenthal KL, Clark DA, Befus AD, Bienenstock J. Intraepithelial leukocytes contain a unique subpopulation of NK-like cytotoxic cells active in defense of gut epithelium to enteric murine coronavirus. *J Immunol* 1986;136:1548–1553.
34. Ernst PB, Clark DA, Rosenthal KL, Befus AD, Bienenstock J. Detection and characterization of cytotoxic T lymphocytes precursors in the murine intestinal intraepithelial leukocyte populations. *J Immunol* 1986;136:2121–2126.
35. Klein JR. Functional involvement of LFA-1 molecules on murine intestinal intraepithelial lymphocytes with natural killer activity. In: MacDermott RP, ed. *Inflammatory bowel disease: current status and future approach*. New York: Elsevier; 1988:113–118.
36. Guy-Grand, Griscelli C, Vassalli P. The gut-associated lymphoid system: nature and properties of the large dividing cells. *Eur J Immunol* 1974;4:435–443.
36a. Hamad M, Klein JR. Functional heterogeneity of murine intestinal intraepithelial lymphocytes: Implications for route of activation and responsiveness to proliferation induction. (submitted for publication)
37. Marsh MN. Studies of intestinal lymphoid tissues. I: Electron microscopic evidence of "blast transformation" in epithelial lymphocytes of mouse small intestinal mucosa. *Gut* 1975;16:665–670.
38. Sprent J. Fate of H2-activated T lymphocytes in syngeneic hosts. I: Fate in lymphoid tissues and intestines traced with ^{3}H-thymidine, ^{125}I-deoxyuridine and ^{51}chromium. *Cell Immunol* 1976;21:278–288.
39. Lyscom N, Brueton MJ. Intraepithelial, lamina propria and Peyer's patch lymphocytes of the rat small intestine: isolation and characterization in terms of immunoglobulin markers and receptor for monoclonal antibodies. *Immunology* 1982;45:775–783.
40. Klein JR. Ontogeny of the Thy-1 $^-$, Lyt-2 $^+$ murine intestinal intraepithelial lymphocyte: characterization of a unique population of thymus-independent cytotoxic effector cells in the intestinal mucosa. *J Exp Med* 1986;164:306–314.
41. Bonneville M, Janeway CA, Ito K, Haser W, Ishida I, Nakanishi N, Tonegawa S. Intestinal intraepithelial lymphocytes are a distinct set of γδ T cells. *Nature* 1988;336:479–481.
42. Viney JL, MacDonald TT, Kilshaw PJ. T-cell receptor expression in intestinal intraepithelial lymphocyte subpopulations of normal and athymic mice. *Immunology* 1989;66:583–587.
43. Kilshaw PJ, Baker KC. A new antigenic determinant on intra-epithelial lymphocytes and its association with CD45. *Immunology* 1989;67:160–166.
44. Lefrancois L, Goodman T. *In vivo* modulation of cytotoxic activity and Thy-1 expression in TCR-γδ $^+$ intraepithelial lymphocytes. *Science* 1989;243:1716–1718.
45. Viney JL, Kilshaw PJ, Macdonald TT. Cytotoxic α/β $^+$ and γ/δ $^+$ T cells in murine intestinal epithelium. *Eur J Immunol* 1990;20:1623–1626.
46. DeGeus B, Van den Enden M, Coolen C, Nagelkerken L, Van der Heijden P, Rozing J. Phenotype of intraepithelial lymphocytes in euthymic and athymic mice: implications for differentiation of cells bearing a CD3-associated γδ T cell receptor. *Eur J Immunol* 1990;20:291–298.
47. Goodman TG, Chang HL, Esselman WJ, LeCorre R, Lefrancois L. Characterization of the CD45 molecule on murine intestinal intraepithelial lymphocytes. *J Immunol* 1990;145:2959–2966.
48. Bonneville M, Itohara S, Krecko E, et al. Transgeneic mice demonstrate that epithelial homing of γ/δ T cells is determined by cell lineages independent of T cell receptor specificity. *J Exp Med* 1990;171:1015–1026.

49. Mosley RL, Styre D, Klein JR. CD4$^+$CD8$^+$ murine intestinal intraepithelial lymphocytes. *Int Immunol* 1990;2:361–365.

50. Lefrancois L, Mayo J, Goodman T. Ontogeny of the T cell receptor (TCR) α,β^+ and γ,δ^+ intraepithelial lymphocyte. In: Lotze M, Finn OJ, eds. *Cellular immunity and the immunotherapy of cancer.* New York: John Wiley; 1990:31–40.

51. Mosley RL, Styre D, Klein JR. Differentiation and functional maturation of bone marrow derived intestinal epithelial T cells expressing membrane T cell receptor in athymic radiation chimeras. *J Immunol* 1991;145:1369–1375.

52. Lefrancois L. Phenotypic complexity of intraepithelial lymphocytes of the small intestine. *J Immunol* 1991;147:1746–1751.

53. Murosaki S, Yoshikai Y, Ishida A, et al. Failure of T cell receptor Vβ negative selection in murine intestinal intraepithelial lymphocytes. *Int Immunol* 1991;3:1005–1013.

54. Yoshikai Y, Ishida A, Murosaki S, Ando T, Nomoto K. Sequential appearance of T-cell receptor $\gamma\delta$- and $\alpha\beta$-bearing intestinal intra-epithelial lymphocytes in mice after irradiation. *Immunol* 1991;74:583–588.

55. Mosley RL, Klein JR. Repopulation kinetics of intestinal intraepithelial lymphocytes in murine bone marrow radiation chimeras. *Transplantation* 1992;53:868–874.

56. Kaiserlian D, Vidal K, Revillard JO. Murine enterocytes can present soluble antigen to specific class II-restricted CD4$^+$ T cells. *Eur J Immunol* 1989;19:1513–1516.

57. Jarry A, Cerf-Bensussan N, Brousse N, Selz F, Guy-Grand D. Subsets of CD3$^+$ (T cell receptor α/β or γ/δ) and CD3$^-$ lymphocytes isolated from normal human gut epithelium display phenotypic features different from their counterparts in peripheral blood. *Eur J Immunol* 1990; 20:1097.

58. Ebert EC. Proliferative responses of human intraepithelial lymphocytes to various T-cell stimuli. *Gastroenterology* 1989;97:1372–1381.

59. Fangmann J, Schwinzer R, Wonigeit K. Unusual phenotype of intestinal intraepithelial lymphocytes in the rat: predominance of T cell receptor α/β^+CD2$^-$ cells and high expression of RT6 alloantigen. *Eur J Immunol* 1991;21:753–760.

60. Heijden FLV. Mucosal lymphocytes in the rat small intestine: phenotypic characterization *in situ. Immunology* 1986;59:397–399.

61. Barrett T, Gajewski TF, Danielpour D, Chang EB, Beagley KW, Bluestone JA. Differential function of intestinal intraepithelial lymphocyte subsets. *J Immunol* 1992;149:1124–1130.

62. Maloy KJ, Mowat AM, Samoyska R, Crispe IN. Phenotypic heterogeneity of intraepithelial T lymphocytes from mouse small intestine. *Immunology* 1991;72:555–562.

63. Taguchi T, Aicher WK, Fujihashi K, Yamamoto M, McGhee JR, Bluestone JA, Kiyono H. Novel function for intestinal intraepithelial lymphocytes: murine CD3$^+$, γ/δ TCR$^+$ T cells produce IFN-γ and IL-5. *J Immunol* 1991;147:3736–3744.

64. Aicher WK, Fujihashi K, Taguchi T, et al. Intestinal intraepithelial lymphocyte T cells are resistant to lpr gene-induced T cell abnormalities. *Eur J Immunol* 1992;22:137–145.

65. Takimoto H, Nakamura T, Takeuchi M, Sumi Y, Tanaka T, Nomoto K, Yoshkai Y. Age-associated increase in number of CD4$^+$CD8$^+$ intestinal intraepithelial lymphocytes in rats. *Eur J Immunol* 1992;22:159–164.

66. Parrott DMV, Tait C, MacKenzie S, Mowat AM, Davies MDJ, Micklem HS. Analysis of the effector functions of different mucosal lymphocytes. *New York Acad Sci* 1983;409:307–320.

67. Schmidt-Ullrich R, Eichmann K. Transfection of the CD8α gene restores specific target cell lysis: factors that determine the function and expression of CD8 in a cytotoxic T cell clone. *Int Immunol* 1990;2:247–256.

68. Hori T, Paliard X, de Waal Malefijt R, Ranes M, Spits H. Comparative analysis of CD8 expressed on mature CD4$^+$CD8$^+$ T cell clones cultured with IL-4 and that on CD8$^+$ T cell clones: implication for functional significance of CD8β. *Int Immunol* 1991;3:737–741.

69. Miceli MC, Parnes JR. The roles of CD4 and CD8 in T cell activation. *Semin Immunol* 1991; 3:133–141.

70. Whetsell M, Mosley RL, Whetsell L, Schaefer FV, Miller KS, Klein JR. Comparison of the T cell receptor variable region gamma gene repertoire of intestinal intraepithelial lymphocytes in inbred and wild mice. *FASEB J* 1992;6:1707.

71. Whetsell M, Mosley RL, Whetsell L, Schaefer FV, Miller KS, Klein JR. Rearrangement and junctional-site sequence analyses of T-cell receptor gamma genes in intestinal intraepithelial lymphocytes from murine athymic chimeras. *Mol Cell Biol* 1991;11:5902–5909.

72. Paliard X, de waal Melefijt R, de Vries J, Spits H. Interleukin-4 mediates CD8 induction on human CD4[+] T cell clones. *Nature* 1988;335:642–645.

73. Bandeira A, Mota-Santos T, Itohara S, Degermann S, Heusser C, Tonegawa S, Coutinho A. Localization of γ/δ T cells to the intestinal epithelium is independent of normal microbial colonization. *J Exp Med* 1990;172:239–244.

74. Goodman T, Lefrancois L. Expression of the γ-δ T-cell receptor on intestinal CD8[+] intraepithelial lymphocytes. *Nature* 1988;333:855–858.

75. Hershberg R, Eghtesady P, Sydora B, Brorson K, Cheroutre H, Modlin R, Kronenberg M. Expression of the thymus leukemia antigen in mouse intestinal epithelium. *Proc Natl Acad Sci USA* 1990;87:9727–9731.

76. Goodman T, Lefrancois L. Intraepithelial lymphocytes: anatomical site, not T cell receptor forms, dictates phenotype and function. *J Exp Med* 1989;170:1569–1581.

77. Barrett TA, Delvy ML, Kennedy DM, et al. Mechanism of self-tolerance of γ/δ T cells in epithelial tissues. *J Exp Med* 1992;175:65–70.

78. Goodman T, LeCorre R, Lefrancois L. A T-cell receptor γδ-specific monoclonal antibody detects a Vγ5 region polymorphism. *Immunogenetics* 1992;35:65–68.

79. Fujihashi K, Taguchi T, Aicher WK, McGhee J, Bluestone JA, Eldridge JH, Kiyono H. Immunoregulatory functions for murine intraepithelial lymphocytes: γ/δ T cell receptor-positive (TCR[+]) T cells abrogate oral tolerance, while α/β TCR[+] T cells provide B cell help. *J Exp Med* 1992;175:695–707.

80. Correa I, Bix M, Liao N-S, Zijlstra M, Jaenisch R, Raulte D. Most γδ T cells develop normally in β2-microglobulin-deficient mice. *Proc Natl Acad Sci USA* 1992;89:653–657.

81. Ullrich R, Schieferdecker L, Ziegler K, Reicken EO, Zeitz M. γδ T cells in the human intestine express surface markers of activation and are preferentially located in the epithelium. *Cell Immunol* 1991;128:619–627.

82. Rocha B, Vassalli P, Guy-Grand D. The Vβ repertoire of mouse gut homodimeric α CD8[+] intraepithelial T cell receptor α/β[+] lymphocytes reveals a major extrathymic pathway of T cell differentiation. *J Exp Med* 1991;173:483–486.

83. Takagaki Y, DeCloux A, Bonneville M, Tonegawa S. Diversity of γδ T-cell receptors on murine intestinal intraepithelial lymphocytes. *Nature* 1989;339:712–714.

84. Asarnow DM, Goodman T, LeFrancois L, Allison JP. Distinct antigen receptor repertoires of two classes of murine epithelium-associated T cells. *Nature* 1989;341:60–62.

85. Ota Y, Kobata T, Seki M, et al. Extrathymic origin of Vγ1/Vδ6 T cells in the skin. *Eur J Immunol* 1992;22:595–598.

86. Kyes S, Carew E, Carding SR, Janeway CA, Hayday A. Diversity in T-cell receptor γ gene usage in intestinal epithelium. *Proc Natl Acad Sci USA* 1989;86:5527–5531.

87. Stickney D, Mosley RL, Whetsell M, Whetsell L, Schaefer FV, Miller KS, Klein JR. T cell receptor delta gene repertoire and diversity of intestinal intraepithelial lymphocytes in athymic mice. *Mol Immunol* 1993;30:813–819.

88. Barrett TA, Delvy ML, Kennedy DM, et al. Mechanism of self-tolerance of γ/δ T cells in epithelial tissue. *J Exp Med* 1992;175:65–70.

89. Fichtelius KE. The gut epithelium—a first level lymphoid organ? *Exp Cell Res* 1967;49:87–92.

90. Fichtelius KE, Yunis EJ, Good RA. Occurrence of lymphocytes within the gut epithelium of normal and neonatally thymectomized mice. *Proc Soc Exp Biol Med* 1968;128:185–188.

91. Lefrancois L, Lecorre R, Mayo J, Bluestone JA, Goodman T. Extrathymic selection of TCR γδ[+] T cells by class II major histocompatibility complex molecules. *Cell* 1990;63:333–340.

92. Mosley RL, Klein JR. Peripheral engraftment of fetal intestine into athymic mice sponsors T cell development: direct evidence for thymopoietic function of murine small intestine. *J Exp Med* 1992;176:1365–1373.

93. MacDonald HR, Schreyer M, Howe RC, Bron C. Selective expression of CD8α (Ly-2) subunit on activated thymic γ/δ cells. *Eur J Immunol* 1990;20:927–930.

94. Dembic Z, Haas W, Zamoyska R, Parnes J, Steinmetz M, von Boehmer H. Transfection of the CD8 gene enhances T-cell recognition. *Nature* 1987;326:510–511.

95. Tomonari K, Soencer S. Epitope-specific binding of CD8 regulates activation of T cells and induction of cytotoxicity. *Int Immunol* 1990;2:1189–1194.

96. Eichmann K, Ehrfeld A, Falk I, et al. Affinity enhancement and transmembrane signaling are associated with distinct epitopes on the CD8 αβ heterodimer. *J Immunol* 1991;147:2075–2081.

97. Baume DM, Caligiuri MA, Manley TJ, Daley JF, Ritz J. Differential expression of CD8α and

CD8β associated with MHC-restricted and non-MHC-restricted cytolytic effector cells. *Cell Immunol* 1990;131:352–365.

98. Croitoru K, Bienenstock J, Ernst PB. CD5 negative murine intraepithelial lymphocytes (IEL) represent a thymic-independent lineage with distinct repertoire. *FASEB J* 1992;6:1707.

99. van de Rijn M, Heimfeld S, Spangrude GJ, Weissman IL. Mouse hematopoietic stem-cell antigen Sca-1 is a member of the Ly-6 antigen family. *Proc Natl Acad Sci USA* 1989;86:4634–4647.

100. Dumont FJ, Coker LZ, Habbersett RC, Treffinger JA. Xenogeneic monoclonal antibody to an Ly-6-linked murine cell surface antigen: differential reactivity with T cell subpopulations and bone marrow. *J Immunol* 1985;134:2257–2262.

101. Takei F. Biochemical characterization of H9/25, allospecificity encoded by the Ly-6 region. *Immunogenetics* 1982;16:201–206.

102. Rock K, Yeh EJH, Gramm CF, Haber SI, Reiser H, Benacerraf B. TAP, a novel T cell-activating protein involved in the stimulation of MHC-restricted T lymphocytes. *J Exp Med* 1986;163:315–333.

103. Palacios R, Samaridis J, Thorpe D, Leu T. Identification and characterization of pro-T lymphocytes and lineage-uncommited lymphocyte precursors from mice with novel markers. *J Exp Med* 1990;172:219–230.

104. Dillon SB, MacDonald TT. Functional characterization of Con A responsive Lyt 2 positive mouse small intestine intraepithelial lymphocytes. *Immunology* 1984;59:389–398.

105. Mowat AM, McInnes IB, Parrott DMV. Functional properties of intra-epithelial lymphocytes from mouse small intestine. IV: Investigation of the proliferative capacity of IEL using phorbol ester and calcium ionophore. *Immunology* 1989;66:398–403.

106. MacDonald TT, Spencer J. Evidence that activated mucosal T cells play a role in the pathogenesis of enteropathy in human small intestine. *J Exp Med* 1988;167:1341–1349.

107. June CH, Ledbetter JA, Linsley PS, Thompson CB. Role of the CD28 receptor in T-cell activation. *Immunol Today* 1990;11:211–216.

108. Jung G, Ledbetter JA, Muller-Eberhard HJ. Induction of cytotoxicity in resting human T lymphocytes bound to tumor cells by antibody heteroconjugates. *Proc Natl Acad Sci USA.* 1987;84:4611–4615.

109. Azuma M, Cayabyab M, Buck D, Phillips JH, Lanier LL. CD28 interaction with B7 costimulates primary allogeneic proliferative responses and cytotoxicity mediated by small, resting T cells. *J Exp Med* 1992;175:353–360.

110. Azuma M, Cayabyab M, Buck D, Phillips JH, Lanier LL. Involvement of CD28 in MHC-unrestricted cytotoxicity mediated by a human natural killer leukemia cell line. *J Immunol* 1992;149:1115–1123.

111. June CH, Gillespie MM, Thompson CB. T-cell proliferation involving the CD28 pathway is associated with cyclosporine-resistant interleukin 2 gene expression. *Mol Cell Biol* 1987;7:4472–4481.

112. Gross JA, Callas E, Allison JP. Identification and distribution of the costimulatory receptor CD28 in the mouse. *J Immunol* 1992;149:380–388.

113. Mosley RL, Whetsell M, Klein JR. Monoclonal antibody to murine CD28: phenotypic and functional studies reveal perviously undescribed properties of CD28 in mice. *Submitted for publication.*

114. Linsley PS, Clark EA, Ledbetter JA. T-cell antigen CD28 mediates adhesion with B cells by interacting with activation antigen B7/BB-1. *Proc Natl Acad Sci USA* 1990;87:5031–5035.

115. Reiser H, Greeman GJ, Razi-Wolf Z, Gimmi CD, Benacerraf B, Nadler LM. Murine B7 antigen provides an efficient costimulatory signal for activation of murine T lymphocytes via the T-cell receptor/CD3 complex. *Proc Natl Acad Sci USA* 1992;89:271–275.

116. Brunet J-F, Denizot F, Luciani M-F, Roux-Dosseto M, Suzan M, Mattei M-G, Goldstein P. A new member of the immunoglobulin superfamily—CTLA-4. *Nature* 1987;328:267–270.

117. Harper K, Balzano C, Rouvier E, Mattei M-G, Luciani M-F, Goldstein P. CTLA-4 and CD28 activated lymphocyte molecules are closely related in both mouse and human as to sequence, message expression, gene structure, and chromosomal location. *J Immunol* 1991;147:1037–1044.

118. Lefrancois L, Bevan M. Functional modification of cytotoxic T-lymphocyte T200 glycoprotein recognized by monoclonal antibody. *Nature* 1985;314:449–452.

119. Lefrancois L, Goodman T. Developmental sequence of T200 antigen modifications in murine T cells. *J Immunol* 1987;139:3718–3724.

120. Halstensen TS, Scott H, Brandtzaeg P. Human CD8[+] intraepithelial T lymphocytes are mainly CD45RA[−]RB[+] and show increased co-expression of CD45RO in coeliac disease. *Eur J Immunol* 1990;20:1825–1830.

121. McFarland HI, Nahill SR, Maciaszek JW, Welsh RM. CD11b (Mac-1): a marker for CD8[+] cytotoxic T cell activation and memory in virus infection. *J Immunol* 1992;149:1326–1333.

122. Budd RC, Cerottini J-C, Horvath C, Bron C, Pedrazzani T, Howe RC, MacDonald HR. Distinction of virgin and memory T lymphocytes: stable acquisition of the Pgp-1 glycoprotein concomitant with antigenic stimulation. *J Immunol* 1987;138:3120–3129.

123. Holcombe HR, Tonkonogy SL. Murine intestinal intraepithelial lymphocytes contain CD8[+] cells that produce IL-2 and IFN-γ but not IL-4. *FASEB J* 1991;5:1781.

124. Tedder TF, Penta AC, Levine HB, Freedman AS. Expression of the human leukocyte adhesion molecule, LAM1: identity with TQ1 and Leu-8 differentiation antigens. *J Immunol* 1990;144:532–540.

125. Dustin ML, Springer T. Role of lymphocyte adhesion receptors in transient interactions and cell locomotion. *Annu Rev Immunol* 1991;9:27–66.

126. Picker L, Butcher EC. Physiological and molecular mechanisms of lymphocyte homing. *Annu Rev Immunol* 1992;10:561–591.

127. Schmitz M, Nunez D, Butcher EC. Selective recognition of mucosal lymphoid high endothelium by gut intraepithelial leukocytes. *Gastroenterology* 1988;94:576–581.

128. Dustin ML, Staunton DE, Springer TA. Supergene families meet in the immune system. *Immunol Today* 1988;9:213–215.

129. Kilshaw PJ, Murant SJ. A new surface antigen on intraepithelial lymphocytes in the intestine. *Eur J Immunol* 1990;20:2201–2207.

130. Kilshaw PJ, Murant SJ. Expression and regulation of β7(βp) integrins on mouse lymphocytes: relevance to the mucosal immune system. *Eur J Immunol* 1991;21:2591–2597.

131. Schieferdecker HL, Ullrich R, Weiss-Breckwoldt AN, Schwarting R, Stein H, Riecken E-O, Zeitz M. The HML-1 antigen of intestinal lymphocytes is an activation antigen. *J Immunol* 1990;144: 2541–2549.

132. Cerf-Bensussan N, Guy-Grand D, Lisowska-Grospierre B, Griscelli C, Bhan AK. A monoclonal antibody specific for rat intestinal lymphocytes. *J Immunol* 1986;136:76–82.

133. Yuan Q, Jiang W, Hollander D, Leung E, Watsson JD, Krissansen W. Identity between the novel integrin β7 subunit and an antigen found highly expressed on intraepithelial lymphocytes in the small intestine. *Biochem Biophys Res Commun* 1991;176:1443–1449.

134. Yuan Q, Jiang W, Krissansen GW, Watson JD. Cloning and sequence analyses of a novel β2-related integrin transcript from T lymphocytes: homology of integrin cysteine-rich repeats to domain III of laminin β chains. *Int Immunol* 1990;2:1097–1108.

135. Bland PW, Warren LG. Antigen presentation by epithelial cells of the rat small intestine. I: Kinetics, antigen specificity and blocking by anti-Ia antisera. *Immunology* 1986;58:1–7.

136. Mayer L, Shlien R. Evidence for function of Ia molecules on gut epithelial cells in man. *J Exp Med* 1987;166:1471–1483.

137. Kaiserlian D, Vidal K, Revillard J-P. Murine enterocytes can present soluble antigen to specific class II-restricted CD4[+] T cells. *Eur J Immunol* 1989;19:1513–1516.

138. Wu M, Kaer LV, Itohara S, Tonegawa S. Highly restricted expression of thymus leukemia antigens on intestinal epithelial cells. *J Exp Med* 1991;174:213–218.

139. Bleicher PA, Balk SP, Hagen SJ, Blumberg RS, Flotte TJ, Terhorst C. Expression of CD1 on gastrointestinal epithelium. *Science* 1990;250:679–682.

140. Guy-Grand D, Malassis-Seris M, Briottet C, Vassalli P. Cytotoxic differentiation of mouse gut thymodependent and independent intraepithelial T lymphocytes is induced locally: correlation between functional assays, presence of perforin and granzymes transcripts, and cytotoxic granules. *J Exp Med* 1991;173:1549–1552.

141. Splitter GA, McGuire TC, Davis WC. The differentiation of bone marrow cells to functional T lymphocytes following implantation of thymus graft and thymic stroma in nude and ATxBM mice. *Cell Immunol* 1977;34:93–103.

142. Davies MDJ, Parrott DMV. Cytotoxic T cells in small intestine epithelial, lamina propria and lung lymphocytes. *Immunology* 1981;44:367–371.

143. Klein JR, Kagnoff MF. Nonspecific recruitment of cytotoxic effector cells in the intestinal mucosa of antigen primed mice. *J Exp Med* 1984;160:1931–1936.

144. Klein JR, Lefrancois L, Kagnoff MF. A murine cytotoxic T lymphocyte clone from the intestinal mucosa that is antigen specific for proliferation and displays broadly reactive inducible cytotoxic activity. *J Immunol* 1985;135:3697–3703.

145. Klein JR, Kagnoff MF. Spontaneous *in vitro* evolution of lytic specificity of cytotoxic T lymphocyte clones isolated from murine intestine epithelium. *J Immunol* 1987;138:58–62.

146. London SD, Cebra JJ, Rubin DH. Intraepithelial lymphocytes contain virus-specific, MHC-restricted cytotoxic cell precursors after gut mucosal immunization with reovirus serotype 1/Lang. *Regional Immunol* 1989;2:98–102.
147. Offit PA, Dudzik K. Rotavirus-specific cytotoxic T lymphocytes appear at the intestinal mucosal surface after rotavirus infection. *J Virol* 1989;63:3507–3512.
148. Offit PA, Cunningham SL, Dudzik KI. Memory and distribution of virus-specific cytotoxic T lymphocytes (CTLs) and CTL precursors after rotavirus infection. *J Virol* 1991;65:1318–1324.
149. Panwala C, Eghtesady P, Kronenberg M. Specificity of mouse intestinal epithelial lymphocytes that express a γδ T-cell antigen receptor. *FASEB J* 1992;6:1408.
150. Arnaud-Battandier F, Bundy AM, O'Neill M, Bienenstock J, Nelson DL. Cytotoxic activities of gut mucosal lymphoid cells in gunea pigs. *J Immunol* 1978;121:1059–1065.
151. Flexman JP, Shellam GR, Mayrhofer G. Natural cytotoxicity, responsiveness to interferon and morphology of intra-epithelial lymphocytes from the small intestine of the rat. *Immunology* 1983;48:733–741.
152. Ortaldo JR, Herberman RB. Heterogeneity of natural killer cells. *Annu Rev Immunol* 1984;2:359–394.
153. Croitoru K, Ernst PB, Bienenstock J, Padol I, Stanisz AM. Selective modulation of the natural killer activity of murine intestinal intraepithelial leukocytes by the neuropeptide substance P. *Immunology* 1990;71:196–201.
154. Mowat AM, Tait RC, MacKenzie S, Davies MDJ, Parrott DMV. Analysis of natural killer effector and suppressor activity by intraepithelial lymphocytes from mouse small intestine. *Clin Exp Immunol* 1983;52:191–198.
155. Bienenstock J, Befus AD, McDermott M, Miraski S, Rosenthal K, Tagliabue A. The mucosal immunologic network: compartmentalization of lymphocytes, natural killer cells, and mast cells. *New York Acad Sci* 1983;83:164–170.
156. Nauss KM, Pavlina TM, Kumar V, Newberne PM. Functional characteristics of lymphocytes isolated from the rat large intestine. *Gastroenterology* 1984;86:468–475.
157. Tice DG. Ontogeny of natural killer activity in rat small bowel. *Transplant Proc* 1990;22:2458–2459.
158. Cohn SM, Roth KA, Birkenmeier EH, Gordon JI. Temporal and spatial patterns of transgene expression in aging adult mice provide insights about the origins, organization, and differentiation of the intestinal epithelium. *Proc Natl Acad Sci USA* 1991;88:1034–1038.
159. Roth KA, Hermiston ML, Gordon JI. Use of trangeneic mice to infer the biological properties of small intestinal stem cells and to examine the lineage relationships of their descendents. *Proc Natl Acad Sci USA* 1991;88:9407–9411.
160. Koyama K, Hosokawa T, Aoike A. Aging effect of the immune functions of murine gut-associated lymphoid tissues. *Dev Comp Immunol* 1990;14:465–473.

Mucosal Immunology: Intraepithelial Lymphocytes,
edited by H. Kiyono and J. R. McGhee.
Raven Press, Ltd., New York © 1993.

4

Differentiation and TCR Selection of Intestinal Intraepithelial Lymphocytes

Leo Lefrançois

University of Connecticut Health Center, Department of Medicine, Farmington, CT.

THYMIC INFLUENCE OF IEL MATURATION

As evidenced by the current volume, intestinal intraepithelial lymphocytes (IEL) have become the subject of intense scientific scrutiny. The reasons for this are manifold. Not the least of these was the realization that IEL as a population comprise a large proportion of the immune system and, of course, an even larger percentage of the mucosal immune system. In addition, the demonstration that a major population of cells utilizing the γδ T cell antigen receptor (TCR) reside in the IEL compartment sparked renewed interest in this T cell population (1,2). However, the primary characteristic that distinguishes most, if not all, IEL from other T cells is their ability to mature in the absence of a thymus (3–13). This is certainly true of IEL expressing the γδ TCR, although sufficient data have not been gathered to determine whether *all* γδ TCR IEL normally mature extrathymically.

In the case of αβ TCR IEL, there has been some controversy concerning their potential to differentiate extrathymically. While nude mice and rats have been reported to contain few αβ TCR IEL (12–14), significant numbers of donor-derived αβ TCR IEL can be found in ATX mice rescued with bone marrow or with fetal liver (4,8,9). We examined TCR expression in individual IEL preparations from eight 20-week-old nude mice from two strains (Table 1). In two C3H/HeJ mice high percentages of αβ TCR IEL were present. In one of these animals the αβ TCR IEL were primarily CD4$^+$8$^+$ (animal #4). Low percentages of αβ TCR IEL were found in the four C57BL/6 nude mice tested.

Percoll-fractionated IEL were stained for Thy1, CD4, CD8, αβ TCR or γδ TCR (15) and analyzed by fluorescence flow cytometry. Thy1 expression did not correlate with the presence of αβ TCR IEL as expected since γδ TCR and αβ TCR IEL are composed of Thy1$^-$ and Thy1$^+$ cells. These results indicate that variable generation of αβ TCR IEL occurs in 20-week-old nude mice. In contrast, several studies using ATX mice reconstituted with bone marrow or fetal liver report apparent consistent reconstitution of the αβ TCR IEL subset. There are several possibilities for

TABLE 1. *IEL TCR expression in nude mice*

Strain and animal number	Percentage of cells expressing				
	Thy1	CD4⁻8⁺	CD4⁺8⁺	γδ TCR	αβ TCR
C3H 1	58	94	<1	34	51
2	6	91	<1	72	2
3	8	86	4	52	5
4	35	67	22	64	31
BL/6 1	64	99	<1	84	3
2	29	94	<1	82	3
3	35	90	<1	75	6
4	17	89	<1	62	2

the dichotomy in αβ TCR IEL generation. On the one hand, a defect in nude mouse αβ TCR T cell generation may exist beyond that due to the absence of a thymus. Perhaps nude mouse intestinal epithelium is unable to support αβ TCR IEL differentiation due to an undescribed cryptic defect. On the other hand, the irradiation used in reconstitution experiments has profound effects on intestinal epithelial cell differentiation. In effect, lethal irradiation results in complete epithelial cell turnover and nascent epithelial cell production from crypt progenitors. This may result in the production of cellular and/or soluble factors that are necessary for αβ TCR IEL homing or production

An alternative explanation is that αβ TCR IEL are thymus-dependent. In one scenario, IEL precursors would mature in the fetal or neonatal thymus and travel to the bone marrow, where they would reside throughout adult life. Thus, reconstitution with adult bone marrow would result in population of the αβ TCR IEL compartment. Why then does fetal liver taken prior to thymus formation work in reconstitution? One would have to assume that IEL precursors in fetal liver are able to colonize gut in the absence of thymic influence, while bone marrow precursors are unable to do so. This is not as improbable as it may seem, considering that fetal liver stem cells, but not adult bone marrow stem cells, are able to generate Vγ3⁺ cells in fetal thymus while neither stem cell population is able to generate Vγ3⁺ cells in adult thymus (16). Thus, two important points must be taken into account in interpreting the nude mouse versus reconstitution of irradiated recipient experiments: the *original* source of stem cells and the receptivity of the intestine to IEL precursors.

IEL RECIRCULATION

Another factor that must be included when considering intestinal colonization is that of IEL trafficking and recirculation. We have employed parabiotic mice to study normal IEL recirculation. In this system, two mice are surgically joined and approximately one week after surgery their circulatory systems become common via formation of anastomoses. In order to determine the source of the cells being an-

TABLE 2. *Trafficking of IEL in parabiotic mice*

Animal	2 weeks postsurgery % of donor cells	
	IEL	LN
A	4.3	45
B	2.2	43

Animal	4 weeks postsurgery % of donor cells	
	IEL	LN
A	13	51
B	12	45

alyzed, Ly5.1 and Ly5.2 C57BL/6 congenic mice were parabiosed. We analyzed lymph node (LN) and IEL from these animals at various times after surgery (Table 2). At 2 weeks postsurgery approximately half of LN cells were derived from the partner animal (herein "donor") indicating that complete mixing of recirculating lymphocytes had occurred. In contrast, less than 5% of IEL were derived from the donor. At four weeks postsurgery half of LN cells and approximately 15% of IEL were donor-derived. Similar results have recently been reported (9). Donor and host lymphocytes were distinguished by flow cytometry using Ly5.1- and Ly5.2-specific mAbs. A and B represent two Ly5.1 mice paired to Ly5.2 mice.

At 4 weeks and beyond it is not possible to distinguish between bone-marrow production of IEL precursors and continued low-level recirculation. However, IEL analysis 8 weeks postsurgery indicated that the percentage of donor IEL remained at about 15%. This suggests a low level of bone-marrow chimerism, which is responsible for regenerating a subset of IEL. Moreover, TCR analysis revealed that the majority of donor IEL were $\alpha\beta$ TCR$^+$ (data not shown). These results suggest that: (a) Minimal $\alpha\beta$ TCR$^+$ IEL recirculation occurs under normal circumstances; (b) IEL are long-lived and have a low turnover rate; (c) IEL appear to represent "tissue" lymphocytes designed to survey their local milieu. It should be noted that alternatives exist to explain our results. For example, a self-renewing IEL precursor may reside in the intestine that does not itself recirculate. Thus, the 85% of IEL that are not renewed could be derived from such a precursor.

EFFECT OF MICROBIAL COLONIZATION ON TCR EXPRESSION

In addition to the above described elements that may influence IEL composition, the effect of antigenic stimulation must be taken into account. We have examined IEL from germ-free mice to determine whether bacterial and/or viral colonization of the gut alters IEL makeup (Table 3). IEL from five Swiss (NIH) germ-free mice were tested for TCR expression. While all animals contained substantial numbers of

TABLE 3. *IEL TCR expression in germ-free mice*

Strain and animal number		Percentage of cells expressing		
		Thy1	γδ TCR	αβ TCR
C3H	1	13	66	8
	2	9	76	6
	3	8	68	6
	4	11	64	7
	5	10	74	4

γδ TCR IEL, low percentages of αβ TCR IEL were found. In addition, as we have previously shown, low numbers of Thy1$^+$ IEL were detected (17). These results are in contrast to those obtained with IEL from normal mice or from germ-free mice that have been introduced to standard housing conditions where approximately 50% of cells are αβ TCR$^+$ and Thy1$^+$ (ref. 17 and data not shown). The effect of microbial colonization of the gut may be manifested in the IEL TCR repertoire. Recent reports suggest that human αβ TCR IEL may express oligoclonal TCRs perhaps as a result of reactivity to a limited set of nonpolymorphic antigens (19,20). It remains to be shown whether microbial colonization of the gut results in an expansion of resident IEL or in the recruitment of cells from elsewhere.

DYNAMICS OF αβ TCR IEL SELECTION

Since positive and negative selection of peripheral T cell precursors occurs in the thymus, one potential result of extrathymic αβ TCR IEL maturation may be alterations in the IEL TCR selection profile as compared to other T cells. Indeed, IEL expressing some V regions that are not expressed by LN T cells have been described (5,6,9). These results have been used further to support the ability of αβ TCR IEL to mature extrathymically. The majority of IEL expressing such "forbidden" V regions were reported to be CD4$^-$, CD8αα$^+$. CD8αα cells comprise approximately one-third of CD4$^-$8$^+$ αβ TCR IEL and the majority of CD4$^+$8$^+$ IEL (18). For this reason we compared αβ TCR V-region usage of CD4$^+$, CD8αα$^+$ IEL, CD4$^-$8$^+$ IEL, and LN T cell subsets (Table 4). Three mouse strains were used that are H-2^k but differ at Mls: AKR/J, Mls-1^{a}2^b; C3H/HeJ, Mls-1^{b}2^a; and C57BR/cdJ, Mls-1^{b}2^b. We examined CD4$^+$8$^+$ IEL TCR expression in several cases in which forbidden V-regions were expressed by CD4$^-$8$^+$ IEL. Two examples are shown in Table 4. Whereas Vβ3$^+$ cells were absent from LN T cells of CD4 and CD8 phenotype, a variable percentage of CD4$^-$8$^+$ IEL were Vβ3$^+$ (8.1 ± 7.1). Most but not all of these cells were CD8αα (21). However, Vβ3$^+$ cells were largely deleted from CD4$^+$, CD8αα$^+$ IEL. Similarly, Vβ6$^+$ cells were absent from AKR/J LN T cells and CD4$^+$8$^+$ IEL but were detectable in CD4$^-$8$^+$ IEL.

Examination of TCR selection in the CD4$^+$8$^+$ IEL subset revealed other examples of subset-specific TCR expression including examples of negative selection. In

TABLE 4. αβ *TCR selection of CD4$^+$8$^+$ IEL*

Strain	V region	Biased expression of "forbidden" TCRs to CD4−8+ IEL: lack of correlation with CD8β chain expression			
		LN subset		IEL subset	
		CD4	CD8	CD4−8+	CD4+8+
C3H/HeJ		1.0 ± 0.4	0.7 ± 0.2	8.1 ± 7.1	1.3 ± 2.0
	Vβ3				
AKR/J		0.5 ± 0.4	0.5 ± 0.2	4.7 ± 2.5	0.5 ± 0.4
	Vβ6				

Strain	V region	Tissue and subset-specific negative selection			
		LN subset		IEL subset	
		CD4	CD8	CD4−8+	CD4+8+
C57BR		8.2 ± 4.2	12.9 ± 0.8	12.1 ± 4.5	0.6 ± 0.4
	Vβ14				

Strain	V region	Tissue and subset-specific positive selection			
		LN subset		IEL subset	
		CD4	CD8	CD4−8+	CD4+8+
C57BR		9.1 ± 2.1	7.2 ± 1.9	12.4 ± 9.2	40.4 ± 7.4
	Vβ3				

C57BR/cdJ mice, lymph nodes and CD4$^-$8$^+$ IEL contained about 10% Vβ14$^+$ cells, but Vβ14$^+$ cells were essentially absent from the CD4$^+$8$^+$ IEL subset. This important result demonstrates that intestine-specific TCR negative selection can occur. Alternatively, a specific positive expansion or selection of the Vβ14$^+$ cells was occurring in the other populations but not in the CD4$^+$8$^+$ subset.

Based on TCR selection by Mls antigens, these results imply that the CD4 molecule of CD4$^+$8$^+$ IEL was involved in negative selection and that the CD8αα dimer may not be able to mediate TCR–MHC interactions that result in negative selection.

Positive selection of CD4$^+$8$^+$ IEL was also observed in C57BR/cdJ mice. Much greater percentages of Vβ3$^+$ cells (40.4 ± 7.4) were found in CD4$^+$8$^+$ IEL than in other IEL or LN subsets. This finding indicates that either a positive selection event occurred during differentiation of IEL precursors into CD4$^+$8$^+$ mature IEL or that antigenic stimulation in the gut caused selective expansion or influx of Vβ3$^+$ CD4$^+$8$^+$ cells. It should be noted that C57BR/cdJ IEL contain unusually high percentages of CD4$^+$8$^+$ cells for as yet unexplained reasons, but selective expansion as just discussed is a potential explanation.

SUMMARY

The results presented indicate that the interplay of multiple contributing factors affects the composition and TCR expression profile of αβ TCR IEL. These factors include (a) the source of IEL precursors and the developmental stage and status of the intestinal target tissue (e.g., nude mouse versus irradiated epithelium), (b) the lack of recirculation of IEL under normal circumstances, and (c) the composition of the intestinal microflora.

In regard to the composition of intestinal microflora, microbial colonization of the gut may not only result in expansion or influx of $\alpha\beta$ TCR IEL, but in all likelihood will affect the TCR V-region usage pattern at any given time. Our results demonstrating subset- and tissue-specific TCR selection support this contention. Alternatively, if $\alpha\beta$ TCR IEL mature from TCR$^-$ precursors within the gut, then the resultant TCR repertoire may be the result of selection of TCRs during differentiation on a set of peptides that are distinct from those in the thymus. In such a scenario, those peptides may be generated from a set of endogenous proteins present in intestinal epithelium that are distinct or only partially overlapping with those selected upon in the thymus and thus would not be dependent on microbial antigen. Nevertheless, without intestinal flora, minimal numbers of $\alpha\beta$ TCR IEL are found. It will be of interest to compare the TCR usage of the few $\alpha\beta$ TCR IEL present in germ-free mice with that of normal mice.

The discovery of CD4$^+$8$^+$ T cells outside of the thymus suggested the possibility that $\alpha\beta$ TCR IEL matured extrathymically via cellular intermediates analogous to those in the thymus (18,22). However, CD4$^+$8$^+$ IEL express mature T cell levels of TCR, suggesting that if these cells were CD4$^-$8$^+$ IEL precursors, a selection mechanism distinct from that in the thymus was in place. The results presented here make it even more unlikely that CD4$^+$8$^+$ IEL are precursors to other IEL subsets. This conclusion is made on the basis of the demonstration of CD4$^+$8$^+$ IEL-specific negative and positive selection. Unless the TCR expression profile of CD4$^+$8$^+$ IEL changes after differentiation into CD4$^-$8$^+$ IEL, it appears unlikely that CD4$^+$8$^+$ IEL are precursors to single positive IEL. This is particularly obvious in the case of negative selection of CD4$^+$8$^+$ IEL expressing certain V regions in the absence of deletion of such cells from other IEL subsets. Thus, CD4$^+$8$^+$ IEL appear to represent a unique gut-specific lineage of mature $\alpha\beta$ TCR T cells with unknown function.

The complexity of the immune system is nowhere more evident than in the intestinal mucosa. With its various compartments, the workings of the intestinal mucosal immune system have defied principles adhered to in defining the extraintestinal immune system. This is exemplified by the ability of some IEL to mature without thymic influence. Controversy aside concerning the extrathymic maturation of $\alpha\beta$ TCR IEL, the IEL compartment constitutes an isolated immune system with as yet poorly defined functional capabilities.

ACKNOWLEDGMENTS

I thank Tom Goodman, Gloria Badiner, and Dawn Ecker for their help in completing these studies. I thank Drs. Elina Donskoy and Irving Goldschneider for their help in producing the parabiotic mice.

REFERENCES

1. Goodman T, Lefrançois L. Expression of the $\gamma\delta$ T cell receptor on intestinal CD8$^+$ intraepithelial lymphocytes. *Nature* 1988;333:855–858.

2. Bonneville M, Janeway CA, Ito N, Haser W, Ishida I, Nakanishi N, Tonegawa S. Intestinal intra-epithelial lymphocytes are a distinct set of γδ T cells. *Nature* 1988;336:479–481.
3. Lefrançois L, LeCorre R, Mayo J, Bluestone JA, Goodman T. Extrathymic selection of Tcr γ,δ⁺ T cells by class II major histocompatibility molecules. *Cell* 1990;63:333–340.
4. Lefrançois L, Mayo JM, Goodman T. Ontogeny of T cell receptor (TCR) α,β⁺ and γ,δ⁺ intra-epithelial lymphocytes (IEL). In: Lotze M, Finn OJ, eds. *Cellular immunity and the immunotherapy of cancer, UCLA symposium on molecular and cellular biology.* New York: Wiley Liss; 1990:31–40.
5. Rocha B, Vassalli P, Guy-Grand D. The Vβ repertoire of mouse gut homodimeric α CD8⁺ intra-epithelial T cell receptor α/β⁺ lymphocytes reveals a major extrathymic pathway of T cell differentiation. *J Exp Med* 1991;173:483–486.
6. Murosaki S, Yoshikai Y, Ishida A, et al. Failure of T cell receptor Vβ negative selection in murine intestinal intra-epithelial lymphocytes. *Int Immunol* 1991;3:1005–1013.
7. Lefrançois, L. Extrathymic differentiation of intraepithelial lymphocytes: generation of a separate and unequal T cell repertoire? *Immunol Today* 1991;12:436–438.
8. Whetsell M, Mosley RL, Whetsell L, Schaefer FV, Miller KS, Klein JR. Rearrangement and junctional-site sequence analyses of T-cell receptor gamma genes in intestinal intraepithelial lymphocytes from murine athymic chimeras. *Mol Cell Biol* 1991;11:5902.
9. Poussier P, Edouard P, Lee C, Binnie M, Julius M. Thymus-independent development and negative selection of T cells expressing T cell receptor α/β in the intestinal epithelium: evidence for distinct circulation patterns of gut- and thymus-derived T lymphocytes. *J Exp Med* 1992;176:187–199.
10. Mosley RL, Styre D, Klein JR. Differentiation and functional maturation of bone marrow-derived intestinal epithelial T cells expressing membrane T cell receptor in athymic radiation chimeras. *J Immunol* 1990;145:1369–1375.
11. Bandeira A, Itohara S, Bonneville M, Burlen-Defranoux O, Mota-Santos T, Coutinho, A, Tonegawa S. Extrathymic origin of intestinal intraepithelial lymphocytes bearing T-cell antigen receptor γδ. *Proc Natl Acad Sci* 1990;88:43–47.
12. De Geus B, Van den Enden M, Coolen C, Nagelkerken L, Van der Heijden P, Rozing J. Phenotype of intraepithelial lymphocytes in euthymic and athymic mice: implications for differentiation of cells bearing a CD3-associated γδ T cell receptor. *Eur J Immunol* 1991;20:291–298.
13. Bonneville M, Itohara S, Krecko EG, et al. Transgenic mice demonstrate that epithelial homing of γ/δ T cells is determined by cell lineages independent of T cell receptor specificity. *J Exp Med* 1990;171:1015–1026.
14. Vaage JT, Dissen E, Ager A, Roberts I, Fossum S, Rolstad B. T cell receptor-bearing cells among rat intestinal intraepithelial lymphocytes are mainly α/β⁺ and are thymus independent. *Eur J Immunol* 1990;20:1193–1196.
15. Goodman T, Lefrançois L. Intraepithelial lymphocytes: anatomical site not T cell receptor form dictates phenotype and function. *J Exp Med* 1989;170:1569–1581.
16. Ikuta K, Kina T, Macneil I, Uchida N, Peault B, Chien Y-h, Weissman I. A developmental switch in thymic lymphocyte maturation potential occurs at the level of hematopoietic stem cells. *Cell* 1990;62:863–874.
17. Lefrançois L, Goodman T. *In vivo* modulation of cytolytic activity and Thy 1 expression in TCR -γδ⁺ intraepithelial lymphocytes. *Science* 1989;243:1716–1718.
18. Lefrançois, L. Phenotypic complexity of intraepithelial lymphocytes of the small intestine. *J Immunol* 1991;147:1746–1751.
19. Balk SP, Ebert EC, Blumenthal RL, McDermott FV, Wucherpfennig KW, Landau SB, Blumberg RS. Oligoclonal expansion and CD1 recognition by human intestinal intraepithelial lymphocytes. *Science* 1991;253:1411–1415.
20. Van Kerckhove C, Russell GJ, Deusch K, Reich K, Bhan AK, DerSimonian H, Brenner MB. Oligoclonality of human intestinal intraepithelial T cells. *J Exp Med* 1991;175:57–63.
21. Badiner G, Goodman TG, Lefrançois L. Selection of intestinal intraepithelial lymphocyte T cell receptors: evidence for a dynamic tissue-specific process. *Int Immunol* 1993;5:223–226.
22. Mosley RL, Styre D, Klein JR. CD4⁺ CD8⁺ murine intestinal intraepithelial lymphocytes. *Int Immunol* 1990;2:361–365.

Mucosal Immunology: Intraepithelial Lymphocytes,
edited by H. Kiyono and J. R. McGhee.
Raven Press, Ltd., New York © 1993.

5

Antigen Receptor Diversity and Putative Specificity of γδ TCR⁺ Intraepithelial Lymphocytes

Marc Bonneville

Inserm U211, Institut de Biologie, Nantes, France.

?Antigen (Ag) recognition by T lymphocytes is accomplished via highly variable surface receptors, the T-cell receptors (TCR), composed of either αβ or γδ subunits structurally homologous to immunoglobulin chains (1). Although specificity and function of lymphocytes expressing αβ TCR are relatively well understood, numerous aspects of γδ TCR⁺ T-cell physiology remain thus far unclear. In recent years, several important features of this lymphocyte subset have been described; among these, restricted repertoire and marked epitheliotropism of γδ TCR⁺ T cells are probably the most salient ones (2,3). However the physiological significance of these observations and, in particular, the antigen specificity and precise function of γδ TCR⁺ intraepithelial lymphocytes (γδ TCR⁺ IEL) are still a matter of controversy. The present review summarizes our current knowledge about the repertoire and specificity of murine and human γδ TCR⁺ T cells, and I propose on the basis of structural and functional evidences that the primary function of γδ TCR⁺ IEL is to regulate immune responses and/or maintain epithelium integrity through recognition of a highly restricted set of endogenous ligands, presumably expressed at specific cell activation stages.

TISSUE DISTRIBUTION AND REPERTOIRE OF MURINE AND HUMAN γδ TCR⁺ T CELLS

Tissue Distribution

In mouse and human, γδ TCR⁺ T cells constitute a minor fraction of mature T lymphocytes in adult thymus and peripheral lymphoid organs (range 0.3 to 10%) (2,4). In contrast, they are enriched in several epithelial sites, where they sometimes represent the majority [e.g., in gut epithelium of young mice (5,6–8)] or even the totality [e.g., in murine epidermis (9–11)] of CD3⁺ T cells. However, although in most species studied thus far, γδ TCR⁺ T cells are preferentially located in close association with epithelial layers covering internal or external surfaces of the body, it is noteworthy that their tissue distribution and enrichment level in a given epithelium greatly vary from one species to another, or within a given species depending on age or environmental conditions. For instance, the epidermis is densely populated with $\gamma\delta$ TCR$^+$ T cells in the mouse (9–11) but virtually devoid of lymphoid cells in humans (12). In the case of intestinal mucosa, both human and murine $\gamma\delta$ TCR$^+$ T cells show a marked tropism for this epithelia (5,6,12); but in humans, their proportion among CD3$^+$ cells is not increased in this site in comparison to peripheral blood (13). Moreover, proportions of $\gamma\delta$ TCR cells among CD3$^+$ intestinal IEL are usually much lower in specific pathogen-free when compared with axenic (or germ-free) mice or in young versus adult individuals (14,15). This demonstrates the dramatic influence of environmental factors on the $\gamma\delta/\alpha\beta$ ratio in a given peripheral site, which might account in part for the above interspecies differences.

RESTRICTED REPERTOIRE OF PERIPHERAL $\gamma\delta$ TCR$^+$ T CELLS

Combinatorial diversity of $\gamma\delta$ TCR is naturally limited by the small number of V genes that can be rearranged to form a functional TCR chain [at most 6 Vγ in the mouse, 9 Vγ in humans, and below 10 Vδ in both species (2,16)]. TCR diversity seems further restricted by TCR dependent and independent processes (see below), leading to preferential use of a highly restricted set of V genes by $\gamma\delta$ TCR$^+$ T cells in a given tissue (Table 1). Throughout this section, the nomenclatures proposed by Heilig and Tonegawa (17) and Elliott et al. (18) are used for the murine Vγ and Vδ genes respectively, and those by Lefranc and Rabbitts (16) and Takihara et al. (19) for their human counterparts.

Murine $\gamma\delta$ TCR$^+$ T Cells

Murine $\gamma\delta$ TCR$^+$ T cells can be divided into two major types, differing in the extent of their TCR structural diversity.

Type I Cells

These lymphocytes are derived from $\gamma\delta$ TCR$^+$ thymic subsets that predominate at fetal and perinatal stages (9,20–22). Their most striking feature is the complete lack of diversity of their expressed TCR chains, even though they are encoded by rearranged γ and δ genes (9,22). Thus far, two (perhaps three) subsets have been described; these subsets differ by their Vγ gene use and tissue distribution (Table 1). Cells expressing TCR with Vγ5 and Vδ1 regions are mainly located in the epidermis (9,20), where they are also referred to as Thy-1 positive dendritic epidermal cells (DEC) due to their peculiar morphology. Vγ5Vδ1 cells might be enriched in lactating mammary gland as well (23). A second subset expressing the same δ chain and a γ chain comprising a distinct V region (Vγ6) but a junctional sequence

TABLE 1. *Human and murine γδ TCR+ T cell subsets*

Species	Expressed V genes		Diversity	Developmental pathway	Tissue distribution	Specificity
Mouse	Vγ5	Vδ1	0	early fetal thymus	epidermis (lactating mammary gland ?)	stressed keratinocytes
	Vγ6	Vδ1	0	late fetal thymus	uterus, vagina, and tongue epithelia	unknown
	Vγ4	Vδs	+ + +	postnatal thymus extrathymic ?	blood, lymph nodes, spleen	diverse (MHC class I, II, Ib, etc.)
		Vδ6	+ + +	postnatal (thymus ?)	lung	bacterial HSP ?
		Vδ4	0	fetal thymus ?	mammary gland	unknown
	Vγ7	Vδ4 Vδ6	+ + +	extrathymic (intestine ?)	epithelia gastro-intestinal tract	unknown
	Vγ1	Vδs	+ + +	postnatal thymus/extra-thymic ?	spleen	unknown
		Vδ6	+/ + + +	late fetal thymus extra-thymic (liver ?)	liver, epidermis, intestinal mucosa	conserved Ag (HSP 65 ?)
Humans	Vγ9	Vδ2	+/ + + +	fetal/postnatal thymus extrathymic	fetal intestinal epithelium, blood	Daudi cells, mycobacterial Ag
	Vγl	Vδ1	+ + +	late fetal/postnatal thymus	adult intestinal epithelium, spleen	diverse (MHC class I, II, Ib, etc.)

identical to the DEC γ chain predominates in mucosal epithelia of uterus, vagina, and tongue (21). Finally in one study (23), cells expressing structurally homogeneous TCR comprising Vγ4 and Vδ4 regions have been derived from lactating mammary glands, but additional experiments are required to confirm the existence of this third subset in several mouse strains.

Type II Cells

These lymphocytes are thought to appear at later stages of ontogeny (4,24) and, unlike type I cells, can develop in extrathymic sites (8,25). Although they use a restricted set of Vγ and Vδ genes in a given location, their TCR chains exhibit significant V(D)J junctional diversity. Cells expressing, the Vγ4 gene together with a wide array of Vδ genes (always distinct from Vδ1) predominate in peripheral lymphoid organs such as spleen and lymph nodes (26,27), and might also be enriched in the lung, where they preferentially use the Vδ6 gene (28). Moreover, Vγ4-expressing cells are reproducibly detected in intestinal epithelium but always constitute a minor fraction of γδ TCR+ IEL in this site (usually below 10%) (7,29).

Lymphocytes using the Vγ7 gene are found almost exclusively in the epithelium of the gastrointestinal tract, where they represent the majority of γδ TCR$^+$ cells (5,6,30). They preferentially use the Vδ4 and Vδ6 genes (7,25,30–32), unlike the few Vγ7$^+$ thymocytes analysed thus far (26 and our own unpublished observations). Finally, the tissue distribution of Vγ1-expressing cells is quite diverse, and different Vδ genes seem preferentially used in distinct locations. For instance, Vγ1Vδ6 lymphocytes are found predominantly in liver (31), in the epidermis of several mouse strains (25,33), and, in some studies, have been described in the intestinal epithelium (25,31). Vγ1-expressing cells also represent a significant fraction of splenic γδ TCR$^+$ T cells (27), but unlike those derived from liver or epidermis, they seem to use a larger set of Vδ genes in general distinct from Vδ6 (31) (Table 1). While the majority of Vγ7$^+$ cells are thought to develop in extrathymic sites [perhaps in the gut epithelium itself (34)], Vγ1$^+$ and Vγ4$^+$ cells might comprise both thymus dependent and independent subsets (25,27).

Human γδ *TCR*$^+$ *T Cell Subsets*

No equivalent of type I lymphocytes has been described in humans. However, restricted TCR combinatorial diversity still remains the hallmark of γδ TCR$^+$ T cells in a given tissue. The most clearcut restriction of V gene use is seen in adult peripheral blood, where 60 to 95% of γδ T cells use Vγ9 and Vδ2 genes to form their TCR (35–37). A similar Vγ/Vδ set is used by most intestinal IEL during fetal life and early after birth (38,39). At later stages, Vγ9Vδ2 intestinal IEL are progressively replaced (or diluted out) by γδ TCR$^+$ cells expressing preferentially Vδ1 gene and Vγ genes distinct from Vγ9 (13) (Table 1).

ORIGIN OF TISSUE-DEPENDENT RESTRICTED V GENE USE BY γδ TCR$^+$ T CELLS

Antigen-Independent Restriction

In vitro thymus organ culture experiments suggest that type I and type II γδ TCR$^+$ cells are derived from distinct precursor cells. Indeed, although both fetal liver and adult bone marrow precursor cells could give rise to Vγ4-expressing cells *in vitro*, only the former could generate Vγ5-expressing cells (and probably type I cells in general) (40). Differentiation of fetal liver cells into Vγ5$^+$ lymphocytes could occur only in fetal (but not adult) thymic lobes (40), which is in full agreement with studies demonstrating a strict fetal thymus-dependency of DECs, which are absent in nude mice epidermis but are restored after grafting with fetal thymic lobes (41). In contrast, it seems clear that, unlike DECs, development of several type II cells is thymus-independent (8,15,25) and, in fact, might occur *in situ* (31,34). Taken together, these observations suggest that tissue-dependent repertoire restriction might be explained, at least in part, by targeted rearrangement and expression of specific

V genes in precursors with specific homing properties [e.g., in the case of type I cells that migrate from thymus to peripheral sites as suggested by the above results (41)] or whose development might occur locally [e.g., in the case of intestinal IEL (34) or liver cells (31)]. Transgenic studies indicate that tissue specificity of these sublineages cannot be dictated merely by the variable regions of the expressed TCR. For instance, in mice carrying transgenes encoding the TCR chains expressed by DEC (i.e., Vγ5Vδ1), cells bearing "wrong" (transgenic) TCR were found in gut epithelium (8). Therefore, one should postulate the existence of specific TCR-unrelated homing receptors, whose expression would be differently regulated in each γδ TCR sublineage.

Antigen-Dependent Restriction

Combinatorial or pairing constraints alone cannot explain the restricted repertoire of γδ TCR$^+$ T cells in a given peripheral tissue location since, apart from type I cells, different Vδ genes are preferentially used by lymphocytes expressing the same Vγ gene in distinct tissues (e.g., see skin versus spleen-derived Vγ1$^+$ cells in the mouse or thymus- versus peripheral blood-derived Vγ9$^+$ cells in humans, Table 1, and refs 31,32,42). It is therefore likely that the γδ TCR$^+$ T cell repertoire is profoundly shaped by TCR-dependent selection events occurring *in situ*. Evidence for such a local Ag-driven selection has come from human studies, which showed that proportions of Vγ9$^+$Vδ2$^+$ lymphocytes among γδ TCR$^+$ PBL gradually increased during the first years following birth, but remained stable and low in the thymus during the same time (43). Moreover, peripheral amplification of the Vγ9Vδ2 subset was accompanied by a parallel increase in the percent of cells expressing the so-called "memory" marker CD45R0 (43,44). Together, these observations strongly suggest that restricted TCR combinatorial diversity seen among human γδ TCR$^+$ PBL is a direct consequence of a postnatal amplification process, presumably driven by peripheral recurrent ligands.

REPERTOIRE SIZE AND ANTIGEN SPECIFICITY OF γδ TCR$^+$ T CELLS

Restricted V-Gene Use Probably Reflects Selection by a Small Set of Structurally Related Ligands

Apart from murine DECs and γδ TCR$^+$ cells from reproductive organ mucosa (9,21,22), TCR diversity of peripheral γδ TCR$^+$ T cell subsets is extensive. They are, however, mostly confined to the junctional regions of the TCR chains since, in general, cells in a given tissue express identical Vγ or Vγ/Vδ genes (Table 1). On the basis of current three-dimensional models of TCR/MHC/peptide interaction (1,45), it has recently been proposed that limited combinatorial but extensive junctional diversity of TCR expressed in peripheral sites would result from a local selection by structurally diverse antigens, presented in the context of the same restriction element (46,47). In fact, data drawn from αβ TCR⁺ T cell studies strongly suggest that diversity of the recognized antigens would not be as extensive as initially proposed and hence that the repertoire size of type II γδ TCR⁺ cells might be dramatically overestimated. Indeed, it is well known that αβ TCR directed against structurally unrelated peptides presented by the same restriction element differ not only in their junctional sequences [as predicted by Davis and Bjorkman's model (1)], but also almost systematically in their V region composition. This lack of correlation between TCR V-gene usage and the ability to recognize unrelated peptides in a specific MHC context is probably due to peptide-induced conformational modifications of the MHC regions thought to interact with V-specific residues (48,49). This would therefore explain why selection for a particular Vβ (50,51), Vα (52), or both Vβ/Vα (e.g., 53–56) region(s) was observed in most instances among T lymphocytes with specificity for the same or closely related MHC/peptide complexes.

For similar reasons, it is likely that restricted Vγ or Vγ/Vδ gene use by peripheral γδ TCR⁺ T cells, regardless of their TCR junctional diversity, results from a local selection by a highly restricted set of ligands, which would be either superantigens or closely related peptides presented in the context of the same restriction element. Since it has been shown that the extent of combinatorial and junctional diversity of αβ TCR with the same fine specificity could vary greatly from one case to another (perhaps due to different structural constraints depending on the positioning of the TCR relative to its ligand) (50–56), one could imagine that γδ TCR diversity might be variable from one tissue to another (e.g., between intestinal IEL and DEC), although in all cases the number of selecting antigens would remain low.

Antigen Specificity and Possible Functions

According to the above hypothesis, γδ TCR⁺ T cells belonging to a V-defined subset that is locally overrepresented must have been selected *in vivo* by a unique antigen or at most by closely related ligands. Moreover these ligands should be conserved and/or presented in a monomorphic context, since the same Vγ or Vγ/Vδ genes are used by cells in a peripheral site in most individuals of a given species. In support of this assumption, two major human and murine γδ TCR⁺ T cell subsets expressing TCR with similar V regions but diverse junctional sequences (namely, murine Vγ1Vδ6 and human Vγ9Vδ2 lymphocytes) were recently shown to recognize a very restricted set of philogenetically conserved antigens (33,57–62). In both cases, these ligands were recognized in a non-MHC restricted fashion (or in the context of a nonpolymorphic molecule) (57,59–62) and might be related to stress proteins (57,59,62), although this issue remains controversial (33,63). Regardless of their precise nature, the common feature of the above antigens, as well as those recognized by another important murine γδ TCR subset, the Vγ5Vδ1 DECs (64), is their expression on activated, transformed, or stressed cells. Moreover, the fact that proportions of lymphocytes reactive to these conserved antigens was much higher among Vγ9Vδ2 PBL (i.e., derived from a site where this subset predominates, presumably following local antigen-driven selection) than among Vγ9Vδ2 thymocytes (which are presumably enriched for "naive," nonselected cells) (our own unpublished observations) supports the physiological relevance of these antigens or closely related ones in the *in vivo* expansion of this subset.

Therefore, on the basis of these findings, I propose that, more generally, γδ TCR⁺ T cells showing restricted V-gene expression in a given location, and in particular most γδ TCR⁺ IEL, are selected *in vivo* by a specific set of highly conserved activation or differentiation molecules. Through recognition of such ligands, these cells would take part in the regulation of endogenous processes, such as cell transformation or immune response regulation, rather than playing a direct role as a first line of defense via recognition and elimination of exogenous pathogens. A similar hypothesis was previously proposed to account for the monospecificity of type I IEL (9,46), but in the present case, these functions would be extended to all γδ TCR⁺ T cells showing antigen-driven TCR combinatorial restriction, regardless of their TCR junctional diversity. This hypothesis would fit in particular with the fact that murine intestinal γδ TCR⁺ IEL, despite their peculiar location and TCR diversity, are not amplified but rather diluted out by αβ TCR⁺ IEL following exposure to a microbial environment (14). It would also be in agreement with the proposed involvement of murine γδ TCR⁺ IEL in the regulation of oral tolerance (65).

Nonetheless, it is important to mention that the present hypothesis does not necessarily rule out a possible recognition by γδ TCR of diverse antigens presented in a polymorphic context, as suggested by several reports (66–68). However, it is assumed that these reactivities are secondary, perhaps because they are redundant with respect to αβ TCR specificities. To illustrate this notion, analysis of antigen specificity of human Vγ9Vδ2 cells revealed that these lymphocytes were not only reactive to the conserved ligands mentioned above but also that they could recognize in a clonal fashion tetanus toxoid peptide in the context of a polymorphic HLA product (DRw52) in some pathological situations (66). In the present case, it seems clear that the latter specificity does not give any insight into the primary function of the Vγ9Vδ2 subset, since most Vγ9Vδ2 PBL of normal individuals were nonreactive to this peptide/MHC complex (66). Because of this observation, it is difficult to make a conclusion about the significance of the reactivities of isolated human and murine γδ TCR⁺ T cell clones to a variety of antigens, including allogeneic MHC molecules (67,68), peptide/MHC complexes (69), and even weakly polymorphic MHC class Ib molecules (70–72).

ACKNOWLEDGMENTS

I would like to thank Drs. H. Vié and F. Lang for helpful discussions.

REFERENCES

1. Davis MM, Bjorkman PJ. T-cell antigen receptor gene and T-cell recognition. *Nature* 1988; 334:395–402.

2. Raulet DH. The structure, function, and molecular genetics of the γ/δ T cell receptor. *Annu Rev Immunol* 1989;7:175–207.
3. Tonegawa S, Berns A, Bonneville M, Farr A. Diversity, development, ligands, and probable functions of γ/δ T cells. *Cold Spring Harbor Symp Quant Biol* 1989;LIV:31–44.
4. Itohara S, Nakanishi N, Kanagawa O, Kubo R, Tonegawa S. Monoclonal antibodies specific to native murine T-cell receptor γδ: analysis of gamma delta T cells during thymic ontogeny and in peripheral lymphoid organs. *Proc Natl Acad Sci USA* 1989;86:5094–5098.
5. Bonneville M, Janeway CA Jr, Ito K, Haser W, Ishida I, Nakanishi N, Tonegawa S. Intestinal intraepithelial lymphocytes are a distinct set of γδ T cells. *Nature* 1988;336:479–481.
6. Goodman T, Lefrançois L. Expression of the γ-δ T-cell receptor on intestinal CD8⁺ intraepithelial lymphocytes. *Nature* 1988;333:855–858.
7. Goodman T, Lefrançois K. Intraepithelial lymphocytes. Anatomical sites, not T cell receptor form, dictate phenotype and function. *J Exp Med* 1989;170:1569–1581.
8. Bonneville M, Itohara S, Krecko EG, et al. Transgenic mice demonstrate that epithelial homing of γ/δ T cells is determined by cell lineages independent of T cell receptor specificity. *J Exp Med* 1990;171:1015–1026.
9. Asarnow DM, Kuziel WA, Bonyhadi M, Tigelaar RE, Tucker PW, Allison JP. Limited diversity of γδ antigen receptor genes of Thy-1⁺ dendritic epidermal cells. *Cell* 1988;55:837–847.
10. Konig F, Stingl G, Yokoyama WM, et al. Identification of a T3-associated γδ T cell receptor on Thy-1⁺ dendritic epidermal cell lines. *Science* 1987;236:834–837.
11. Kuziel WA, Takashima A, Bonyhadi M, et al. Regulation of T-cell receptor γ-chain RNA expression in murine Thy-1⁺ dendritic epidermal cells. *Nature* 1987;328:263–266.
12. Groh V, Porcelli S, Fabbi M, et al. Human lymphocyte bearing T cell receptor γ/δ are phenotypically diverse and evenly distributed throughout the lymphoid system. *J Exp Med* 1989; 169:1277–1294.
13. Spencer J, Isaacson PG, Diss TC, MacDonald TT. Expression of disulfide-linked and non-disulfide-linked forms of the T cell receptor γ/δ heterodimer in human intestinal intraepithelial lymphocytes. *J Immunol* 1989;19:1335–1338.
14. Bandeira A, Mota-Santos T, Itohara S, et al. Localization of γ/δ T cells to the intestinal epithelium is independent of normal microbial colonization. *J Exp Sci Med* 1990;172:239–244.
15. Bandeira A, Ithohara S, Bonneville M. Extrathymic origin of intestinal intraepithelial lymphocytes bearing T-cell antigen receptor γ/δ. *Proc Natl Acad Sci USA* 1991;88:43–47.
16. Lefranc MP, Rabbitts TH. *Res Immunol* 1990;141:267–270.
17. Heilig JS, Tonegawa S. Diversity of murine gamma genes and expression in fetal and adult T lymphocytes. *Nature* 1986;322:836–840.
18. Elliott JF, Rock EP, Pattern PA, Davis MM, Chien YH. The adult T-cell receptor δ-chain is diverse and distinct from that of fetal thymocytes. *Nature* 1988;331:627–631.
19. Takihara Y, Tkaduk D, Michalopoulos E, et al. Sequences and organization of the diversity, joining, and constant region genes of the human T-cell δ-chain locus. *Proc Natl Acad Sci USA* 1988; 85:6097–6101.
20. Havran, WL, Allison JP. Developmentally ordered appearance of thymocytes expressing different T-cell antigen receptors. *Nature* 1988;335:443–445.
21. Itohara S, Farr AG, Lafaille JJ, et al. Homing of a γ/δ thymocyte subset with homogeneous T-cell receptors to mucosal epithelial. *Nature* 1990;343:754–757.
22. Lafaille JJ, Decloux A, Bonneville M, Takagaki Y, Tonegawa S. Junctional sequences of T cell receptor γ/δ genes: implications for γ/δ T cell lineages and for a novel intermediate of V-(1)-J joining. *Cell* 1989;59:857–870.
23. Reardon C, Lefrançois L, Farr A, Kubo R, O'Brien R, Born WJ. Expression of γ/δ T cell receptors on lymphocyte from the lactating mammary gland. *J Exp Med* 1990;172:1263–1266.
24. Bluestone JA, Cron RQ, Barrett TA, et al. Repertoire development and ligand specificity of murine TCR γ/δ cells. *Immunol Rev* 1991;120:5–33.
25. Ota Y, Kobata T, Seki M, et al. Extrathymic origin of V gamma 1/V delta 6 T cells in the skin. *Eur J Immunol* 1992;22:595–598.
26. Takagaki Y, Nakanishi N, Ishida I, Kanagawa O, Tonegawa S. T cell receptor-γ and -δ gene preferentially utilized by adult thymocytes for the surface expression. *J Immunol* 1989;142:2112–2121.
27. Bluestone JA, Cron RQ, Barrett TA, et al. Repertoire development and ligand specificity of murine TCR γ/δ cells. *Immunol Rev* 1991;120:5–33.

28. Augustin A, Kubo RT, Simm GK. Resident pulmonary lymphocytes expressing the γ/δ T-cell receptor. *Nature* 1989;340:239–241.
29. Correa I, Bix M, Liao NS, Ziljstra M, Jaenisch R, Raulet DH. Most γ/δ T cells develop normally in beta α-microglobulin-deficient mice. *Proc Natl Acad Sci USA* 1992;89:653–657.
30. Takagaki Y, Decloux A, Bonneville M, Tonegawa S. Diversity of γ/δ a T-cell receptors on murine intestinal intra-epithelial lymphocytes. *Nature* 1989;339:712–714.
31. Ohteki T, Abo T, Seki S, et al. Predominant appearance of γ/δ T lymphocytes in the liver of mice after birth. *Eur J Immunol* 1991;21:1733–1740.
32. Asarnow DM, Goodman T, Lefrançois L, Allison JP. Distinct antigen receptor repertoires of two classes of murine epithelium-associated T cells. *Nature* 1989;341:60–62.
33. Ezquerra A, Wilde DB, McConnell TJ, et al. Mouse autoreactive γ/δ T cells. II: Molecular characterization of the T cell receptor. *Eur J Immunol* 1992;22:491–498.
34. Rocha B, Vassalli P, Guy-Grand D. The extrathymic T-cell development pathway. *Immunol Today* 1992;13:449–454.
35. Triebel F, Faure F, Graziani M, Jitsukawa S, Lefranc MP, Hercend T. A unique V-J-C-rearranged gene encodes a γ protein expressed on the majority of CD3⁺ T cell receptor α/β-circulating lymphocytes. *J Exp Med* 1988;167:694–699.
36. Triebel F, Faure F, Mami-Chouaib F, et al. A novel human V δ gene expressed predominantly in the T_1 γ A fraction of γ/δ⁺ peripheral lymphocytes. *Eur J Immunol* 1988;18:2021–2027.
37. Borst J, Wicherink A, Van Dongen JJM, et al. Non-random expression of T cell receptor γ and δ variable gene segments in functional T lymphocyte clones from human peripheral blood. *Eur J Immunol* 1989;19:1599–1568.
38. Deusch K, Lüling F, Reich K, Classen M, Wagner H, Pfeffer K. A major fraction of human intraepithelial lymphocytes simultaneously expresses the γ/δ T cell receptor, the CD8 accessory molecule and preferentially uses the V δ/gene segment. *J Immunol* 1991;21:1053–1059.
39. McVay LD, Carding SR, Bottomly K, Hayday AC. Regulated expression and structure of T cell receptor γ/δ transcripts in human thymic ontogeny. *EMBO J* 1991;10:83–91.
40. Ikuta K, Kina T, McNeil I, et al. A development switch in thymic lymphocyte maturation potential occurs at the level of hematopoietic stem cell. *Cell* 1990;62:863–874.
41. Havran WL, Allison JP. Origin of Thy-1⁺ dendritic epidermal cells of adult mice from fetal thymic precursors. *Nature* 1990;344:68–70.
42. Casorati G, De Libero G, Lanzavecchia A, Migone N. Molecular analysis of human γ/δ⁺ clones from thymus and peripheral blood. *J Exp Med* 1989;170:1521–1535.
43. Parker CM, Groh V, Band H, et al. Evidence for extrathymic changes in the T cell receptor γ/δ repertoire. *J Exp Med* 1990;171:1597–1612.
44. Miyawaki T, Kasahara Y, Taga K, Yachie A, Taniguchi N. Differential expression of CD45RO (VCHL1) and its functional relevance in two subpopulations of circulating TCR-γ/δ⁺ lymphocytes. *J Exp Med* 1990;171:1833–1838.
45. Chothia C, Boswell DR, Lesk AM. The outline structure of the T-cell α/β receptor. *EMBO J* 1988;7:3745–3755.
46. Janeway CA Jr, Jones B, Hayday A. Specificity and function of T cells bearing γ/δ receptors. *Immunol Today* 1988;9:73–76.
47. Van Kaer L, Wu M, Ichikawa Y, et al. Recognition of MHC TL gene products by γ/δ T cells. *Immunol Rev* 1991;120:89–115.
48. Fremont DH, Matsumnura M, Stura EA, Peterson PA, Wilson IA. Crystal structures of two viral peptides in complex with murine MHC class I H-2Kb. *Science* 1992;257:919–927.
49. Marrack P, Kappler JJW. Atomic structure of a human MHC molecule presenting an influenza virus peptide. *Nature* 1992;360:367–369.
50. Marrack P, Kappler JJW. T cells can distinguish between allogeneic major histocompatibility complex products on different cell types. *Nature* 1988;332:840–843.
51. Boitel B, Ermonval M, Panina-Bordignon P, Mariuzza RA, Lanzavecchia A, Acuto O. Preferential V beta gene usage and lack of junctional sequence conservation among human T cell receptors specific for a tetanus toxin-derived peptide: evidence for a dominant role of a germ line-encoded V region in antigen/major histocompatibility complex recognition. *J Exp Med* 1992;175:765–777.
52. Natarajan K, Burstyn D, Zauderer M. Major histocompatibility complex determinants select T-cell receptor α chain variable region dominance in a peptide-specific response. *Proc Natl Acad Sci USA* 1992;89:8874–8879.

53. Hedrick SM, Engel I, McElligott DL, et al. Selection of amino acid sequences in the β chain of the T cell antigen receptor. *Science* 1988;239:1541–1544.
54. Acha Orbea H, Mitchell DJ, Timmermann L, et al. Limited heterogeneity of T cells receptors from lymphocytes mediating autoimmune encephalomyelitis allows specific immune intervention. *Cell* 1988;54:263–273.
55. Lai MZ, Jang YJ, Chen LK, Gefter ML. Restricted V-(D)-J junctional regions in the T cell response to λ-repressor: identification of residues critical for antigen recognition. *J Immunol* 1990;144:4851–4856.
56. Danska JS, Livingstone AM, Paragas V, Ishihara J, Fathman CG. The presumptive CDR3 regions of both T cell receptor α and β chains determine T cell specificity for myoglobin peptides. *J Exp Med* 1990;172:27–33.
57. O'Brien RL, Happ MP, Dallas A, Palmer E, Kubo R, Born WK. Stimulation of a major subset of lymphocytes expressing T cell receptor γ/δ by an antigen derived from Mycobacterium tuberculosis. *Cell* 1989;57:667–674.
58. Happ MP, Kubto RT, Palmer E, Born WK, O'Brien RL. Limited receptor repertoire in a mycobacteria-reactive subset of γ/δ T lymphocytes. *Nature* 1989;342:696–698.
59. Born W, Hall L, Dallas A, et al. Recognition of a peptide antigen by heat shock—reactive γ/δ T lymphocytes. *Science* 1990;249:67–69.
60. Kabelitz D, Bender A, Prospero T, Wesselborg S, Janssen O, Pechhold K. The primary response of human γ/δ⁺ T cells to *Mycobacterium tuberculosis* is restricted to V γ9-bearing cells. *J Exp Med* 1991;173:1331–1336.
61. De Libero G, Casorati G, Giachino C, et al. Selection by two powerful antigens may account for the presence of the major population of human peripheral γ/δ T cells. *J Exp Med* 1991;173:1311–1322.
62. Fisch P, Malkovsky M, Kovats S, et al. Recognition by human Vγ9/Vδ2 T cells of a Grotl homolog on David Burkitt's lymphoma cells. *Science* 1990;250:1269–1273.
63. Pfeffer K, Schoel B, Plesnila N, et al. A lectin-binding, protease-resistant mycobacterial ligand specifically activates Vγ9⁺ human γ/δ T cells. *J Immunol* 1992;148:575–583.
64. Havran WL, Chien YH, Allison JP. Recognition of self antigens by skin derived T cells with invariant γ/δ antigen receptors. *Science* 1991;252:1430–1432.
65. Fujihashi K, Taguchi T, Aicher WK, et al. Immunoregulatory functions for murine intraepithelial lymphocytes: γ/δ T cell receptor-positive (TCR⁺) T cells abrogate oral tolerance, while α/β TCR⁺ T cells provide B cell help. *J Exp Med* 1992;175:695–707.
66. Holoshitz J, Vila LM, Keroack BJ, McKinley DR, Bayne NK. Oval antigenic recognition by cloned human γ/δ T cells. *J Clin Invest* 1992;89:308–314.
67. Ciccone E, Viale O, Pende D, et al. Specificity of human T lymphocytes expressing a γ/δ T cell antigen receptor. Recognition of a polymorphic determinant of HLA class I molecules by a γ/δ clone. *Eur J Immunol* 1989;19:1267–1271.
68. Bluestone JA, Cron RQ, Cotterman M, Houlden BA, Matis LA. Structure and specificity of T cell receptor γ/δ on major histocompatibility complex antigen-specific CD3⁺, CD4⁻, CD8⁻ T lymphocytes. *J Exp Med* 1988;168:1899–1916.
69. Kozbor D, Trinchieri G, Monos DS, et al. Human TCR-γ⁺/δ⁺, CD8⁺ T lymphocytes recognize tetanus toxoid in an MHC-restricted fashion. *J Exp Med* 1989;169:1847–1851.
70. Matis LA, Cron R, Bluestone JA. Major histocompability complex-linked specificity of γ/δa receptor-bearing T lymphocytes. *Nature* 1987;330:262–264.
71. Ito K, Van Kaer L, Bonneville M, Hsu S, Murphy DB, Tonegawa S. Recognition of the product of a novel HC T1 region gene (27b) by a mouse γ/δ T cell receptor. *Cell* 1990;62:549–561.
72. Porcelli S, Brenner MB, Greenstein JL, Balk SP, Terhorst C, Bleicher PA. Recognition of cluster of differentiation antigens by human CD4-CD8-cytolytic T lymphocytes. *Nature* 1989;341:447–450.

Mucosal Immunology: Intraepithelial Lymphocytes,
edited by H. Kiyono and J. R. McGhee.
Raven Press, Ltd., New York © 1993.

6

Intraepithelial Lymphocyte Lineage and Function

The Interactions Between the Intestinal Epithelium and the Intraepithelial Lymphocyte

Kenneth Croitoru* and Peter B. Ernst†

**Intestinal Disease Research Unit, Department of Medicine, McMaster University,
Hamilton, Ontario, Canada and †Children's Health Research Center,
Department of Pediatrics, University of Texas Medical Branch, Galveston, TX.*

Intraepithelial lymphocytes (IEL) are a heterogeneous population of mononuclear cells that lie within the epithelial lining of the intestine. The intimate anatomical relationship between IEL and intestinal epithelial cells suggests that the function of one is affected by the other in a manner that would have important physiological as well as pathological significance. To understand these interactions, a more complete understanding of IEL biology is required. Recent work has focused on the nature of the intraepithelial T cell, its T cell receptor (TCR) repertoire and its relationship to the thymic-derived T cell lineage. The fact that most IEL contain intracytoplasmic granules has only just begun to attract attention and critical analysis, and the nature of the non-T cell IEL has almost been forgotten. In the search for the biological function of this intriguing population, these issues need to be re-examined. In this review, we re-examine studies on IEL lineage and function in the context of the bidirectional interactions that occur between immune and nonimmune cells.

INFLUENCE OF THE EPITHELIAL ENVIRONMENT ON IEL

Heterogeneity of the Nonepithelial Cell Population

Upon examination of the IEL, it has become evident that these cells are adapted to the epithelial environment in that they express identifiable phenotypes unique to this compartment. In addition to mast cell precursors (1,2), a significant proportion of IEL express T cell markers [reviewed in (3)]. Many IEL contain large, azurophilic, intracytoplasmic granules that are unusual for a T cell population. These granulated cells have been compared to the large granular lymphocytes found in the peripheral blood, which are thought to mediate natural killer (NK) activity. This led to the examination of IEL for NK cell markers and for their ability to mediate cytotoxic activity (4).

From the earliest studies, it had been suggested that IEL were related to T cells since a majority were shown to express a number of T cell markers, such as Thy-1 and CD8 (1,2). However, over half of the CD8$^+$ IEL in the mouse lacked expression of other pan-T cell markers such as Thy-1 and, in both man and mouse, CD5 (Lyt-1/Leu-1) (3). Moreover, the CD8$^+$ IEL could be divided into two distinct subsets, those expressing the CD8 $\alpha\beta$ heterodimer (Ly2/Ly3) and those with the CD8 $\alpha\alpha$ homodimer (Ly2/Ly2) (5–7). The latter subset is rarely found in other tissues and has become one of the hallmarks of the IEL compartment. This heterogeneity of the T cells in the IEL population is also evident in the expression of the T cell receptor, in that both α/β TCR and γ/δ TCR expressing cells are represented (8–10). It is now apparent that a significant proportion of IEL do not require the presence of a thymus for their differentiation: they generate their TCR repertoire extrathymically (11–15).

Finally, a host of *in vitro* functional activities have been described in the IEL. These include antiviral (16) and antitumor NK activity (4), CTL (17–19), CTL precursors (20), regulatory T cell activities involving cytokine production (21,22), and contrasuppressor activity (23).

These observations suggest that the epithelial microenvironment serves to induce and support the development of a widely divergent population of leukocytes. The cellular and molecular bases for this heterogeneity are largely unknown. The possibilities are that the enterocyte contributes to the positive or negative selection of these cells by facilitating the specific traffic of these cells to this location or by modulating the differentiation of precursor cells that arrive at an immature stage of development.

Homing and Traffic

The gut-associated lymphoid tissue (GALT) is part of a larger subset of the immune system referred to as the mucosa-associated lymphoid tissue (MALT). The characteristics of the MALT are the presence of IgA as the predominant antibody and the ability of these mucosal lymphocytes to emigrate, recirculate, and traffic selectively back to mucosal surfaces (24). In fact, T lymphoblasts isolated from Peyer's patch (PP) or mesenteric lymph node reach the thoracic duct lymphatics and reappear in the mucosa, including the epithelium, after adoptive transfer (25,26). This suggests that to some extent the IEL are derived from recirculating T cells perhaps originating in the PP (26). The mechanisms that lead these cells selectively to home to this site are being explored. Recently defined integrin-like molecules have been found on IEL. These include HML-1 in humans and a more recently defined analogous molecule in the mouse (27–29). The thymic-independent IEL, however, have not been shown to recirculate in this manner (30,31).

IEL also express cell surface molecules such as CD2 that can interact with ligands, e.g., LFA-3 present on the intestinal epithelium (32,33). These interactions may be important in the local expansion of IEL given that CD2 activation can lead to a proliferative response in a population normally found to be relatively unresponsive to mitogenic stimuli (32). Needless to say, other such activation molecules will be defined on IEL that may help explain the specific expansion that occurs. Defining the role of these molecules and other adhesion molecules will help our understanding of how IEL home to the gut epithelium.

The observation that the γ/δ TCR is expressed on lymphocytes found in different epithelial surfaces, including the intestinal IEL, suggested that the γ/δ TCR may be responsible for the specific homing of IEL to the epithelium. However, evidence suggests that the CD8[+] IEL can localize to the intestinal epithelium, independently of the expression of TCR (34,35). It may be that this subset arises from the differentiation of precursors already within the intestine. In fact, ligands for the γ/δ TCR include MHC class Ib molecules such as TL antigens (36–38) and CD1 (39). These molecules have been identified on intestinal epithelial cells and may represent a signaling mechanism that results in the positive selection of the unique IEL phenotype (39). Recent studies have shown that γ/δ TCR-[+] T cell hybridomas from IEL appear to have self-reactivity that is not due to heat-shock protein reactivity (40). It must be remembered, however, that evidence from our studies in the SCID mouse and from studies in mice bearing transgenic γ/δ TCR molecules suggest the TCR is not required for the accumulation of granulated, CD8[+] cells in the intestinal epithelium (34,35). At this time we are unable to identify the molecular signals that lead to the local expansion of IEL in the gut.

The striking observation that cells with the morphology, TCR gene usage, or surface antigen phenotype typical of IEL are not found in the adjacent lamina propria or draining lymph suggests that mature IEL do not migrate from the epithelial niche. Several studies of coccidia-infected chickens have shown IEL migrating from the villous epithelium to the adjacent lamina propria (41,42). Electron microscopy shows not only that these cells contain the typical granules of IEL but also that they contain numerous sporozoites, suggesting further that the IEL play a role in the immunity to coccidia. On the other hand, more recent studies of parabiotic mice suggest that PBL do not migrate to the IEL and do not represent a pathway for recirculation of IEL (30). Therefore the fate of IEL as well as their recirculation ability remains controversial.

The Intestinal Epithelial Microenvironment
as an Extrathymic Source of T Cells

The finding that nude rodents have T cells within the IEL but not in the periphery suggests that some IEL may not require thymic processing, i.e., are not classic T cells (6,43,44). In fact, as far back as the late 1960s Fichtelius (45) showed that IEL were present in neonatally thymectomized mice. This has been supported by similar observations in the nude rat and mouse and in experiments in which IEL were reconstituted in thymectomized recipients from T cell depleted bone marrow (13).

Some of the most compelling evidence for thymic independence is the presence of both α/β and γ/δ TCR bearing IEL in animals lacking a thymus (11,14,30, 46,47). In addition, IEL display an atypical TCR repertoire. For example, IEL are one of the few cell populations to use the Vγ7 TCR gene (9). Moreover, IEL can express "forbidden clones," T cells that display a repertoire deleted in the thymus but that exist in the epithelium. This, combined with the observation that RAG1 is expressed in IEL (48), suggests that TCR rearrangement and repertoire selection can occur within the gut under the control of local environmental influences. Although there is no direct evidence that IEL precursors develop within the intestinal epithelium itself, there is substantial evidence that the gut can sponsor the development of extrathymic T cells and affect both positive and negative selection (11,30, 31,47).

In an attempt to define the nature of the thymic-independent IEL, the characteristics of different IEL subsets have been examined more closely. In general terms, the granulated IEL that bear CD3/TCR complex and lack pan-T cell markers such as Thy-1 appear to be thymic independent (6,49). In this regard, Thy-1 is readily inducible on IEL by gut flora and therefore is an unreliable marker of lineage (49,50). Thymic-independent IEL, on the other hand, are characterized by CD8 α/α homodimer, which correlates with the expression of most γ/δ TCR and with those α/β TCR that have escaped thymic deletion (5,6,14). A second major subset of IEL that have been demonstrated in nude mice also lack CD5 expression (2,7). Our studies have shown that most γ/δ TCR IEL and those α/β TCR IEL that escape thymic deletion also lack CD5 (50a).

CD5 is expressed predominantly on T cells and B cells of the "B1" lineage (51). These B cells are interesting in that they represent a lineage distinct from conventional "B2" B cells. Similar to CD5[+] and CD5[-] IEL, the repertoire of B cells which are separable by this marker also differs (52). The function of CD5 is less clear. It has the potential to act in T cell/B cell interactions given that one of its ligands is the B cell marker CD72/Ly2-b (53,54). Since B cells are present in the thymus, this may suggest a mechanism by which B cells have the potential to modulate T cell differentiation (55). The absence of B cells in IEL suggests that intraepithelial T cell/B cell interactions must occur through other mechanisms perhaps involving cytokine secretion (23). The lack of expression of CD5 on thymus-independent IEL T cells not only may be a useful marker that distinguishes the two lineages of IEL but also may help explain some of the unique features of the thymic-independent IEL.

Functional studies suggest that the thymic-independent subset of IEL show a poor proliferative response to TCR activation that can be reversed with exogenous IL-2. This anergic response is not due to the lack of CD5 since the CD5[-] IEL will respond to anti-CD3 stimulation, yet the γ/δ TCR IEL do not (50a). This suggests that the state of anergy seen in the CD5$^-$ thymic-independent IEL may reflect a mechanism that serves to protect the intestine from nondeleted self-reactive T cells (30,46,47). Thus, the self-reactive γ/δ TCR$^+$ IEL recognizing an epithelial ligand and the α/β TCR$^+$ IEl recognizing an endogenous superantigen do not cause intestinal epithelial cell damage in the normal adult mouse. The mechanisms that allow for the intestinal environment to influence the development and selection of this heterogenous population are still not well understood.

The Enterocyte as an Immunological Effector Cell

The recognition that intraepithelial T cells may differentiate *in situ* has led to increased interest in the role of the enterocyte in T cell activation or education. The intestinal environment may play a role in the positive (11,39,47) and negative (14,30) selection of the IEL repertoire. The epithelial cells express MHC class I related antigens such as TL (56,57) and CD1 (58) and MHC class II antigens (59). The molecules may play a pivotal role in the selection of the oligoclonal repertoire seen in human IEL (9,39). It has been proposed that the enterocyte is involved in "antigen presentation" because of their expression of MHC class II antigens (60, 61). Paradoxically, these MHC class II epithelial cells were shown to stimulate CD8$^+$ cells (62,63), which is in keeping with the predominance of CD8$^+$ T cells in the epithelium. Heat-shock proteins have also been shown to act as ligands for γ/δ TCR$^+$ T cells and have been shown to be expressed in the intestinal epithelium (64,64a).

Following the paradigm of lymphocyte/epithelial cell interactions for local IEL differentiation, it is reasonable to consider the possibility that enterocytes may influence IEL development through secretion of soluble factors. Epithelial cells from various tissues have been shown to produce a range of cytokines and growth factors including GM-CSF, IL-6, and IL-8 (65,66). During healing, the epithelium becomes a source for EGF (67), and epithelial cell lines from the gastrointestinal tract have been reported to produce IL-6 (68), IL-8 (Crowe et al., submitted for publication), and possibly TGF-β (69). The influence of these cytokines on IEL differentiation needs to be examined more rigorously.

THE INFLUENCE OF IEL ON THE EPITHELIUM

Cytokine Production by IEL

One of the interesting aspects of IEL function is their ability to produce a wide spectrum of cytokines. This is discussed in more detail elsewhere in this book; however, cytokines are instrumental as mediators of intercellular interactions and merit some discussion here. Reports have suggested that murine IEL can produce IL-2 (70,71) IL-3 (70), IL-5 (22,23), IL-6 (21,22), TNF-α, TGF-β (21), GM-CSF (70), and interferon-γ (21). The IEL T cell has been implicated as the source of many of these cytokines as lectins (70), or antibodies directed toward the T cell receptor (21) can induce their release. Moreover, recent reports of IEL sorted into T cell subsets further support cytokine production by the intraepithelial T cell (21,23). Mast cells have also been shown to produce a number of cytokines (72), and given that IEL contain many mast cell precursors (1,2) one can suggest that mast cell activation may contribute to the local production of cytokines in this environment. It is noteworthy that there are no reports demonstrating cytokine production *in situ*, leaving open the question of whether the different isolation procedures may activate IEL to increase cytokine production.

Influence on Epithelial Cell Proliferation

In view of the ability of IEL to produce cytokines, one can speculate that they can modulate a variety of epithelial functions. Anti-CD3 and PWM-stimulated fetal intestinal explants in humans, in fact, lead to changes in the epithelial cell and crypt cell proliferation (73,74). It is argued in these experiments that the lamina propria cells are responsible for these changes, since activated T cells, as indicated by the presence of IL-2 receptor expression, are seen only in the lamina propria. Nonetheless, it remains possible that the IEL contribute to these changes in the epithelium under conditions in which IEL are activated, such as gluten sensitive enteropathy. Several investigators have also observed that cytokines such as TNF can modulate the proliferation of epithelial cell lines, providing a mechanism for these T cell/ epithelial cell interactions (74a).

Influence on Epithelial Cell Phenotype/Morphology

In addition to modulating proliferation, cytokines from IEL may also modify the gene expression and function of enterocytes. During intestinal inflammation the epithelium often responds with an increase in expression of MHC class II molecules and secretory component. In addition, one can see goblet cell depletion, which can be reproduced in explants in which T cells have been activated (75). These changes could contribute to the host response to luminal antigen.

Cytokines released from IEL and other mucosal T cells may have the potential for influencing these changes in epithelial cells. TNF-α can increase secretory component expression by enterocytes (76), as can IL-4 and interferon-γ (77,78). Interferon-γ has also been shown to alter the barrier function of epithelium, increasing permeability via altering tight junction integrity (79); to increase class II antigen expression by the intestinal epithelium (59); and to alter epithelial ion secretion (80). In addition, IL-1 and IL-3 can stimulate epithelial ion transport (81). Thus, these and other cytokines are probably part of the "immunophysiological axis" and provide the molecular mechanism that accounts for part of the changes in epithelial cell function seen in diseases thought to be due to stimulation of local T cell responses.

It should be highlighted that IEL produce other cytotoxic proteins, including neutral proteases and granule-associated serine proteases such as granzyme and perforin (6), which can be released in response to activation. The ability of these proteases to affect epithelium suggests a mechanism by which IEL deal with damaged or infected epithelial cells.

SUMMARY

IEL have attracted the attention of scientists due to their unusual properties and distinct lineages, yet their biological functions remain unknown. The proximity of IEL to the epithelium implies that interactions between these two cells have important consequences on the physiological homeostasis of the intestine. Unfortunately, the function of IEL in this and other interactions is almost entirely speculative. This, in part, is due to the lack of a model in which IEL are deficient, so that the impact of their absence could be assessed. This alone may suggest that these cells may be critical to host survival. New and very creative technologies will have to evolve to ascertain the role of IEL in intestinal immune and physiological processes.

ACKNOWLEDGMENTS

The work described has been funded by the Medical Research Council of Canada and the Canadian Foundation for Ileitis and Colitis. Kenneth Croitoru is the holder of an Ontario Ministry of Health Career Scientist Award.

REFERENCES

1. Schrader JW, Scollay R, Battye F. Intramucosal lymphocytes of the gut: Lyt2 and Thy1 phenotype of the granulated cells and evidence for the presence of both T cells and mast cell precursors. *J Immunol* 1983;130:558–564.
2. Petit A, Ernst PB, Befus AD, Clark DA, Rosenthal KL, Ishizaka T, Bienenstock J. Murine intestinal intraepithelial lymphocytes. I: Relationship of a novel Thy1-, Lyt1-, Lyt2$^+$, granulated subpopulation to natural killer cells and mast cells. *Eur J Immunol* 1985;15:211–215.
3. Ernst PB, Befus AD, Bienenstock J. Leukocytes in the intestinal epithelium: an unusual immunological compartment. *Immunol Today* 1985;6:50–55.
4. Tagliabue A, Befus AD, Clark DA, Bienenstock J. Characteristics of natural killer cells in the murine intestinal epithelium and lamina propria. *J Exp Med* 1982;155:1785–1796.
5. Parrott DMV, Tait C, Mackenzie S, Mowat AM, Davies MDJ, Micklem HS. Analysis of the effector functions of different populations of mucosal lymphocytes. *Ann NY Acad Sci* 1983;409:307–319.
6. Guy-Grand D, Cerf-Bensussan N, Malissen B, Malassis-Seris M, Briottet C, Vassalli P. Two gut intraepithelial CD8$^+$ lymphocyte populations with different T cell receptors: a role for the gut epithelium in T cell differentiation. *J Exp Med* 1991;173:471–481.
7. Lefrançois L. Phenotypic complexity of intraepithelial lymphocytes of the small intestine. *J Immunol* 1991;147:1746–1751.
8. Goodman T, Lefrançois L. Expression of the γ/δ T-cell receptor on intestinal CD8$^+$ intraepithelial lymphocytes. *Nature* 1988;333:855–858.
9. Bonneville M, Janeway CA, Ito K, Haser W, Ishida I, Nakanishi N, Tonegawa S. Intestinal intraepithelial lymphocytes are a distinct set of γ/δ T cells. *Nature* 1988;336:479–481.
10. Viney JL, Kilshaw PJ, MacDonald TT. Cytotoxic α/β$^+$ and γ/δ$^+$ T cells in murine intestinal epithelium. *Eur J Immunol* 1990;20:1623–1626.
11. Lefrançois L, LeCorre R, Mayo J, Bluestone JA, Goodman T. Extrathymic selection of TCR γ/δ$^+$ T cells by class II major histocompatability complex molecules. *Cell* 1990;63:333–340.
12. Viney JL, MacDonald TT, Kilshaw PJ. T-cell receptor expression in intestinal intra-epithelial lymphocyte subpopulations of normal and athymic mice. *Immunology* 1989;66:583–587.

13. Mosley RL, Styre D, Klein JR. Differentiation and functional maturation of bone marrow-derived intestinal epithelial T cells expressing membrane TCR in athymic radiation chimeras. *J Immunol* 1990;145:1369–1375.

14. Rocha B, Vassalli P, Guy-Grand D. The Vβ repertoire of mouse gut homodimeric α CD8[+] intra-epithelial T cell receptor α/β[+] lymphocytes reveals a major extrathymic pathway of T cell differentiation. *J Exp Med* 1991;173:483–486.

15. Rocha B, Vassalli P, Guy-Grand D. The extrathymic T-cell development pathway. *Immunol Today* 1992;13:449–454.

16. Carman PS, Ernst PB, Rosenthal KL, Clark DA, Befus DA, Bienenstock J. Intraepithelial leukocytes contain a unique subpopulation of NK-like cytotoxic cells active in the defense of gut epithelium to enteric murine coronavirus. *J Immunol* 1986;136:1548–1553.

17. Davies MDJ, Parrott DMV. Cytotoxic T cells in small intestine epithelial, lamina propria and lung lymphocytes. *Immunology* 1981;44:367–371.

18. Klein JR, Kagnoff MF. Non-specific recruitment of cytotoxic effector cells in the intestinal mucosa of antigen-primed mice. *J Exp Med* 1984;160:1931–1939.

19. London SD, Cebra JJ, Rubin DH. Intraepithelial lymphocytes contain virus-specific, MHC-restricted cytotoxic precursors after gut mucosal immunization with reovirus serotype 1/Lang. *Regional Immunol* 1989;2:98–102.

20. Ernst PB, Clark DA, Rosenthal KL, Befus AD, Bienenstock J. Detection and characterization of cytotoxic T lymphocyte precursors in the murine intestinal intraepithelial leukocyte population. *J Immunol* 1986;136:2121–2126.

21. Barrett TA, Gajewski TF, Danielpour D, Chang EB, Beagley KW, Bluestone JA. Differential function of intestinal intraepithelial lymphocyte subsets. *J Immunol* 1992;149:1124–1130.

22. Taguchi T, Aicher WK, Fujihashi K, Yamamoto M, McGhee JR, Bluestone JA, Kiyono H. Novel function for intestinal intraepithelial lymphocytes: murine CD3[+], γ/δ TCR[+] T cells produce IFN-gamma and IL-5. *J Immunol* 1991;147:3736–3744.

23. Fujihashi K, Taguchi T, Aicher WK, McGhee JR, Bluestone JA, Eldridge JH, Kiyono H. Immunoregulatory functions for murine intraepithelial lymphocytes: γ/δ T cell receptor-positive (TCR[+]) T cells abrogate oral tolerance, while α/β TCR[+] T cells provide B cell help. *J Exp Med* 1992;175:695–707.

24. Bienenstock J, McDermott M, Befus D. A common mucosal immune system. In: *Immunology of breast milk*. P.L. Ogra and D. Dayton eds. New York: Raven Press; 1979:91–104.

25. McDermott MR, Horley BA, Warner AA, Bienenstock J. Mesenteric lymphoblast localization throughout the murine small intestine: temporal analysis relating intestinal length and lymphoblast division. *Cell Tissue Kinet* 1985;18:505–519.

26. Guy-Grand D, Griscelli C, Vassalli P. The mouse T lymphocyte, a novel type of T cell: nature, origin, and traffic in mice in normal and graft-versus-host conditions. *J Exp Med* 1978;148:1661–1677.

27. Cerf-Bensussan N, Jarry A, Brousse N, Lisowska-Grospierre B, Guy-Grand D, Griscelli C. A monoclonal antibody (HML-1) defining a novel membrane molecule present on human intestinal lymphocytes. *Eur J Immunol* 1987;17:1279–1285.

28. Parker CM, Cepek KL, Russell GJ, Shaw SK, Posnett DN, Schwarting R, Brenner MB. A family of β7 integrins on human intestinal lymphocytes. *Proc Natl Acad Sci USA* 1992;89:1924–1928.

29. Kilshaw PJ, Murant SJ. Expression and regulation of β7(βp) integrins on mouse lymphocytes: relevance to the mucosal immune system. *Eur J Immunol* 1991;21:2591–2597.

30. Poussier P, Edouard P, Lee C, Binnie M, Julius M. Thymus-independent development and negative selection of T cells expressing T cell receptor α/β in the intestinal epithelium: evidence for distinct circulation patterns of gut- and thymus-derived T lymphocytes. *J Exp Med* 1992;176:187–199.

31. Mosley RL, Klein JR. Peripheral engraftment of fetal intestine into athymic mice sponsors T cell development: direct evidence for thymopoietic function of murine small intestine. *J Exp Med* 1992;176:1365–1373.

32. Ebert EC. Proliferative responses of human intraepithelial lymphocytes to various T-cell stimuli. *Gastroenterology* 1989;97:1372–1381.

33. Trejdosiewicz LK. Intestinal intraepithelial lymphocytes and lymphoepithelial interactions in the human gastrointestinal mucosa. *Immunol Lett* 1992;32:13–20.

34. Bonneville M, Itohara S, Krecko EG, et al. Transgenic mice demonstrate that epithelial homing of gamma/delta T cells is determined by cell lineages independent of T cell receptor specificity. *J Exp Med* 1990;171:1015–1026.

35. Croitoru K, Stead RH, Bienenstock J, et al. Presence of intestinal intraepithelial lymphocytes in mice with severe combined immunodeficiency disease. *Eur J Immunol* 1990;20:645–651.

36. Janeway CA, Jones B, Hayday A. Specificity and function of T cells bearing gamma/delta receptors. *Immunol Today* 1988;9:73–76.
37. Bluestone JA, Matis LA. TCR gamma/delta: minor redundant T cell subset or specialized immune system component. *J Immunol* 1989;142:1785–1788.
38. Tonegawa S, Berns A, Bonneville M, et al. Diversity, development, ligands, and probable functions of γ/δ T cells. *Adv Exp Med Biol* 1991;292:53–61.
39. Balk SP, Ebert EC, Blumenthal RL, McDermott FV, Wucherpfennig KW, Landau SB, Blumberg RS. Oligoclonal expansion and CD1 recognition by human intestinal intraepithelial lymphocytes. *Science* 1991;253:1411–1415.
40. Nagler-Anderson C, McNair LA, Cradock A. Self-reactive, T cell receptor-γ/δ$^+$, lymphocytes from the intestinal epithelium of weanling mice. *J Immunol* 1992;149:2315–2322.
41. Lawn AM, Rose ME. Mucosal transport of *Eimeria tenella* in the cecum of the chicken. *J Parasitol* 1982;68:1117–1123.
42. Fernando MA, Lawn AM, Rose ME, Al-Attar MA. Invasion of chicken caecal and intestinal lamina propria by crypt epithelial cells infected with coccidia. *Parasitology* 1983;86:391–398.
43. de Geus B, Van den Enden M, Coolen C, Nagelkerken L, Van der Heijden P, Rozing J. Phenotype of intraepithelial lymphocytes in euthymic and athymic mice: implications for differentiation of cells bearing a CD3-associated gamma δ T cell receptor. *Eur J Immunol* 1990;20:291–298.
44. Bandeira A, Itohara S, Bonneville M, Burlen-Defranoux O, Mota-Santos T, Coutinho A, Tonegawa S. Extrathymic origin of intestinal intraepithelial lymphocytes bearing T-cell antigen receptor gamma δ. *Proc Natl Acad Sci USA* 1991;88:43–47.
45. Fichtelius KE, Yunis EJ, Good RA. Occurrence of lymphocytes within the gut epithelium of normal and neonatally thymectomized mice. *Proc Soc Exp Biol Med* 1968;128:185–188.
46. Barrett TA, Delvy ML, Kennedy DM, et al. Mechanisms of self-tolerance of γ/δ T cells in epithelial tissue. *J Exp Med* 1992;175:65–70.
47. Rocha B, von Boehmer H, Guy-Grand D. Selection of intraepithelial lymphocytes with CD8 α/α co-receptors by self-antigen in the murine gut. *Proc Natl Acad Sci USA* 1992;89:5336–5340.
48. Guy-Grand D, Vanden Broecke C, Briottet C, Malassis-Seris M, Selz F, Vassalli P. Different expression of the recombination activity gene RAG-1 in various populations of thymocytes, peripheral T cells and gut thymus-independent intraepithelial lymphocytes suggests two pathways of T cell receptor rearrangement. *Eur J Immunol* 1992;22:505–510.
49. Lefrançois L, Goodman T. *In vivo* modulation of cytolytic activity and Thy-1 expression in TCR-gamma/delta intraepithelial lymphocytes. *Science* 1989;243:1716–1718.
50. Bandeira A, Mota-Santos T, Itohara S, Degermann S, Heusser C, Tonegawa S, Coutinho A. Localization of gamma/delta T cells to the intestinal epithelium is independent of normal microbial colonization. *J Exp Med* 1990;172:239–244.
50a. Croitoru K, Bienenstock J, Ernst PB. Intestinal intraepithelial T lymphocytes that express self-reactive α/β T cell receptor lack CD5 expression and are functionally anergic. Submitted for publication.
51. Hayakawa K, Hardy RR, Parks DR, Herzenberg LA. The Ly-1 B cell subpopulation in normal, immunodeficient and autoimmune mice. *J Exp Med* 1983;157:202.
52. Lalor PA, Morahan G. The peritoneal Ly-1 (CD5) B cell repertoire is unique among murine B cell repertoires. *Eur J Immunol* 1990;20:485–492.
53. Van de Velde H, von Hoegen I, Luo W, Parnes JR, Thielemans K. The B-cell surface protein CD72/Lyb-2 is the ligand for CD5. *Nature* 1991;351:662–664.
54. Luo W, Van de Velde H, von Hoegen I, Parnes JR, Thielemans K. Ly-1 (CD5), a membrane glycoprotein of mouse T lymphocytes and a subset of B cells, is a natural ligand of the B cell surface protein Lyb-2 (CD72). *J Immunol* 1992;148:1630–1634.
55. Miyama-Inaba M, Kuma SI, Inaba K, et al. Unusual phenotype of B cells in the thymus of normal mice. *J Exp Med* 1988;168:811.
56. Wu M, Van Kaer L, Itohara S, Tonegawa S. Highly restricted expression of the thymus leukemia antigens on intestinal epithelial cells. *J Exp Med* 1991;174:213–218.
57. Hershberg R, Eghtesady P, Sydora B, Brorson K, Cheroutre H, Modlin R, Kronenberg M. Expression of the thymus leukemia antigen in mouse intestinal epithelium. *Proc Natl Acad Sci USA* 1990;87:9727–9731.
58. Bleicher PA, Balk SP, Hagen SJ, Blumberg RS, Flotte TJ, Terhorst C. Expression of murine CD1 on gastrointestinal epithelium. *Nature* 1990;250:679–682.
59. Cerf-Bensussan N, Quaroni A, Kurnick JT, Bhan AK. Intraepithelial lymphocytes modulate Ia expression by intestinal epithelial cells. *J Immunol* 1984;132:224–225.

60. Bland PW, Warren LG. Antigen presentation by epithelial cells of the rat small intestine. I: Kinetics, antigen specificity and blocking by anti-Ia antisera. *Immunology* 1986;58:1–7.
61. Mayer L, Shlien R. Evidence for function of Ia molecules on gut epithelial cells in man. *J Exp Med* 1987;166:1471–1483.
62. Bland PW, Warren LG. Antigen presentation by epithelial cells of the rat small intestine. II: Selective induction of suppressor T cells. *Immunology* 1986;58:9–14.
63. Mayer L, Eisenhardt D. Lack of induction of suppressor T cells by intestinal epithelial cells from patients with inflammatory bowel disease. *J Clin Invest* 1990;86:1255–1260.
64. Engstrand L, Scheynius A, Påhlson C. An increased number of gamma/δ T-cells and gastric epithelial cell expression of the groEL stress-protein homologue in *Helicobacter pylori*-associated chronic gastritis of the antrum. *Am J Gastroenterol* 1991;86:976–980.
64a. Baca-Estrada ME, Gupta RS, Stead RH, Croitoru K. Intestinal expression and cellular immune responses to human heat-shock protein 60 in Crohn's disease. *Dig Dis Sci* (in press).
65. Standiford TJ, Kunkel SL, Basha MA, et al. Interleukin-8 gene expression by a pulmonary epithelial cell line: a model for cytokine networks in the lung. *J Clin Invest* 1990;86:1945–1953.
66. Ohtoshi T, Vancheri C, Cox G, Gauldie J, Dolovich J, Denburg JA, Jordana M. Monocyte-macrophage differentiation induced by human upper airway epithelial cells. *Am J Respir Cell Mol Biol* 1991;4:255–263.
67. Wright NA, Pike C, Elia G. Induction of a novel epidermal growth factor-secreting cell lineage by mucosal ulceration in human gastrointestinal stem cells. *Nature* 1990;343:82–85.
68. Shirota K, LeDuy L, Yuan S, Jothy S. Interleukin-6 and its receptor are expressed in human intestinal epithelial cells. *Virchows Arch [B]* 1990;58:303–308.
69. Wu, S, Theodorescu D, Kerbel RS, Wilson JKv, Mulder KM, Humphrey LE, Brattain MG. TGF-β1 is an autocrine-negative growth regulator of human colon carcinoma FET cells *in vivo* as revealed by transfection of an antisense expression vector. *J Cell Biol* 1992;116:187–196.
70. Dillon SB, Dalton BJ, MacDonald TT. Lymphokine production by mitogen and antigen activated mouse intraepithelial lymphocytes. *Cell Immunol* 1986;103:326–338.
71. Nagi AM, Babiuk LA. Interleukin-2 production by mitogen-stimulated intestinal mucosal leukocytes from cattle. *Am J Vet Res* 1989;50:1591–1597.
72. Gordon JR, Burd PR, Galli SJ. Mast cells as a source of multifunctional cytokines. *Immunol Today* 1990;11:458–464.
73. MacDonald TT, Spencer J. Evidence that activated mucosal T cells play a role in the pathogenesis of enteropathy in human small intestine. *J Exp Med* 1988;167:1341–1349.
74. Ferreira RDC, Forsyth LE, Richman PI, Wells C, Spencer J, MacDonald TT. Changes in the rate of crypt epithelial cell proliferation and mucosal morphology induced by a T-cell-mediated response in human small intestine. *Gastroenterology* 1990;98:1255–1263.
74a. Shanahan F, Targan SR. Mechanisms of tissue injury in inflammatory bowel disease. In: *Inflammatory bowel disease*. MacDermott RP, Stenson WF eds. New York: Elsevier Science Publishers BV 1992:77–93.
75. Evans CM, Phillips AD, Walker-Smith JA, MacDonald TT. Activation of lamina propria T cells induces crypt epithelial proliferation and goblet cell depletion in cultured human fetal colon. *Gut* 1992;33:230–235.
76. Kvale D, Lovhaug D, Sollid LM, Brandtzaeg P. Tumour necrosis factor-alpha up-regulates expression of secretory component, the epithelial receptor for polymeric Ig. *J Immunol* 1988;140:3086–3089.
77. Phillips JO, Everson MP, Moldoveanu Z, Lue C, Mestecky J. Synergistic effect of IL-4 and IFN-gamma on the expression of polymeric Ig receptor (secretory component) and IgA binding by human epithelial cells. *J Immunol* 1990;145:1740–1744.
78. Sollid LM, Kvale D, Brondtzaeg P, Markussen G, Thorsby E. Interferon-gamma enhances expression of secretory component, the epithelial receptor for polymeric immunoglobulins. *J Immunol* 1987;138:4303–4306.
79. Madara JL, Stafford J. Interferon-gamma directly affects barrier function of cultured intestinal epithelial monolayers. *J Clin Invest* 1989;83:724–727.
80. Holmgren J, Fryklund J, Larsson H. Gamma-interferon-mediated down-regulation of electrolyte secretion by intestinal epithelial cells: a local immune mechanism? *Scand J Immunol* 1989;30:499–503.
81. Chang EB, Musch MW, Mayer L. Interleukins 1 and 3 stimulate anion secretion in chicken intestine. *Gastroenterology* 1990;98:1518–1524.

Mucosal Immunology: Intraepithelial Lymphocytes,
edited by H. Kiyono and J. R. McGhee.
Raven Press, Ltd., New York © 1993.

7

Intraepithelial Lymphocytes

Immunoregulatory Function and Cytokine Production by $\alpha\beta$ TCR$^+$ and $\gamma\delta$ TCR$^+$ T cells for Mucosal Immune Responses

Kohtaro Fujihashi, Masafumi Yamamoto, Jerry R. McGhee, and Hiroshi Kiyono

Departments of Oral Biology and Microbiology, The Mucosal Immunization Research Group, Immunobiology Vaccine Center, University of Alabama at Birmingham, Medical Center, UAB Station.

As in other mucosa-associated tissues, the gastrointestinal (GI) tract is in continuous and direct contact with environmental antigens via the epithelial cell layer. In the columnar epithelium, a population of lymphocytes in addition to epithelial cells was discovered, and is most commonly termed intraepithelial lymphocytes (IELs) (reviewed in 1–3). As the name IELs indicates, these lymphocytes reside between the basolateral surfaces of epithelial cells. It has been estimated that one IEL can be found for every six epithelial cells (3). This indicates that tremendous numbers of lymphocytes are situated in the GI mucosa and these lymphocytes are continuously exposed to orally encountered antigens via the epithelial cell layer, since the total surface area of the GI tract is approximately 80 to 90% of a basketball court (about 400 m^2; 4). It would be logical to consider that these IELs could be important immunocompetent cells that participate in the induction and regulation of mucosal immune responses. In this regard, it has been shown that a subset of IELs, specifically the CD4$^-$, CD8$^+$ T cells, possess cytotoxic functions (1–3; Chapters 2,3,6,9 and 14). Oral immunization of mice with reovirus and rotavirus resulted in the induction of antigen-specific cytotoxic T cells in IELs (5,6). Furthermore, our recent studies demonstrated that a subset of IEL T cells possess a regulatory function for the maintenance of IgA responses in the presence of oral tolerance (7,8). These findings strongly suggest that IELs are an important T cell population for the induction and regulation of mucosal immune responses (Fig. 1). Since the cytolytic function of IELs has been extensively described in Chapters 2,3,6,9 and 14, our focus in this chapter is on the regulatory function and cytokine synthesis by different subsets of IEL T cells.

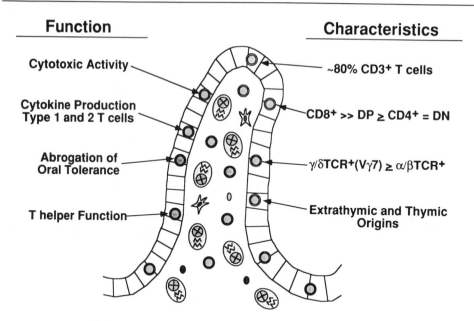

FIG. 1. Unique features of intraepithelial lymphocytes (IEL).

OCCURRENCE OF A UNIQUE T CELL SUBSET DISTRIBUTION BASED ON THE EXPRESSION OF TCR, CD4, AND CD8

In general, greater than 80 to 90% of human and mouse IELs are classified as T cells since these lymphocytes express CD3 peptides in association with the TCR (1–3). Further, other T cell related surface molecules, including Thy-1 and Lyt-1 (CD5), are expressed on subpopulations of IEL T cells. For example, it was shown that 90% of IELs were Thy-1$^+$, and 70% were Lyt-1$^+$ (CD5$^+$) (9), whereas others found much lower numbers of Thy-1$^+$, CD5$^-$ IELs (10,11). Concerning IEL T cell expression of MHC class I and II recognition molecules, CD8 and CD4, respectively, it has been shown that a majority of the cells bear CD8 molecules (1–3). Further, although about 75 to 80% of IELs are CD8$^+$, a substantial number of cells (about 15 to 20%) can be grouped as CD4-bearing cells including CD4$^+$, CD8$^-$ and CD4$^+$, CD8$^+$ (double positive: DP) (7,11–14). The occurrence of increased numbers of CD8$^+$ T cells in IELs is distinctively different from T cells that reside in the other lymphoid tissues. Finally, most IELs express either γ/δ or α/β heterodimer chains of TCR, and it is now generally agreed that an approximately equal number of γ/δ TCR$^+$ and α/β TCR$^+$ T cells are seen in IELs of young adult mice (8,13–18); however, it was originally reported that large numbers of CD3$^+$ T cells in IELs are γ/δ TCR bearing cells (15,16). Thus, IELs are also considered to be an enriched source for γ/δ TCR$^+$ T cells when compared with peripheral T cells. IELs are characterized as TCR-CD3$^+$ mature T cells that harbor unique and distinct characteristics in comparison to T cells residing in other lymphoid organs (Fig. 1).

Because of the fact that IELs are immunologically and physiologically situated in distinct environments when compared with peripheral T cells, various environmental factors, including the gastrointestinal microflora and age, have been suggested to influence the development of different T cell subsets in IELs. Thus, before we describe the study of immunobiological functions of IEL T cells, we have defined the T cell subsets present in murine IELs (e.g., 8 to 12-week old C3H/HeN mice). When IELs were examined for the expression of CD3, CD4, CD8, and TCR, the vast majority of IELs expressed CD3, and these CD3 bearing T cells were separated into four distinct subsets based on the expression of CD4 and CD8 (7,14). The major population in CD3$^+$ IELs was CD4$^-$, CD8$^+$ T cells, comprising approximately 75% of IELs (region I of Fig. 2). The CD4$^+$, CD8$^-$ (region IV) and CD4$^-$, CD8$^-$ (double negative; DN) (region III) subsets were smaller fractions (5 to 8%), and approximately 10% of IELs were DP T cells (region II) (8,14). Similar results have also been reported for IEL T cells isolated from other strains of mice commonly used in immunological studies (e.g., BALB/c and C57BL/6 mice) (12,13).

These four subsets of CD3$^+$ IELs were assessed for the frequency of α/β TCR and γ/δ TCR bearing cells in each subset by using monoclonal antibodies (mAbs) for α/β TCR (H57-597) and γ/δ TCR (GL-3 or UC7-13D5). By simple double-labeling experiments using mAbs anti-α/β TCR and anti-γ/δ TCR, it was shown that no overlapping population of T cells occurred (8,14). Among the CD3$^+$ IELs, the CD4$^-$, CD8$^+$ T cell subset generally contained more γ/δ TCR$^+$ than α/β TCR$^+$ cells; however, the frequency of γ/δ TCR$^+$ cells varied between 45 and 65%

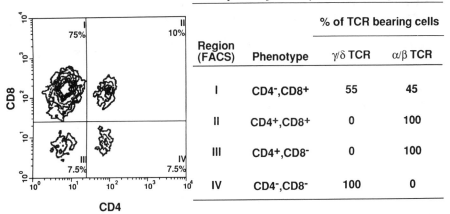

Frequency of α/β TCR and γ/δ TCR

Region (FACS)	Phenotype	% of TCR bearing cells	
		γ/δ TCR	α/β TCR
I	CD4-,CD8+	55	45
II	CD4+,CD8+	0	100
III	CD4+,CD8-	0	100
IV	CD4-,CD8-	100	0

FIG. 2. Occurrence in murine intestinal IELs of four distinct T cell subsets based upon CD4 and CD8 expression and their association with either the α/β TCR or γ/δ TCR.

(average 55%) (Fig. 2). The striking result from the analysis of other T cell subsets was the finding that all $CD4^+$, $CD8^-$ and DP T cell subsets were α/β TCR bearing cells, while the DN IEL T cell subset was essentially γ/δ TCR$^+$ T cells (8,14). To this end, γ/δ TCR$^+$ T cells occurred only in the $CD4^-$, $CD8^+$ (region I) and DN (region III) IEL subsets (Fig. 2). In contrast, T cells in DP (region II) and $CD4^+$, $CD8^-$ (region IV) expressed the α/β TCR but not γ/δ TCR (Fig. 2). These results suggested that CD4 expression is associated with α/β TCR usage and imply that γ/δ TCR$^+$ T cells, which are always $CD4^-$, do not recognize foreign peptide in association with class II MHC. Furthermore, this difference reflects their biological function as discussed later in this chapter.

In summary, IEL T cells consist of four distinct subsets represented by 75% of $CD4^-$, $CD8^+$ T cells followed by DP T cells (10%), $CD4^+$, $CD8^-$ T cells (7.5%) and DN T cells (about 7.5%). The dominant T cell fraction—namely, $CD4^-$, $CD8^+$ T cells contains higher numbers of γ/δ TCR$^+$ T cells (45 to 65%) than α/β TCR$^+$ T cells. In the case of DP and $CD4^+$, $CD8^-$ T cells, all of these IEL T cells express the α/β TCR. Finally, DN T cells are characterized as γ/δ TCR$^+$ cells. In the following sections, the distinct functions and profiles of cytokine production by these different subsets of IELs are concisely summarized and discussed from the standpoint of their contribution in the mucosal immune system.

IMMUNOREGULATORY FUNCTIONS OF γ/δ TCR$^+$ AND α/β TCR$^+$ T CELLS IN IELS

Inasmuch as high numbers of both γ/δ TCR$^+$ and α/β TCR$^+$ T cells are distributed over the entire intestinal epithelium as IELs, it is important to understand their potential role as effector T cells in the mucosal immune system. Although intensive studies have focused on the ontogeny of γ/δ TCR and α/β TCR bearing IELs, the precise biological functions of IEL T cell subsets remain to be elucidated, other than the fact that $CD8^+$ T cells, with either form of TCR, are capable of providing cytolytic function (see Chapters 2 and 3). In this section, we summarize our recent findings, which provide new evidence for possible immunological functions of γ/δ TCR$^+$ and α/β TCR$^+$ T cells in the mucosal immune system, including IgA immune responses.

Role of γ/δ TCR$^+$ IELs in the Maintenance of Mucosal IgA Responses in the Presence of Oral Tolerance

For the induction of antigen-specific IgA responses in the mucosal effector tissues (e.g., the GI tract), oral immunization has been shown to be an effective and practical immunization route (Chapter 1). However, orally administered antigen induces two distinctively opposite types of antigen-specific responses in mucosal effector tissues and in systemic lymphoid tissues in order to maintain appropriate immunological and physiological homeostasis to orally encountered antigens. Following oral administration with a high dose of soluble protein antigens or with continuous oral administration of particulate protein antigens, the mucosal immune system generates and maintains an antigen-specific secretory IgA (S-IgA) response in the mucosal effector tissues while unresponsiveness to these orally encountered antigens is induced in the systemic lymphoid tissues (19–21). This immunologically unique and important concept has been termed *oral tolerance* (OT) (22). In order to maintain these opposite immune responses to orally administered antigens, one could envision that a subset of regulatory T cells in IgA effector tissues may play an important role in the maintenance of antigen-specific S-IgA responses in the presence of systemic unresponsiveness.

Besides induction and maintenance of oral tolerance, the GI tract can be characterized as an environment of suppression that avoids development of inflammatory and hyperimmune responses to the myriad of gut environmental antigens and mitogens. One may speculate that in order to maintain S-IgA responses at mucosal sites such as the lamina propria (LP) regions of the GI tract, where an overall environment of suppression normally exists, IELs contain T cells that function in the immune response and, in effect, maintain this compartment for continued immune responses to orally encountered antigens. Thus, a subset of T cells that resides in the basolateral surfaces between intestinal epithelial cells—especially γ/δ TCR$^+$ T cells, which represent a large percentage of IELs in this tissue—may provide important functions in the maintenance of mucosal IgA immune responses.

To test the hypothesis that γ/δ TCR$^+$ IELs possess unique immunoregulatory functions to support or maintain antigen-specific S-IgA immune responses in IgA effector sites independent of the influence of systemic unresponsiveness and environmental suppression, a well characterized murine OT model was used (23–26). This murine system determines the ability of T cells derived from mucosa-associated tissues, including IELs of mice given T cell dependent (TD) antigens (e.g., sheep erythrocytes, SRBC) by the oral route, to counter the effect of systemic unresponsiveness (or OT) and allow antigen-specific immune responses including those of the IgA isotype (Fig. 3; 7,8). To test directly whether γ/δ TCR bearing T cells in IELs possess an immunoregulatory function for the maintenance of a balance between S-IgA responses and systemic unresponsiveness, purified CD3$^+$ IELs from mice orally immunized with SRBC were separated into γ/δ TCR$^+$ and α/β TCR$^+$ fractions by FACS using anti-γ/δ TCR and anti-α/β TCR mAbs. When purified, γ/δ TCR$^+$ and α/β TCR$^+$ IELs were adoptively transferred to mice orally tolerized with SRBC, a conversion of systemic unresponsiveness to IgM, IgG1, IgG2b, and IgA anti-SRBC responses was seen only in mice that received γ/δ TCR$^+$ cells and the homologous antigen (Fig. 4). On the other hand, the α/β TCR$^+$ IEL T cell fraction did not abrogate systemic unresponsiveness (7,8). This finding was the first demonstration that γ/δ TCR$^+$ T cells possess biological functions in the regulation of mucosal antibody responses. Our most recent study also demonstrated that γ/δ TCR$^+$ T cells from IELs of mice orally immunized with more relevant antigens such as tetanus toxoid (TT) and diphtheria toxoid (DT) possessed the ability to maintain TT- or DT-specific IgA responses in the LP of the gut while systemic

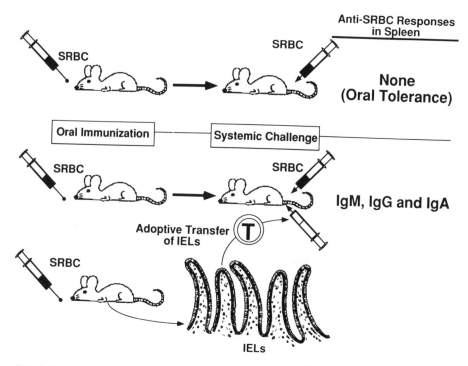

FIG. 3. Induction and abrogation of oral tolerance: an *in vivo* system used for the characterization of regulatory functions of IELs. One group of mice was orally immunized with TD antigen (e.g., SRBC) for prolonged periods (e.g., 28 days), which led to systemic unresponsiveness; i.e., these mice were unable to respond to systemically administered SRBC. However, mucosal IgA responses were maintained in these mice in the presence of systemic unresponsiveness. In order to examine regulatory functions of IELs, different subsets of T cells were isolated from IELs of mice orally immunized with SRBC and then adoptively transferred back to mice with oral tolerance. If a subset of IEL T cells (e.g., γ/δ TCR$^+$ T cells) is essential for the maintenance of the IgA response in the GI tract in the presence of oral tolerance, one might expect abrogation of systemic unresponsiveness to immune responses upon adoptive transfer to orally tolerized mice.

immune responses to these soluble antigens were inhibited (K. Fujihashi et. al., manuscript in preparation). Taken together, one can visualize that γ/δ TCR$^+$ T cells that reside in the gut epithelium can provide regulatory functions for the maintenance of an appropriate immunological balance between local S-IgA response and systemic unresponsiveness in mucosa-associated and systemic lymphoid tissues, respectively.

Based on the studies of others and our own work (8,13,14,27), γ/δ TCR$^+$ T cells are associated with the CD4$^-$, CD8$^+$, and DN IEL fractions (Fig. 2). Thus, CD4$^-$, CD8$^+$, γ/δ TCR$^+$ or DN, γ/δ TCR$^+$ IELs were isolated from mice orally immunized with SRBC, and their ability to abrogate systemic unresponsiveness was examined (8). As we described above, the CD4$^-$, CD8$^+$ IEL T cell population contains 45 to 65% γ/δ TCR$^+$ T cells, and all of the DN IELs express the γ/δ heterodimer

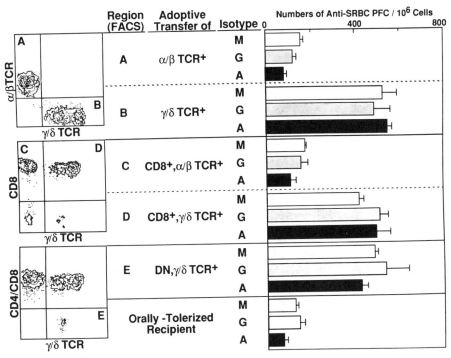

FIG. 4. The γ/δ TCR$^+$ T cells with phenotypes of CD4$^-$, CD8$^+$ and DN from IELs of mice orally immunized with SRBC possess the ability to abrogate unresponsiveness to immune responses including IgA isotype.

chain of TCR (Figs. 2 and 4). When these two subsets of γ/δ TCR$^+$ IELs were isolated from mice given SRBC by the oral route and then adoptively transferred to OT mice, the conversion of systemic unresponsiveness to IgM, IgG1, IgG2b, and IgA anti-SRBC plaque forming cell (PFC) responses was seen. In contrast, the CD4$^-$, CD8$^+$, α/β TCR$^+$ T cell fraction did not reverse unresponsiveness to SRBC-specific immune responses (8). These findings further identified the precise subsets of γ/δ TCR$^+$ T cells, namely CD4$^-$, CD8$^+$ T cells and DN T cells, which possess immunoregulatory function for the protection of S-IgA responses from the influence of systemic suppression. This type of immunoregulatory function has been considered to be one form of "contrasuppression," which was originally advocated by Gershon and his colleagues (28 and reviewed in 29).

Since γ/δ TCR$^+$ IELs from mice orally immunized with protein antigens can support antigen-specific immune responses in the presence of systemic unresponsiveness, an alternative possibility is that these γ/δ TCR$^+$ T cells are a family of "helper cells" or "super helper cells." In this regard, it was recently shown that γ/δ TCR$^+$ T cells from freshly isolated IELs are capable of producing type 1 (e.g., IFN-γ) and type 2 (e.g., IL-5 and IL-6) cytokines (14; see below). To examine this possibility, γ/δ TCR$^+$ T cells from IELs of mice orally administered SRBC were cocultured with the same antigen in Peyer's patch (PP) or spleen (SP) B cell cultures. As a positive control, α/β TCR bearing T cells with CD4[+], CD8[-] T cells from PP and spleen (SP) of the same mice were used as a source of typical Th cells. Although CD4[+], CD8[-], α/β TCR[+] T cells supported antigen-specific B cell responses in PP or SP B cell cultures, γ/δ TCR[+] IELs did not provide any helper functions under similar conditions (8). In contrast, addition of an aliquot of these γ/δ TCR[+] T cells to cultures containing SP cells from orally tolerized mice resulted in the abrogation of unresponsiveness to SRBC-specific responses. When CD4[+], CD8[-], α/β TCR[+] T cells from PP or SP were added to identical cultures, no B cell responses were induced. Thus, γ/δ TCR[+] IEL T cells including both CD4[-], CD8[+] and DN subsets, which maintain IgA responses in the presence of systemic suppression, are an independent population of regulatory T cells and are separate from classical Th cells.

It is generally considered that CD4[+] Th cells in the underlying LP regions of the GI tract induce the terminal differentiation of surface IgA[+] (sIgA[+]) B cells into IgA-producing plasma cells (see Chapter 2). In this regard, our recent studies have shown that high numbers of Th2-type CD4[+] T cells, which produce essential cytokines such as IL-5 and IL-6 for the terminal differentiation of sIgA[+] B cells to become high IgA-producing cells, are seen in the LP regions of the GI tract when compared with other tissues (30,31). In addition, it was shown that γ/δ TCR[+] T cells in the intestinal epithelium may provide another form of cells with regulatory functions to further sustain appropriate IgA immune responses primarily supported by CD4[+] Th2 type cells in the presence of systemic unresponsiveness. Taken together, the anatomical proximity of CD4[-], CD8[+] and DN, γ/δ TCR[+] T cells in IELs and CD4[+] Th cells (e.g., type 2 Th cells) at IgA effector sites would make immunological and physiological sense, since this would provide a suitable environment for the maintenance of efficient IgA responses for the protection of mucosal surfaces.

To further characterize γ/δ TCR[+] T cells in IELs, the γ/δ TCR[+] T cells from mice orally immunized with SRBC were separated into *Vicia villosa* lectin adherent and nonadherent fractions, since it has been shown that both splenic and PP DN T cells that possess the ability to abrogate systemic unresponsiveness have a strong affinity for this plant lectin (23–25,29). When these two fractions of γ/δ TCR[+] IELs were adoptively transferred to mice with systemic unresponsiveness, only the *V. villosa*-adherent fraction of γ/δ TCR[+] T cells abrogated systemic tolerance to SRBC-specific immune responses (8). These results provided the first evidence that γ/δ TCR[+] IELs, which share common characteristics of contrasuppressor cells, i.e., the property of binding to *V. villosa* (29), can provide a regulatory function for the abrogation of systemic unresponsiveness.

In order to prove directly that γ/δ TCR[+] T cells in IELs of orally tolerized mice are responsible for supporting antigen-specific IgA responses in mucosa-associated tissues in the presence of systemic unresponsiveness, γ/δ TCR[+], *V. villosa*-adherent and nonadherent T cells were isolated from IELs and SP of mice given SRBC for 28 days by the oral route; separate experiments with mice from this group showed that the animals were unresponsive to the antigen. Each T cell subset from

IELs or SP of these mice with OT were then adoptively transferred to syngeneic mice rendered systemically unresponsive. Only the γ/δ TCR$^+$, *V. villosa*-adherent T cells from IELs abrogated systemic unresponsiveness (8). On the other hand, the γ/δ TCR$^+$, *V. villosa*-nonadherent IEL T cells, as well as the *V. villosa*-adherent and nonadherent splenic T cells from the same mice, did not convert unresponsiveness to immune responses (8). These findings showed that γ/δ TCR$^+$, *V. villosa*-adherent T cells in IELs were the only T cell fraction capable of abrogating systemic unresponsiveness. Furthermore, this would suggest that these γ/δ TCR$^+$ IEL T cells were indeed functioning in the intestinal epithelium of mice that were receiving toleragenic doses of antigen. It would also suggest that this subset of γ/δ TCR$^+$ T cells in IELs may play an important role in the maintenance of IgA responses in the presence of suppression in the gut.

When cytokine secretion and mRNA levels (e.g., IFN-γ and IL-5) by γ/δ TCR$^+$ *V. villosa*-adherent cells were analyzed, this subset with the ability to abrogate systemic unresponsiveness exhibited low IFN-γ and IL-5 levels, although these cells were fully capable of producing cytokines. Among the *V. villosa*-adherent cells that were secreting IFN-γ and IL-5, at least 50% were shown to produce both cytokines simultaneously (double cytokine producers) (8). These features are clearly distinct from classical Th cell clones, which can be separated into IFN-γ producing type 1 and IL-5 secreting type 2 Th cells (32). These results have also provided compelling evidence that, although these γ/δ TCR$^+$ IEL T cells can produce type 1 and type 2 cytokines, γ/δ TCR$^+$ IELs with the ability to support IgA responses in OT are not a special form of classical Th cells. Furthermore, addition of different doses of a prominent IgA cytokine, i.e., IL-5, into the cultures containing SP cells from mice orally tolerized with SRBC, did not result in conversion of suppression to IgA synthesis (33). On the other hand, γ/δ TCR$^+$ *V. villosa*-adherent IELs from orally tolerized mice supported SRBC-specific IgA B cell responses under similar culture conditions. These findings indicated that cell-to-cell interactions among γ/δ TCR$^+$ IELs, CD4$^+$ Th cells, and sIgA$^+$ B cells would be essential for the induction of antigen-specific IgA responses in mucosal effector tissues in the presence of systemic responsiveness.

It was important to determine the cellular and molecular aspects of the precise cell-to-cell interactions among *V. villosa*-adherent γ/δ TCR$^+$ T cells (including CD4$^-$, CD8$^+$, and DN T cells), CD4$^+$, α/β TCR$^+$ Th2 type cells, and sIgA$^+$ B cells for the maintenance of appropriate IgA responses in mucosa-associated effector tissues in the presence of suppression (Fig. 5). Based on our findings, γ/δ TCR$^+$ T cells may require direct cell-to-cell contact with CD4$^+$ Th cells in order to provide their regulatory signals for enhancement or protection of CD4$^+$ Th cell functions in the presence of suppression (Fig. 5). In this regard, it is possible that γ/δ TCR$^+$ T cells may recognize the TCR idiotype expressed by the V region of α/β TCR on CD4$^+$ Th cells. The γ/δ TCR$^+$ IELs may also interact with CD4$^+$ Th cells via the CD1 molecule, since it has been shown that γ/δ T cells isolated from immunodeficient patients recognized a CD1$^+$ target T cell line (34,35). Alternatively, γ/δ TCR$^+$ IELs may communicate with CD4$^+$, α/β TCR$^+$ T cells via a heat-shock

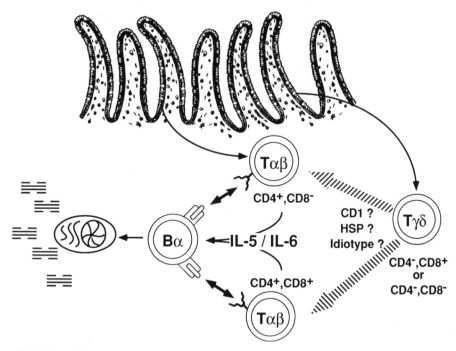

FIG. 5. Possible interactions of IEL γ/δ TCR⁺ T cells, type 2 CD4⁺ Th cells, and sIgA⁺ B cells for the induction and regulation of IgA responses in mucosal effector sites.

protein-like molecule expressed on activated subsets of the latter cell type. It is possible that CD8⁺, γ/δ TCR⁺ T cells may interact with antigen-presenting cells, including B cells, in an MHC class II-peptide restricted fashion. Thus, CD8⁺, γ/δ TCR⁺ IELs have been shown to exhibit MHC class II-restricted antigen recognition (36). In addition, the selection of a certain family of V_δ genes ($V_\delta 4$) was always associated with a distinct haplotype of I-E expression (36). Moreover, it has been shown that antigen-specific γ/δ TCR⁺ T cells can respond to tetanus toxoid antigen in a class II-restricted manner (37). Although our studies have provided novel features of γ/δ TCR⁺ T cells in IELs, the exact cellular and molecular mechanisms for the abrogation of systemic unresponsiveness by this subset of regulatory T cells remains to be further elucidated.

CD4⁺ T Cells in α/β TCR⁺ IELs Exhibited Helper Functions

In contrast to γ/δ TCR⁺ IELs from mice orally immunized with TD protein antigens (e.g., SRBC, TT, or DT), the α/β TCR⁺ T cell fraction contains CD4 bearing T cells that can support antigen-specific B cell responses (8). When α/β TCR⁺ T cells were isolated from IELs of mice orally immunized with SRBC and

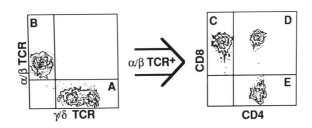

Region (FACS)	TCR Expression	Phenotype	Helper Function in B Cell Cultures	Cytokine Production				
				Type 1		Type 2		
				IFN-γ	IL-2	IL-4	IL-5	IL-6
A	γ/δ TCR+	—	−	±	±	±	±	±
B	α/β TCR+	—	++++	+	+	++	+++	++
C	α/β TCR+	CD4⁻,CD8+	−	±	±	±	±	±
D	α/β TCR+	CD4+,CD8+	++++	+	+	++	+++	++
E	α/β TCR+	CD4+,CD8⁻	++++	+	+	++	+++	++

FIG. 6. The α/β TCR⁺ T cells from IELs of mice orally immunized with TD antigen contain effector cells that can provide helper functions.

cocultured with SP or PP B cells in the presence of the same antigen, elevated numbers of SRBC-specific antibody secreting cells including those of the IgA isotype were noted (Fig. 6). As positive controls, CD4⁺ T cells expressing α/β TCR were isolated from PP and SP of mice orally primed with SRBC. Both PP and SP CD4⁺, α/β TCR⁺ T cells provided helper function for SRBC-specific B cell responses. The α/β TCR⁺ T cells isolated from IELs, PP, or SP of nonimmunized mice failed to support SRBC-specific B cell differentiation. These findings were the first results to demonstrate that α/β TCR⁺ IELs contain T cell subsets with helper activity for the induction of antigen-specific B cell differentiation to Ig producing cells (8).

The α/β TCR⁺ T cells isolated from IELs could be separated into three subsets according to the expression of CD4 and CD8 (8,38). As described above, the α/β TCR⁺ T cells comprise almost half (approximately 45%) of the CD3⁺ IELs (8,14,17). Among these α/β TCR⁺ IELs, the CD4⁺, CD8⁻ and DP T cells represent about 15% and about 20% of the α/β TCR⁺ T cells, respectively, while the rest (about 65%) consist of CD4⁻, CD8⁺ T cells. In order to elucidate the subsets of α/β TCR⁺ IEL T cells that provide helper functions, these three subsets of IEL T cells were isolated from mice orally primed with SRBC and examined for their ability to support SRBC-specific B cell responses. As one might expect, CD4⁺,

CD8$^-$ T cells supported IgM, IgG, and IgA anti-SRBC PFC responses in PP B cell cultures, while CD4$^-$, CD8$^+$ T cells did not (38). DP T cells provided helper activity in these B cell cultures. Thus, this study provided important new evidence that DP T cells in IELs exhibit effector functions similar to helper T cells expressing the classical phenotype of CD4$^+$, CD8$^-$ (Fig. 6). In general, during T cell development in the thymus, DP T cells mainly occur as immature cortical thymocytes, which become mature CD4$^+$, CD8$^-$ or CD4$^-$, CD8$^+$ T cells (39). However, our findings suggested that DP T cells in IELs might not be precursors for CD4$^+$, CD8$^-$ or CD4$^-$, CD8$^+$ T cells because of their ability to provide a mature effector function, i.e., helper activity. Thus, DP T cells in IELs could be considered as a family of CD4 bearing Th cells.

The view that DP T cells in IELs are a mature functional Th cell subset was further supported by the analysis of cytokine profiles using IFN-γ, IL-2-, IL-4-, IL-5-specific RT-PCR and ELISPOT assays. In this study, DP T cells from IELs of mice orally immunized with SRBC were incubated with feeder cells and SRBC for 5 to 7 days. An aliquot of antigen-stimulated DP T cells was then examined for type 1 (IFN-γ and IL-2) and type 2 (IL-4 and IL-5) Th cell cytokine production by the respective cytokine-specific ELISPOT assay (38,40,41). Upon antigen-stimulation, both type 1 and type 2 cytokine producing cells were noted in DP T cells. Further, cytokine-specific RT-PCR analysis revealed that messages for both type 1 (IFN-γ and IL-2) and type 2 (IL-4 and IL-5) Th cell cytokines were present in RNA isolated from the other aliquot of antigen-pulsed DP T cells from IELs of mice orally immunized with SRBC (38). These findings clearly indicated that DP T cells in IELs are mature, functional helper T cells. In contrast to antigen-stimulated DP T cells, unstimulated cells harbored mRNA messages for IFN-γ, and IL-5, but not IL-2 or IL-4. Furthermore, these cells produced only the former three cytokines when examined by the cytokine-specific ELISPOT assay. This pattern of cytokine profile was also seen by IEL DP T cells freshly isolated from normal mice (see Chapter 1, 42). However, stimulation of DP T cells via TCR-CD3 complex resulted in the synthesis of an array of both type 1 (IFN-γ and IL-2) and type 2 (IL-4, IL-5, and IL-6) cytokines. Thus, antigen stimulation signals delivered via the TCR-CD3 complex appear to turn on all of the cytokine-specific gene promoters (38,42).

In addition to DP T cells, when antigen-stimulated CD4$^+$, CD8$^-$ T cells from IELs of mice orally immunized with SRBC were examined for both type 1 and type 2 Th cell cytokine synthesis, IFN-γ, IL-2, IL-4, IL-5, and IL-6 producing T cells were noted by the respective cytokine-specific ELISPOT assay (Fig. 6). Furthermore, analysis of cytokine-specific mRNA by RT-PCR revealed that RNA isolated from antigen-activated CD4$^+$, CD8$^-$ T cells contained mRNA messages for both type 1 (IFN-γ and IL-2) and type 2 (IL-4, IL-5, and IL-6) cytokines (38). This cytokine profile analysis at the mRNA and protein levels confirmed our functional studies in which CD4$^+$, CD8$^-$ T cells were shown to possess helper function, and to support B cell differentiation to Ig producing cells *in vitro*. Thus, IELs contain at least two different types of regulatory T cells, which include CD4$^-$, CD8$^+$ or DN

γ/δ TCR$^+$ T cells capable of maintaining IgA responses in the presence of systemic unresponsiveness (contrasuppressors) and CD4$^+$, CD8$^-$ or DP α/β TCR$^+$ T cells supporting B cell responses including the IgA isotype (helpers). Taken together, the IELs are important members of a regulatory T cell network for induction and maintenance of IgA responses in mucosal effector tissues such as the intestinal LP in the GI tract.

CYTOKINE PRODUCTION BY γ/δ TCR$^+$ IELS

One of the major functions for effector T cells, including Th cells, is the production of an array of regulatory cytokines upon antigen stimulation. In this regard, CD3$^+$, CD4$^+$, CD8$^-$ T cell clones may be divided into two subsets, designated helper type 1 and type 2 cells according to the assortment of cytokines produced (32,43). Type 1 Th cells selectively produce IL-2, IFN-γ, and TNF-β (or lymphotoxin) following activation with processed antigen and MHC class II on antigen presenting cells via recognition by TCR-CD3 complex on the Th cell surface, while IL-4, IL-5, IL-6, and IL-10 are exclusively secreted by type 2 helper T cells (see Chapter 2). However, recent studies have also indicated that a subset of CD8 bearing T cells can also produce some type 1 and type 2 cytokines (14,44–46). Since IEL T cells consist of at least four different subsets based upon the expression of CD4 and CD8 (7,12–14), the exact nature of cytokine profiles in these different T cell subsets was examined. Thus, we have used type 1 (IFN-γ and IL-2) and type 2 (IL-2, IL-5, and IL-6) cytokine specific ELISPOT assays and RT-PCR for the characterization of cytokine production by IELs (40,41) (see also Chapter 1).

To better understand the immunobiological function of IELs, which includes the relationship between IELs and LP lymphocytes (LPLs) as well as the reciprocal influence between IELs and epithelial cells in the mucosa-associated tissues, it is important to characterize the exact profiles of their cytokine production. Our initial studies showed that when freshly isolated IELs were subjected to the IFN-γ and IL-5 specific ELISPOT assays, approximately 1 to 3% of lymphocytes spontaneously produced both of these cytokines (31). As we described in the analysis of T cell subsets in IEL earlier in this text, the CD3$^+$ T cell fraction contains both γ/δ TCR$^+$ and α/β TCR$^+$ IELs, and we next characterized these two subsets for cytokine production. CD3$^+$ IELs were separated into γ/δ TCR$^+$ and α/β TCR$^+$ T cell fractions by FACS and examined for synthesis of IFN-γ and IL-5. It was of interest that CD3$^+$, γ/δ TCR$^+$ T cells, like α/β TCR$^+$ T cells in comparison with CD3$^-$ IEL, showed that only the CD3$^+$ populations produced IFN-γ and IL-5. Furthermore, the cytokines were produced *de novo*, since treatment with cycloheximide blocked cytokine-specific SFC by 85 to 90%. Thus, this finding demonstrated that in addition to the α/β TCR$^+$ T cells, the γ/δ TCR$^+$ IELs contain T cells that can produce both type 1 and 2 cytokines, namely IFN-γ and IL-5 (14).

Since the dominant T cell fraction of IELs, i.e., CD4$^-$, CD8$^+$ T cells, contained both α/β TCR$^+$ and γ/δ TCR$^+$ T cells (Fig. 2), the CD4$^-$, CD8$^+$ IELs were separated into α/β TCR$^+$ (approximately 45%) and γ/δ TCR$^+$ (approximately 55%) T cells for the analysis of cytokine production. Both CD8$^+$, γ/δ TCR$^+$ and CD8$^+$, α/β TCR$^+$ IELs produced these two cytokines as assayed by cytokine-specific ELISPOT assays; however, higher numbers of IFN-γ and IL-5 SFC were associated with α/β TCR$^+$ T cells. This was the first study showing that mouse CD8$^+$ T cells, regardless of TCR usage, produce IL-5. Furthermore, both γ/δ TCR$^+$ and α/β TCR$^+$ IEL T cells in the CD8$^+$ fraction produce IFN-γ (14). Thus, a unique and potentially important finding in this study was that CD3$^+$, CD8$^+$ IELs, which express either γ/δ TCR or α/β TCR, produce the cytokines IFN-γ and IL-5 (14). To ensure that the production of these cytokines by CD3$^+$, CD8$^+$ T cells were expressed at the gene level, mRNA was isolated from different subsets of IELs and hybridized with IFN-γ and IL-5 specific cDNA probes. When mRNA isolated from CD3$^+$, γ/δ TCR$^+$ and CD3$^+$, α/β TCR$^+$ IEL fractions were hybridized with these probes, high levels of IFN-γ and IL-5 specific message were seen in both IEL T cell subsets (14). Furthermore, the occurrence of IFN-γ and IL-5 specific messages in these IEL T cell fractions was also confirmed by using cytokine-specific RT-PCR. It is also important to note that Southern blot analysis of PCR amplified IFN-γ and IL-5 mRNA specifically hybridized with the cDNA probe for IFN-γ and IL-5, respectively (Fujihashi, K. and Yamamoto, M., unpublished data). These results clearly showed that the mRNA in both CD8$^+$, γ/δ TCR$^+$ and α/β TCR$^+$ IEL T cells contained messages for both IFN-γ and IL-5.

It is well established that CD3$^+$, CD8$^+$, α/β TCR$^+$ CTLs produce IFN-γ in response to class I MHC-mediated recognition of target cells (44,47). Thus, it was recently shown that IFN-γ production could be correlated with antigen-specific CTL activity in human CD4$^-$, CD8$^+$ T cells isolated from peripheral blood mononuclear cells of influenza-vaccinated subjects (48). CD3$^+$, CD4$^-$, CD8$^+$ T cells in human IELs have been shown to be capable of producing IFN-γ upon stimulation of CD2 or lectin binding molecules expressed on T cells (45). The presence of IFN-γ producing cells in IELs was recently shown by immunohistochemical analysis *in situ* using anti-human IFN-γ antibody (49). Therefore, it was not surprising to discover IFN-γ producing T cells in the major CD4$^-$, CD8$^+$ IEL T cell subset. However, until our results were obtained, no evidence had emerged that IEL CD4$^-$, CD8$^+$ T cell expressing γ/δ TCR also produce IFN-γ (14). In addition to IEL CD4$^-$, CD8$^+$, γ/δ TCR$^+$ T cells, previous studies have shown that MHC antigen (H-2^k) specific, CD3$^+$, DN T cell clones that express γ/δ TCR produced IFN-γ upon antigen stimulation (50). Furthermore, splenic CD3$^+$, DN, γ/δ TCR$^+$ T cells were also capable of producing IFN-γ upon stimulation with anti-CD3 mAb (51). Taken together, these findings have shown that γ/δ TCR$^+$ T cells in IEL and other lymphoid tissues produce cytokines such as IFN-γ.

Even more striking was the observation that γ/δ TCR$^+$ IELs also produce IL-5. Most past studies in mice had shown that IL-5 production is most often associated with type 2 CD4$^+$ T cells that exhibit helper function (43,44). Thus, our study was the first to show that γ/δ TCR$^+$ T cells reside in mucosa-effector tissues, such as intestinal epithelium, and produce IL-5, and its production is associated with the

CD4$^-$, CD8$^+$ IEL subset. Since our most recent as well as separate studies have provided new evidence that γ/δ TCR$^+$ T cells in IgA effector sites (e.g., salivary glands) harbor high levels of IL-5-specific mRNA and produce this cytokine (Hiroi, T. et al., manuscript in preparation), it is possible that the occurrence of IL-5 producing γ/δ TCR$^+$ T cells in these IgA effector tissues may contribute to the predominance of IgA plasma cells.

Because our studies have shown that CD8$^+$, γ/δ TCR$^+$ IEL T cells can produce cytokines, it was important to determine whether these T cells produce both IFN-γ and IL-5 simultaneously, or only one cytokine, which would be more reminiscent of type 1 and type 2 T cells, which produce IFN-γ and IL-5, respectively. To this end, distinct subsets of CD3$^+$ T cells freshly isolated from IEL were added to wells coated with both anti-IFN-γ and anti-IL-5 mAbs, and SFC were developed either with anti-IFN-γ or anti-IL-5 or with both antibodies simultaneously (8,14). With this type of analysis, about 30% of CD3$^+$, γ/δ TCR$^+$ T cells produced both cytokines (cytokine double producers). Furthermore, T cells that produce either IFN-γ or IL-5 (single producers) in the γ/δ TCR$^+$ IEL subset comprised 60 to 80%. However, in the α/β TCR$^+$ subset, most of the T cells were single producers, and only about 8% of cells produced both cytokines. These results showed that γ/δ TCR$^+$ IEL contain a higher frequency of cytokine double producer cells when compared with the α/β TCR$^+$ fraction (14). The appearance of high numbers of γ/δ TCR$^+$ cytokine double producers suggested that these cells may be precursors for γ/δ TCR$^+$ T cells that produce either IFN-γ or IL-5, analogous to the postulated type 0 cells that can develop into either type 1 or type 2 cells (32). Thus, γ/δ TCR$^+$ T cells may also be separated into three subsets of T cells (e.g., type 0, type 1, and type 2) on the basis of the profile of cytokine synthesis.

NATURE OF CYTOKINE PRODUCING IELS

In addition to CD4$^-$, CD8$^+$ T cells expressing γ/δ TCR and α/β TCR$^+$ IELs, as described above, our most recent study has demonstrated that CD4 bearing α/β TCR$^+$ IELs, including both CD4$^+$, CD8$^-$ and DP, contain T cells capable of producing type 1 and type 2 cytokines (42; see Chapter 1). Other recent studies also showed that α/β TCR$^+$ and γ/δ TCR$^+$ IELs synthesize a large repertoire of cytokines including IL-2, IL-3, IL-6, IFN-γ, TNF-α, and TGF-β (46). Since these different subsets of α/β TCR$^+$ and γ/δ TCR$^+$ T cells, which include CD4$^+$, CD8$^-$ T cells, CD4$^-$, CD8$^+$ T cells, and DP T cells, possess the ability to secrete regulatory cytokines including type 1 (IFN-γ and IL-2) and type 2 (IL-4, IL-5, and IL-6), it is now logical to consider that IEL T cells are an important family of effector cells that could involve all aspects of cell-to-cell interactions for the induction and regulation of mucosal immune responses. In spite of these provocative findings, the exact characteristics of these cytokine producing IELs remain to be determined.

To understand the exact nature of type 1 (e.g., IFN-γ) and type 2 (e.g., IL-5) cytokine producing T cells in murine IELs, cytokine-specific mRNA analysis and

ELISPOT assay, as well as flow cytometry cell cycle analysis, were used to characterize cytokine producing γ/δ TCR$^+$ and α/β TCR$^+$ IEL T cells (52). Since IELs contained relatively higher numbers of *in situ* cytokine producing cells in comparison to splenic T cells, an obvious hypothesis would be that IEL T cells could be in a more activated stage of the cell cycle, while the majority of splenic T cells are in the resting phase.

When aliquots of freshly isolated IELs and splenic lymphocytes (SPLs) were stained for CD3, γ/δ TCR or α/β TCR expression with respective fluorescence-conjugated mAbs and further reacted with propidium iodide for DNA analysis using flow cytometry, it was surprising to note that a similar pattern of cell cycle was seen in both IELs and SPLs. The majority of CD3$^+$ T cells in both IELs and SPLs were in the G_0 to G_1 phase and less than 5% of lymphocytes were in mid-cell cycle (S/G$_2$ + M) (52). In IELs, no difference was noted between α/β TCR$^+$ and γ/δ TCR$^+$ T cells in their cell cycle stage. However, when other aliquots of IELs and SPLs were tested for cytokine production by using IFN-γ and IL-5 specific ELISPOT assays, IELs contained substantially higher numbers of IFN-γ and IL-5 producing cells ($\sim$150–250 SFC/10^4 cells) when compared with SPLs (0–20 SFC/10^4 cells) (52). This finding indicated that although IELs and SPLs were in similar cell cycle stages, the former lymphocytes contained cytokine producing cells but the latter did not.

In general, activated blast cell (low density) populations are characterized by the occurrence of increased numbers of cells in G_1 and S/G$_2$ + M phases, while resting cells (high density) contain high numbers of cells mainly in G_0 and small numbers in the G_1 phase of cell cycle (53). Further, activated blasts and resting cells are generally found in the layers of low and high density fractions upon separation by the discontinuous cell density gradients, respectively. Thus, freshly isolated IELs were separated into two fractions according to their cell density by using discontinuous Percoll® gradients. Approximately two thirds of the cells were present in the low density fraction while the remainder separated into the high density fraction. The CD3$^+$, γ/δ TCR$^+$ and α/β TCR$^+$ IELs were then examined for their respective cell cycle stages (52). Among these different T cell subsets in both high and low density fractions, essentially no differences in the stages of cell cycle were seen (Table 1). Regardless of cell density and TCR expression, the majority of cells (95–98%) were in the G_0 + G_1 phase in IELs (52).

However, when levels of RNA content were assessed in these two fractions, a significant difference was noted (Fig. 7). In this experiment, high and low density IELs were treated with acridine orange in order to stain both DNA and RNA, and then analyzed by flow cytometry. The G_1 phase of IELs in the low density fraction possessed a higher RNA content in comparison to high density IELs and SPLs (Fig. 7). This finding was more obvious when histograms of flow cytometry RNA analysis were examined (Fig. 7). A distinct shift to higher RNA content was observed with the low density fraction when compared with high density IELs and SPLs. In contrast to the low density fraction of IELs, high density IELs revealed an identical pattern of RNA content with SPLs (Fig. 7). These findings suggested that, although both high and low density IELs were in G_0 + G_1 stages of cell cycle, the latter

TABLE 1. Characterization of cytokine production by γ/δ TCR+ and α/β TCR+ IELs

TCR Expression	Cell Density by Discontinuous Percoll Gradient	Cytokine Producing Cells (/10⁶Cells) by ELISPOT		Cytokine mRNA Analysis by PCR			Cell Cycle Stage (%)	
		IFN-γ	IL-5	IL-5	IFN-γ	β-actin	G_0+G_1	S/G_2+M
γ/δ TCR	Low	32,500	32,000	(243→)	(460→)	(349→)	97	3
	High	5,200	3,250				94	6
α/β TCR	Low	33,000	32,250	(243→)	(460→)	(349→)	96	4
	High	5,000	4,000				96	4

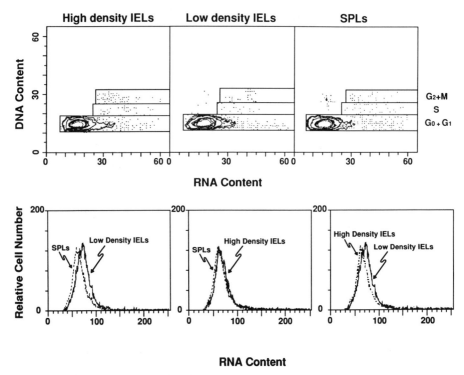

FIG. 7. Analysis of DNA and RNA content in low- and high-density IELs. Murine IELs were separated into low- and high-density cells by discontinuous Percoll gradients. Lymphocytes were permeabilized with Tritron x-100 solution and then reacted with acridine orange for DNA and RNA staining. Cells were then analyzed by flow cytometry. (A) DNA and RNA contents of low- and high-density IELs. (B) Levels of total RNA in the $G_0 + G_1$ phase of low- and high-density IELs.

fraction of cells were in the G_1 stage and may have contained cells actively secreting cytokines. In order to test this assumption, low and high density fractions of freshly isolated α/β TCR$^+$ and γ/δ TCR$^+$ IELs were tested for IFN-γ and IL-5 production by cytokine-specific ELISPOT assay. IFN-γ and IL-5 producing cells were predominantly found in the low-density fraction of α/β TCR$^+$ and γ/δ TCR$^+$ IELs, and smaller numbers of cytokine secreting cells were associated with the high-density IELs (52). This finding further supports the idea that low-density α/β TCR$^+$ and γ/δ TCR$^+$ IELs are in G_1 and are producing cytokines.

This view was further reinforced by cytokine specific mRNA analysis using mRNA-cDNA dot-blot hybridization and RT-PCR (52). When mRNA was isolated from low- and high-density fractions of IELs and then hybridized with the IFN-γ and IL-5 specific cDNA probes, higher levels of these cytokine specific messages were observed in the former population than in the high-density subset. To further confirm this finding, cytokine-specific RT-PCR analysis was also performed. In these studies, mRNA preparations were obtained from these two fractions of α/β TCR$^+$ and γ/δ TCR$^+$ IELs, reverse transcribed, and amplified by using IFN-γ and IL-5 specific 5' and 3' primers. Following 35 cycles of amplification, distinct messages for IFN-γ and IL-5 were noted in the low-density fraction (52). On the other hand, very low messages were seen in high-density IELs (Table 1). These findings provided evidence that γ/δ TCR$^+$ and α/β TCR$^+$ T cells in IELs were capable of producing the type 1 and type 2 cytokines, IFN-γ and IL-5, respectively. Furthermore, γ/δ TCR$^+$ and α/β TCR$^+$ T cells in IELs that were separated in low-density fractions and that were in the G_1 phase of cell cycle were responsible for the spontaneous production of these cytokines.

Another important finding was that the low-density fraction, which consists of IFN-γ and IL-5 producing cells, contained an approximately equal frequency of γ/δ TCR$^+$ and α/β TCR$^+$ T cells. On the other hand, the high-density fraction was represented mainly by α/β TCR$^+$ T cells with low numbers of γ/δ TCR T cells (52). This fraction of IEL T cells did not produce IFN-γ or IL-5. However, our most recent as well as separate studies have shown that T cells with high density were able to respond to activation signals via the CD3-TCR complex and subsequently pass through cell cycle and become cytokine-producing cells (56; see below). Taken together with the fact that γ/δ TCR$^+$ T cells in IELs are committed to programmed cell death (apoptosis) (54), one can suggest that the G_1 phase of T cells in the low-density fraction will undergo apoptosis upon completion of cytokine production. On the other hand, T cells in the high-density fraction could respond to lumenal antigens and/or mitogens and then become activated T cells that could produce cytokines and replace neighboring cells that had undergone programmed cell death. These possibilities are further discussed in the next section together with our newly generated results.

BIOLOGICAL CONSEQUENCES OF CYTOKINE SYNTHESIS AND APOPTOSIS BY IELs

IELs have been shown to contain α/β TCR$^+$ and γ/δ TCR$^+$ cells that are capable of producing both type 1 (IFN-γ and IL-2) and type 2 (IL-4, IL-5, and IL-6) cytokines (14,31,38,42). It was also shown that in addition to type 1 and type 2 cytokines, α/β TCR$^+$ and γ/δ TCR$^+$ IELs produce TNF-α and TGF-β (46). A wide variety of cytokine production by IEL T cells (14,31,38,42,45,46,55) suggested that IEL T cells are an important population of effector cells, which could be involved in all aspects of cell-to-cell interactions including T-B cells, T-T cells, and T-epithelial cells for the induction and regulation of mucosal immune responses. Thus, it is important to examine the exact life cycle (activation $\rightarrow$ proliferation $\rightarrow$ cytokine secretion $\rightarrow$ apoptosis) of these cytokine-producing T cells in IELs for an understanding of the immunobiological contributions of different IEL T cell subsets in the mucosal immune system.

Exposure to antigens in the natural milieu is an initial step for the activation of resting T cells and the priming of naive T cells to develop memory and/or effector T cells. In comparison to T cells that reside in systemic lymphoid tissues that are anatomically isolated from direct and continuous burdens of environmental antigens, IEL T cells are continuously exposed to uncountable numbers of antigens in the GI tract. This consistent antigen exposure could explain the development of several immunologically unique countenances of IELs when compared with systemic T cells. For example, it was recently demonstrated that IELs and SPLs behave in a completely different manner in response to stimulation signals delivered by T cell mitogen and mAbs anti-TCR and anti-CD3 (56). Elevated DNA replication was noted in culture containing SPLs and these stimuli, while IELs did not respond to Con A or to mAbs specific for the TCR-CD3 complex. Thus, this result completely agreed with the previous finding by others that IELs are unresponsive to proliferation signals provided by T cell mitogen, phorbol myristate acetate and calcium ionophores, and mAbs anti-TCR and anti-CD3 (17,57,58). However, our recent study has produced new findings that two different activation stages of α/β TCR$^+$ and γ/δ TCR$^+$ T cells can be isolated from IELs which respond distinctively to stimulation signals delivered to cytoplasma of T cells via the TCR-CD3 complex. (56).

As described in the above section, freshly isolated IELs can be separated into high- and low-density fractions. When these two fractions of IEL T cells were stimulated with solid phase mAbs specific for CD3, γ/δ TCR, and α/β TCR molecules, the former subset of IELs was responsible for stimulation signals delivered via the TCR-CD3 complex (56). Furthermore, large numbers of high-density cells entered into cell cycle of $S/G_2 + M$ phase in response to mAbs specific for TCR-CD3 molecules. By contrast, low-density IELs were unable to respond to proliferation signals (56). This observation was the first demonstration that a subpopulation of IEL T cells was capable of responding to proliferation signals transmitted through the TCR-CD3 complex (Fig. 8).

In the human system, IELs have been shown to respond to proliferative stimulation signals delivered via the CD2 molecule expressed on T cells (59). Cultivation of IELs freshly isolated from human intestine together with anti-T11 (CD2) mAb or SRBC resulted in a level of DNA replication comparable to that of T cells obtained from human peripheral blood. Taken together, these findings suggested that, although as a whole IELs respond poorly to T cell specific stimuli, IELs contain a subpopulation of T cells such as high-density IELs that are able to respond to activation signals transmitted through the TCR-CD3 complex and T cell specific surface molecule (e.g., CD2).

It was interesting to note that stimulation of high-density IELs via the TCR-CD3 complex led to the induction of cytokines (56). Thus, anti-CD3, anti-α/β TCR, and anti-γ/δ TCR treatments augmented the numbers of IFN-γ and IL-5 cytokine producing cells in the high-density fraction of IELs (Fig. 8). When mRNA isolated from these stimulated high-density IELs via the TCR-CD3 complex were examined for IFN-γ and IL-5 messages by RT-PCR, the levels of the respective cytokine specific mRNA were increased (56). Based on these findings, one could postulate that high-density IELs could respond to stimulation signals provided by gut environ-

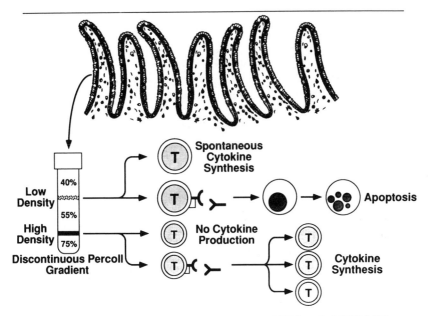

FIG. 8. Cytokine production and apoptosis by α/β TCR⁺ and γ/δ TCR⁺ IELs.

mental antigens that result in their entrance into the cell cycle and progression to the M phase and subsequent proliferation. Furthermore, these activated high-density T cells will become cytokine (e.g., IFN-γ and IL-5) producing cells (Fig. 8).

In contrast to IELs in the high-density fraction, the low-density T cells are distinguished by differences in response to stimulation signals transmitted through the TCR-CD3 complex. Activation of low-density IELs with different mAbs to TCR-CD3 antigens did not cause any alteration of their cell cycle stage or lead to induction of any DNA replication (56). As expected, this treatment did not elevate the number of IFN-γ or IL-5 producing cells. These findings suggested two possibilities to explain the behavior of low-density T cells upon activation via TCR-CD3 complex. First, the majority of low-density T cells could be in a form of anergy where the T cells persist and are capable of providing effector functions but are unresponsive to stimuli. Inasmuch as T cells in the intestinal epithelium are chronically exposed to an array of environmental antigens, persistence of these antigens in the gut lumen may involve the development of T cell anergy in IELs.

As a second possibility, the low-density IEL T cells may contain high numbers of T cells that are in the process of programmed cell death. In this regard, earlier histological studies showed that IELs possess histological features of apoptosis such as cytoplasmic blebbing and pyknotic nuclei (60,61). It was demonstrated that γ/δ TCR⁺ T cells isolated from IELs underwent apoptosis *in vitro* when compared with α/β TCR⁺ T cells (54). Our recent study also showed that low-density T cells in IELs that were unable to respond to DNA replication signals transmitted through the

TCR-CD3 complex exhibited T cells undergoing DNA fragmentation. Thus, gel analysis of DNA from anti-CD3 and anti-TCR mAb treated low-density IELs resulted in a ladder-like endogenous nucleotide fragmentation (56). Furthermore, by analysis of nuclei of anti-CD3 stimulated low-density IEL T cells, the fraction was enriched for apoptotic cells. In contrast, similarly treated high-density IEL T cells contained much lower numbers of apoptotic cells in comparison to low density T cells (56). Thus, it is plausible to postulate that, following the high expression of cytokine-specific mRNA and subsequent protein synthesis, these cells in the low-density IELs undergo programmed cell death (Fig. 8).

SUMMARY

Intestinal IELs including both γ/δ TCR$^+$ and α/β TCR$^+$ T cells reside in the gut epithelium, where trafficking of orally encountered antigens from the intestinal lumen into the host occurs. Furthermore, underneath the epithelium, a large number of IgA antibody producing B cells and effector T cells, which play a major role in mucosal immunity, are presumably interacting with neighboring cells including epithelial cells and IELs for the formation of an immune network to prevent microbial infections. Thus, IELs could potentially provide various T cell functions for the mucosal immune system. CD3$^+$ T cells in IELs were separated into four subsets based on the expression of CD4 and CD8 in which CD4$^-$, CD8$^+$ T cells were the dominant fraction (approximately 75%), followed by DP T cells (approximately 10%), CD4$^+$, CD8$^-$ T cells (approximately 7.5%), and DN T cells (approximately 7.5%). In terms of γ/δ TCR and α/β TCR usage in these four subsets, the γ/δ TCR$^+$ T cells comprised 100% of the DN T cell subset and 45 to 65% of the CD4$^-$, CD8$^+$ T cell fraction, while α/β TCR$^+$ T cells were all CD4$^+$, CD8$^-$ T cells and DP T cells. Inasmuch as IEL T cells harbor these unique T cell subset distributions in comparison to peripheral T cells, it was important to examine the immunobiological contributions of different T cell subsets in mucosal immune responses.

Concerning the immunological contribution of different subsets of IEL T cells (e.g., γ/δ TCR and α/β TCR bearing cells) in IgA responses, these two subsets of T cells could be crucial regulatory T cells for the induction and maintenance of appropriate IgA immune responses in GI environments where two opposite immune reactions simultaneously occur, e.g., where continuous activation by lumenal antigens and suppression of inflammatory reactions takes place. In this regard, our work has provided new evidence that subsets of γ/δ TCR$^+$ and α/β TCR$^+$ T cells possess distinctively different immunoregulatory functions. The γ/δ TCR bearing CD4$^-$, CD8$^+$ T cells and DN T cells seem to be important effector T cells that can maintain IgA responses in the presence of a major form of suppression termed oral tolerance. Thus, it was shown that these two subsets of γ/δ TCR$^+$ T cells isolated from IELs (CD4$^-$, CD8$^+$ T cells and DN T cells) of mice orally tolerized with TD antigens were capable of abrogating systemic unresponsiveness to immune responses including those of the IgA isotype. In contrast to γ/δ TCR$^+$ IELs, α/β TCR bearing CD4$^+$,

CD8$^-$ T cells and DP T cells were capable of producing type 1 (IFN-γ and IL-2) and type 2 (IL-4, IL-5, and IL-6) Th cell cytokines at the level of both protein and mRNA. Thus, addition of these α/β TCR$^+$ T cells in B cell cultures resulted in the induction of B cell differentiation to IgA producing cells as well as other isotypes. Further, α/β TCR$^+$, CD4$^+$, CD8$^-$ T cells, and DP T cells also supported TD-antigen-specific B cell responses. Upon antigenic stimulation via the TCR-CD3 complex, α/β TCR bearing CD4$^+$, CD8$^-$ and DP T cells produce type 1 and 2 Th cell cytokines and provide classical T helper functions.

In terms of the biological nature and consequence of cytokine producing IELs, T cells can be separated into two different stages of cell cycle. Although the cell cycle characterization revealed that most CD3$^+$ T cells in IELs were very similar to splenic T cells where greater than 95% of T cells were in the G$_0$–G$_1$ phase of the cell cycle, both α/β TCR$^+$ and γ/δ TCR$^+$ T cells in the low-density fraction contained cells spontaneously producing cytokines (e.g., IFN-γ and IL-5). Transmission of activation signals to these low-density α/β TCR$^+$ and γ/δ TCR$^+$ T cells leads to the induction of DNA fragmentation, which indicated entrance into apoptosis. In contrast to the low-density IELs, α/β TCR$^+$ and γ/δ TCR$^+$ T cells in the high-density fraction did not contain any cytokine producing cells. When stimulation signals were transduced through the TCR-CD3 complex, both α/β TCR$^+$ and γ/δ TCR$^+$ T cells entered into the cell cycle stage of S/G$_2$ + M phase, which resulted in DNA replication. Following cell proliferation, stimulated α/β TCR$^+$ and γ/δ TCR$^+$ T cells in the high-density fraction became cytokine-producing T cells. Thus, stimulation of high- and low-density IELs via the TCR-CD3 complex by gut environmental antigens could provide two opposing effects, such as cytokine synthesis and apoptosis, respectively. This subtle balance may play an important role in the maintenance of an appropriate immunological homeostasis in IEL T cell regulated mucosal immune responses in the gut epithelium and lamina propria regions.

ACKNOWLEDGMENTS

The results summarized in this chapter were supported in part by U.S. Public Health Service Contract AI 15128, and Grants DK 44240, AI 30366, DE 09837, AI 18958, DE 04217, and DE 08228. Dr. H. Kiyono is the recipient of the NIH Research Career Development Award, DE 00237. We thank Ms. Sheila Weatherspoon for preparation of this chapter. We are indebted to Drs. Dennis McGee and Katherine Merrill for their critical review of this manuscript.

REFERENCES

1. Croitoru K, Ernst PB. Leukocytes in the intestinal epithelium: an unusual immunological compartment revisited. *Reg Immunol* 1992;4:63–69.
2. Lefrançois L. Intraepithelial lymphocytes of the intestinal mucosa: curiouser and curiouser. *Semin Immunol* 1991;3:99–108.
3. Ernst PB, Befus AD, Bienenstock J. Leukocytes in the intestinal epithelium: an unusual immunologic compartment. *Immunol Today* 1985;6:50–55.

4. McGhee JR, Kiyono H. Mucosal immunity to vaccines: current concepts for vaccine development and immune response analysis. *Adv Exp Med Biol* 1992;327:3–12.
5. London SD, Cebra JJ, Rubin DH. Intraepithelial lymphocytes contain virus-specific, MHC restricted cytotoxic T cell precursors after gut mucosal immunization with reovirus serotype 1/lung. *Reg Immunol* 1989;2:98–102,
6. Offit PA, Dudzik KI. Rotavirus-specific cytotoxic T lymphocytes appear at the intestinal mucosa surface after rotavirus infection. *J Virol* 1989;63:3507–3512.
7. Fujihashi K, Taguchi T, McGhee JR, et al. Regulatory function for intraepithelial lymphocyte: two subsets of CD3$^+$, T cell receptor-1$^+$ intraepithelial lymphocyte T cells abrogate oral tolerance. *J Immunol* 1990;145:2010–2019.
8. Fujihashi K, Taguchi T, Aicher WK, et al. Immunoregulatory function for murine intraepithelial lymphocytes: γ/δ T cells abrogate oral tolerance, while α/β TCR$^+$ T cells provide B cell help. *J Exp Med* 1992;175:695–707.
9. Guy-Grand D, Griscelli C, Vassalli P. The mouse gut T lymphocytes, a novel type of T cell: nature, origin, and traffic in mice in normal and graft-versus-host conditions. *J Exp Med* 1978;148:1661–1677.
10. Petit A, Ernst PB, Befus AD, Clark DA, Rosenthal KL, Ishizaka T, Bienenstock J. Murine intestinal intraepithelial lymphocytes. I: Relationship of a novel Thy-1$^-$, Lyt-1$^-$, Lyt-2$^+$ granulated subpopulation to natural killer cells and mast cells. *Eur J Immunol* 1985;15:211–215.
11. Lefrançois L. Phenotypic complexity of intraepithelial lymphocytes of the small intestine. *J Immunol* 1991;147:1746–1751.
12. Mosley RL, Styre D, Klein JR. CD4$^+$ CD8$^+$ murine intestinal intraepithelial lymphocytes. *Int Immunol* 1990;2:361–365.
13. Aicher WK, Fujihashi K, Taguchi T, et al. Intestinal intraepithelial lymphocyte T cells are resistant to lpr gent-induced T cell abnormalities. *Eur J Immunol* 1992;22:137–145.
14. Taguchi T, Aicher WA, Fujihashi K, Yamamoto M, McGhee JR, Bluestone JA, Kiyono H. Novel function for intestinal intraepithelial lymphocytes: murine CD3$^+$, γ/δ TCR$^+$ T cells produce IFN-γ and IL-5. *J Immunol* 1991;147:3736–3744.
15. Goodman T, Lefrançois L. Expression of the γ-δ T cell receptor on intestinal CD8$^+$ intraepithelial lymphocytes. *Nature* 1988;333:855–858.
16. Bonneville M, Janeway CA Jr, Ito K, Haser W, Ishida I, Nakanishi N, Tonegawa S. Intestinal intraepithelial lymphocytes are distinct set of γδ T cells. *Nature* 1988;336:479–481.
17. Mosley RL, Whetsell M, Klein JR. Proliferative properties of murine intestinal intraepithelial lymphocytes (IEL): IEL expressing TCR αβ or TCR γδ are largely unresponsive to proliferative signals mediated via conventional stimulation of the CD3-TCR complex. *Int Immunol* 1991;3:563–569.
18. Guy-Grand D, Cerf-Bensussan N, Malissen B, Malassis-Seris M, Briottet C, Vassalli P. Two gut intraepithelial CD8$^+$ lymphocyte populations with different T cell receptors: a role for the gut epithelium in T cell differentiation. *J Exp Med* 1991;173:471–481.
19. Challacombe SJ, Tomasi TB Jr. Systemic tolerance and secretory immunity after oral immunization. *J Exp Med* 1980;152:1459–1472.
20. Kiyono H, McGhee JR, Wannemuehler MJ, Michaleck SM. Lack of oral tolerance in C3H/HeJ mice. *J Exp Med* 1982;155:605–610.
21. Mowat AM. The regulation of immune responses to dietary protein antigens. *Immunol Today* 1987;8:93–98.
22. Tomasi TB Jr. Oral tolerance. *Transplantation* 1980;29:353–356.
23. Suzuki I, Kiyono H, Kitamura K, Green DR, McGhee JR. Abrogation of oral tolerance by contrasuppressor T cells suggests the presence of regulatory T-cell networks in the mucosal immune system. *Nature* 1986;320:451–454.
24. Suziki I, Kitamura K, Kiyono H, Kurita T, Green DR, McGhee JR. Isotype-specific immunoregulation: evidence for a distinct subset of T contrasuppressor cells for IgA responses in murine Peyer's patches. *J Exp Med* 1986;164:501–516.
25. Kitamura K, Kiyono H, Fujihashi K, Eldridge JH, Green DR, McGhee JR. Contrasuppressor cells that break oral tolerance are antigen-specific T cells distinct from T helper (L3T4$^+$), T suppressor (Lyt-2$^+$) and B cells. *J Immunol* 1987;139:3251–3259.
26. Fujihashi K, Kiyono H, Aicher WK, et al. Immunoregulatory function of CD3$^+$, CD4$^-$ and CD8$^-$ T cells: γδ TCR-positive T cells from nude mice abrogate oral tolerance. *J Immunol* 1989;143:3415–3422.

27. Bonneville M, Itohara S, Krecko EG, et al. Transgenic mice demonstrate that epithelial homing of γ/δ T cells is determined by cell linages independent of T cell receptor specificity. *J Exp Med* 1990;171:1015–1026.
28. Gershon RK, Eardley DD, Durum S, et al. Contrasuppression: a novel immunoregulatory activity. *J Exp Med* 1981;153:1533–1546.
29. Kiyono H, Green DR, McGhee JR. Contrasuppression in the mucosal immune system. *Immunol Res* 1988;7:67–81.
30. Beagley KW, Eldridge JH, Lee F, et al. Interleukins and IgA synthesis: human and murine interleukin 6 induce high rate IgA secretion in IgA-committed B cells. *J Exp Med* 1989;169:2133–2148.
31. Taguchi T, McGhee JR, Coffmann RL, et al. Analysis of Th1 and Th2 cells in murine gut-associated tissue: frequencies of CD4$^+$ and CD8$^+$ T cells that secrete IFN-γ and IL-5. *J Immunol* 1990;145:68–77.
32. Mosmann TR, Coffman RL. TH1 and TH2 cells: different patterns of lymphokine secretion lead to different functional properties. *Annu Rev Immunol* 1989;7:145–173.
33. Fujihashi K, Yamamoto M, McGhee JR, et al. Intraepithelial T lymphocytes and cytokines for the maintenance of oral tolerance. *Adv Exp Med Biol* 1993;*in press.*
34. Porcelli S, Brenner MB, Greenstein JL, Balk SP, Therhorst C, Bleiche PA. Recognition of cluster of differentiation 1 antigens by human CD4$^-$, CD8$^-$ cytolytic T lymphocytes. *Nature* 1989;341:447–450.
35. Faure F, Jitsukawa S, Miossec C, Hercend T. CD1c as a target recognition structure for human T lymphocytes: analysis with peripheral bood γ/δ cells. *Eur J Immunol* 1990;20:703–706.
36. Lefrançois L, LeCorre R, Mayo J, Bluestone JA, Goodman T. Extrathymic selection of TCR γδ$^+$ T cells by class II major histocompatibility complex molecules. *Cell* 1990;63:333–340.
37. Kozbor D, Trinchieri G, Monos DS, et al. Human TCR-γ$^+$/δ$^+$, CD8$^+$ T lymphocytes recognize tetanus toxoid in an MHC-restricted fashion. *J Exp Med* 1989;169:1847–1851.
38. Fujihashi K, Yamamoto M, McGhee JR, Kiyono H. α/β TCR$^+$ IELs with CD4$^+$, CD8$^-$ and CD4$^+$, CD8$^+$ phenotypes from orally-immunized mice possess type 2 helper function for B cell responses; *J Immunol.*
39. von Boehmer H. The developmental biology of T lymphocytes. *Ann Rev Immunol* 1988;6:309–326.
40. Taguchi T, McGhee JR, Coffman RL, Beagley KW, Eldridge JH, Takatsu K, Kiyono H. Detection of individual mouse splenic T cells producing IFN-γ and IL-5 using the enzyme-linked immunospot (ELISPOT) assay. *J Immunol Methods* 1990;128:65–73.
41. Fujihashi K, McGhee JR, Beagley KW, McPherson DT, McPherson SA, Huan C-M, Kiyono H. Cytokine-specific ELISPOT assay: single cell analysis of IL-2, IL-4, and IL-6 producing cells. *J Immunol Methods* 1993;160:181–189.
42. Fujihashi K, Yamamoto M, Beagley KW, McGhee JR, Kiyono H. Function of intraepithelial lymphocytes: α/β TCR bearing CD4$^+$, CD8$^-$ and CD4$^+$, CD8$^+$ T cells possess helper activity. *Intern Immunol* 1993; in press.
43. Street NE, Mosmann TR. Functional diversity of T lymphocytes due to secretion of different cytokine patterns. *FASEB J* 1991;5:171–177.
44. Prystowsky MB, Ely JM, Beller DI, et al. Alloactive cloned T cell line. VI: Multiple lymphokine activities secreted by helper and cytolytic cloned T lymphocytes. *J Immunol* 1982;129:2337–2344.
45. Ebert EC. Intra-epithelial lymphocytes: interferon-gamma production and suppressor/cytotoxic activities. *Clin Exp Immunol* 1990;82:81–85.
46. Barrett TA, Gajewski TF, Danielpour D, Chang EB, Beagley KW, Bluestone JA. Differential function of intestinal intraepithelial lymphocyte subsets. *J Immunol* 1992;149:1124–1130.
47. Kelso A, Glasebrook AL. Secretion of interleukin 2, macrophage-activating factor, interferon and colony-stimulating factor by alloreactive T lymphocyte clones. *J Immunol* 1984;132:2924–2931.
48. DiFabio S, Mbawuike IN, Kiyono H, Fujihashi K, Couch RB, McGhee JR. Quantitation of human-influenza-virus specific CTLs: correlation of cytotoxicity and perforin synthesis with increased numbers of interferon gamma producing CD8$^+$ T cells; *submitted for publication.*
49. Al-Dawoud A, Nakshabendi I, Foulis A, Mowat AM. Immunohistochemical analysis of mucosal gamma interferon production in coeliac disease. *Gut* 1992;33:1482–1486.
50. Bluestone JA, Cron RQ, Cotterman M, Houlden BA, Matis LA. Structure and specificity of T cell receptor γ/δ on major histocompatibility complex antigen-specific CD3$^+$, CD4$^-$, CD8$^-$ T lymphocytes. *J Exp Med* 1988;168:1899–1916.
51. Cron RQ, Gajewski TF, Sharrow SO, Fitch FW, Matis LA, Bluestone JA. Phenotypic and func-

tional analysis of murine CD3[+], CD4[−], CD8[−] TCR[−] γ/δ expressing peripheral T cells. *J Immunol* 1989;142:3754–3762.

52. Yamamoto M, Fujihashi K, Beagley KW, McGhee JR, Kiyono H. Cytokine synthesis by intestinal epithelial lymphocytes (IELs): both γ/δ TCR[+] and α/β TCR[+] T cells in the G1 phase of cell cycle produce IFN-γ and IL-5. *J Immunol* 1993;150:106–114.

53. Cross F, Roberts J, Weintraub H. Simple and complex cell cycles. *Annu Rev Cell Biol* 1989;5:341–396.

54. Viney JL, MacDonald TT. Selective death of T cell receptor γ/δ[+] intraepithelial lymphocytes by apoptosis. *Eur J Immunol* 1990;20:2809–2812.

55. Dillon SB, Dalton BJ, MacDonald TT. Lymphokine production by mitogen and antigen activated mouse intraepithelial lymphocytes. *Cell Immunol* 1986;103:326–338.

56. Yamamoto M, Fujihashi K, Amano M, McGhee JR, Beagley KW, Kiyono H. Cytokine synthesis and apoptosis by intestinal intraepithelial lymphocytes: signaling of high density α/β TCR[+] and γ/δ TCR[+] T cells via the TCR-CD3 complex results in IFN-γ and IL-5 production, while low density T cells undergo DNA fragmentation;*submitted for publication.*

57. Mowat AM, MacKenzie S, Baca ME, Felstein MV, Parrott DM. Functional characteristics of intraepithelial lymphocytes from mouse small intestine. II: *In vivo* and *in vitro* responses of intraepithelial lymphocytes to mitogenic and allogenic stimuli. *Immunology* 1986;58:627–634.

58. Mowat AM, McInnes IB, Parrott DM. Functional properties of intra-epithelial lymphocytes from mouse and small intestine I.V. Investigation of the proliferative capacity of IELs using phorbol ester and calcium ionophore. *Immunology* 1989;66:398–403.

59. Ebert EC. Proliferative responses of human intraepithelial lymphocytes to various T-cell stimuli. *Gastroenterology* 1989;97:1372–1381.

60. Andrew W, Andrew V. Mitotic division and degeneration of lymphocytes within the cells of intestinal epithelium in the mouse. *Anat Rec* 1945;93:251–277.

61. Shields J, Touchon R, Dickinson D. Quantitative studies on small lymphocyte disposition in epithelial cells. *Am J Pathol* 1969;54:129–145.

Mucosal Immunology: Intraepithelial Lymphocytes,
edited by H. Kiyono and J. R. McGhee.
Raven Press, Ltd., New York © 1993.

8

Tolerance of Intraepithelial Lymphocytes in the Intestine

Terrence A. Barrett, Ann M. Koons, Jeffrey A. Bluestone*, and
Stephen D. Hurst

*Department of Medicine, Section of Gastroenterology, Lakeside Veterans' Medical Center
and Northwestern University Medical School, 303 E. Chicago Ave.,
Med/GI S207, Chicago, IL, and *Ben May Institute and Department of Pathology,
University of Chicago, Chicago, IL.*

Several groups have demonstrated that potentially self-reactive T cells can be detected in the intestinal epithelial compartment (1–4). In these studies intraepithelial lymphocytes (IELs) were shown to develop in an extrathymic pathway and thus were not subject to normal clonal deletion mechanisms in the thymus (1–4). This suggests that maturation and regulation of regional self-tolerance for IELs may be distinct from previously demonstrated thymic mechanisms. There are several possible reasons for these differences. First, the antigen presenting cell (APC) populations in these two locations may be different. Although thymic T cells interact with bone marrow–derived APCs capable of mediating clonal deletion, intestinal IELs may interact with antigens presented on "nonprofessional" APCs such as epithelial cells. Second, there may be a different profile of lymphokines produced in these locations. It has been demonstrated that lymphokines are involved in the regulation of thymic T cell development (5). In the intestine, the profile of lymphokines as well as their effect on T cell development may be unique. Third, thymic T cell selection is dependent on T cell receptor (TCR) interactions with major histocompatibility complex (MHC) plus self-peptides (6). The APCs involved in IEL development may present a different spectrum of self-peptides, which may influence selection of the IEL TCR repertoire. Finally, compared to thymic development, extrathymic T cell maturation has not been well characterized. The phenotypic and functional properties that distinguish immature from mature IELs are largely unknown. Intraepithelial lymphocytes may interact with self-Ag at a different stage of development compared to thymic T cells. This variable has made it difficult to discriminate between IELs that are unresponsive due to incomplete maturation and those that have undergone tolerance induction. Several model systems have been analyzed which help delineate the similarities and distinctions between thymic and extrathymic mechanisms of tolerance.

TOLERANCE IN THE INTESTINE

The extrathymic pathway of intestinal IEL development was initially examined by Mayerhofer in athymic rats (7). These early findings have been confirmed and expanded in athymic nude mice. These mice are athymic due to a genetic defect and subsequently lack a normal population of T cells in the spleen and lymph nodes. However, CD8$^+$, TCR$^+$ IELs are present in large numbers in the intestine of nude mice. Recently, it has been shown that this lineage of T cells in nude mice uniformly expresses the $\alpha\alpha$ homodimeric form of CD8 (CD8$\alpha\alpha^+$) (3). In contrast, the intestines of normal euthymic mice possess IELs expressing either CD8$\alpha\alpha$ or CD8$\alpha\beta$ isoforms. This observation has suggested that the CD8$\alpha\alpha$ IEL lineage is extrathymically-derived.

The induction of tolerance for $\alpha\beta$ TCR IELs was first examined in Mls-1^a, I-E$^+$ DBA/2 mice based on the approaches used to demonstrate negative selection in the thymus (8–17). In DBA/2 mice, T cells expressing Vβ6, Vβ8.1 (reactive to Mls-1^a), and Vβ11 (reactive to I-E plus self-antigen) are deleted in the thymus and absent in the spleen and lymph nodes. Unexpectedly, these potentially self-reactive TCRs were detected among the CD8$\alpha\alpha^+$ IELs of the intestine. These findings suggest that extrathymically-derived CD8$\alpha\alpha^+$ IELs had bypassed negative selection in the thymus. Furthermore, examination of CD8$\alpha\beta^+$ and CD4$^+$/CD8$^-$ IEL subsets failed to reveal T cells expressing the potentially self-reactive TCRs. The absence of the potentially self-reactive IELs among these subsets may be explained by thymic or extrathymic deletion as described by Poussier et al. (2).

Another approach to examining tolerance in the gut has utilized the TCR transgenic (Tg) mouse specific for the male HY antigen in the context of H-2D^b. In male Tg$^+$ mice, the T cells expressing the self-reactive Tg$^+$ TCR were deleted during thymic development and therefore were absent in the spleen and lymph nodes (8). In the intestine of HY-expressing male Tg$^+$ mice, significant numbers of potentially self-reactive CD8$\alpha\alpha^+$ Tg$^+$ IELs were detected (4). These results provide further evidence that potentially self-reactive IELs may be detected in the CD8$\alpha\alpha^+$ subset.

Recent studies by Poussier et al. (2) have suggested that normal IEL populations can be divided into four distinct phenotypic subsets based on CD4, CD8$\alpha\alpha$, and CD8$\alpha\beta$ expression. Furthermore, potentially self-reactive IELs in CB6F1 (Vβ11$^+$) and DBA/1 (Vβ6$^+$) strains were detected in the CD4$^+$/CD8$\alpha\alpha^+$ and CD4$^-$/CD8$\alpha\alpha^+$ subsets. To test the functional responsiveness of the four subsets, cells were isolated and sorted into four purified populations of $\alpha\beta$ TCR IELs. Each subset was stimulated with anti-$\alpha\beta$TCR mAb (H57-597) or with Con-A. The CD4$^+$/CD8$^-$ and CD4$^-$/CD8$\alpha\beta^+$ subsets proliferated in response to TCR-mediated activation, whereas the CD8$\alpha\alpha^+$ subsets were refractory to TCR-mediated activation. The functional integrity of these four subsets was verified by their ability to proliferate in response to Con-A. Thus, it appeared that the self-reactive IELs detected in CD4$^+$/CD8$\alpha\alpha^+$ and CD4$^-$/CD8$\alpha\alpha^+$ subsets were either nonfunctional or required stimulation other than the TCR for activation.

Next, to examine tolerance within the extrathymically-derived IEL populations, Poussier and coworkers prepared thymectomized, irradiated chimeras. Irradiated

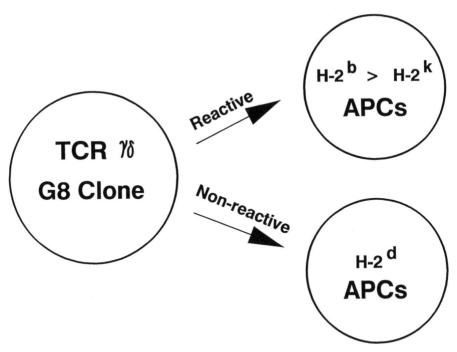

FIG. 1. The γδ TCR G8 clone is alloreactive to an MHC class I, TL gene product expressed by H-2^b and H-2^k, but not H-2^d strains of mice.

Mls-1^b, I-E$^+$ hosts were reconstituted with fetal liver from B6 donor mice (Mls-1^b, I-E$^-$). By flow cytometry these fetal liver chimeras were found to contain all four subsets of gut IELs originally identified in normal animals. Self-reactive Vβ-expressing IELs where not detected in the functional subsets (CD4$^+$, CD8αβ$^+$), which demonstrated that these IELs were deleted in the extrathymic pathway. However, the potentially self-reactive Vβ6 and 11$^+$ IELs were present in the two nonfunctional CD8αα$^+$ subsets. Future studies are needed to resolve whether potentially self-reactive αβ TCR$^+$ IELs were functionally unresponsive due to tolerance induction or immaturity.

γδ TCR TRANSGENIC MICE

In peripheral epithelial tissues, T cells may express the γδ T cell receptor (γδ TCR). These cells comprise a T cell lineage separate from αβ TCR cells and appear to undergo thymic and extrathymic developmental pathways. To examine γδ TCR cell development, Dent et al. (18,19) generated TCR transgenic (Tg) mice expressing an alloreactive γδ TCR. The genes were isolated from an alloreactive BALB/c-derived H-2^d T cell clone (G8) specific for an MHC class I gene product encoded in the TL region of the MHC of H-2^k and H-2^b strains of mice (Fig. 1). This antigen

TABLE 1. *Self-reactive transgenic (Tg) IEL but not splenic T cells can be detected in Ag-bearing mice. Flow cytometry analysis of spleen at 6 weeks and IEL from $Tg^{d/d}$ and $Tg^{b/d}$ mice at 6 weeks and 20 weeks of age. Transgenic cells were not detected in splenic tissue of $Tg^{b/d}$ mice at 20 weeks of age. Quadrants were determined on the basis of control staining with irrelevant hamster FITC and rat PE mAbs. The percentage of positive cells is shown.*

Population	$Tg^{d/d}$	$Tg^{b/d}$
Spleen		
% Tg^+	72	0
% $CD8^+$	8	0
IELs (6 wk)		
% Tg^+	95	75
% $CD8^+$	34	37
IELs (20 wk)		
% Tg^+	91	37
% $CD8^+$	10	45

is expressed ubiquitously in all tissues, including those present in the intestine. Transgenic mice were generated by injecting productively rearranged γ TCR ($V\gamma2/J\gamma1/C\gamma1$) and δ TCR ($V\alpha11/D\delta2/J\delta1/C\delta1$) genomic DNA clones into (C57BL/6 $\times$ BALB/c)F_2 embryos. As shown in Table 1, transgene-expressing (Tg^+) $\gamma\delta$ TCR cells constituted a major component of the spleen of transgenic H-2^d ($Tg^{d/d}$) mice. Transgenic cells in the thymus and spleen of these animals expressed the CD4$^-$/CD8$^-$ phenotype of the G8 $\gamma\delta$ TCR clone. The transgenic receptor was detected using a Vγ2-specific monoclonal antibody, UC3-10A6 (20). Transgenic $\gamma\delta$ TCR splenocytes in these $Tg^{d/d}$ mice could be activated by alloantigen-bearing spleen cells in a pattern similar to the original G8 clone (18).

THE LOCALIZATION OF $\gamma\delta$ TCR TRANSGENIC CELLS IN THE INTESTINE

The pattern of peripheral localization displayed by some subsets of $\gamma\delta$ TCR cells appears to correlate with the expression of selection Vγ regions. Intestinal IELs express Vγ5 at an increased frequency compared to $\gamma\delta$ TCR IELs in other tissues (21 and reviewed by Lefrançois in this text). In the G8 $\gamma\delta$ TCR transgenic mice, a homogeneous population of Vγ2-expressing $\gamma\delta$ TCR cells was examined (22). In previous reports, Vγ2$^+$ $\gamma\delta$ TCR cells have been detected in splenic sinusoidal areas but not commonly among IELs of normal mice (23). Thus, this $\gamma\delta$ TCR transgenic model allowed us to examine whether Vγ2-expressing $\gamma\delta$ TCR cells preferentially localized to selected lymphoid and nonlymphoid compartments in the intestine. The data show that Vγ2$^+$ cells were capable of localizing to all lymphoid compartments of the intestine in $Tg^{d/d}$ mice.

Peyer's patch lymphoid tissue is organized into T cell-dependent and non-T cell dependent areas. Populations of APCs such as B cells and macrophages are present in the non-T cell dependent areas. In Figure 2E, the T cell dependent area of a Peyer's patch from a $Tg^{d/d}$ animal is identified by the high concentration of cells staining with an anti-CD3 mAb. In Fig. 2F, a serial section was stained for transgenic cells using the anti-Vγ2 mAb. The staining pattern suggests that Tg^+ cells are present in the non-T cell area of the Peyer's patch. These data are similar to previously reported localization patterns in the spleen, where $\gamma\delta$ TCR cells have been shown to localize to sinusoidal (non-T cell dependent) areas (23). These cells may have homed to the non-T cell dependent areas in these tissues because they are involved in the initial response to antigen. The precise nature of this involvement, however, is unknown. We have previously shown that activated $\gamma\delta$ TCR IELs produce transforming growth factor β (TGF-β) (24). Studies have shown that TGF-β can initiate Ig class switching, from IgM to IgA (an important immunoglobulin isotype in the intestine) (25). Therefore, one possible role of $\gamma\delta$ TCR cells in intestinal lymphoid tissue may be to regulate antibody responses.

In Fig. 2 at B and D, Tg^+ cells are demonstrated in both the lamina propria and epithelial compartments of duodenal (Fig. 2B) and ileal (Fig. 2D) tissues. Thus, a population of $\gamma\delta$ TCR cells expressing a homogeneous Vγ2$^+$ transgenic TCR was able to home to mucosal surfaces in the intestine. This homing pattern has also been observed in another $\gamma\delta$ TCR Tg model (25). In this $\gamma\delta$ TCR transgenic model, Tg^+ cells were greatly enriched in the intraepithelial compartment. By flow cytometry, the percentage of Tg^+ IELs was found to be typically greater than 90% (Table 1). Transgenic IELs from $Tg^{d/d}$ mice were Thy-1$^+$ and could be divided into CD4$^-$/CD8$\alpha\alpha^+$ and CD4$^-$/CD8$^-$ subsets (1). The high percentage of Tg^+ cells in the epithelial compartment was in contrast to TCR expression observed in splenic and other intestinal lymphoid compartments of $Tg^{d/d}$ mice. This is consistent with the notion that $\gamma\delta$ TCR cells preferentially home to epithelial surfaces. Regardless of the mechanism, these results confirm previous reports (26) that homing to the epithelial compartment is not dependent on expression of a specific V region (e.g., Vγ5 for intestinal IELs) (26).

TOLERANCE OF $\gamma\delta$ TCR CELLS IN G8 TRANSGENIC MICE

To examine tolerance in G8 transgenic mice, Tg^+ founders were bred to Ag-bearing, H-2^b mice, and offspring were screened for the presence of the transgenic construct. As initially reported by Dent et al. (19), transgenic H-2$^{b/d}$ ($Tg^{b/d}$) mice demonstrated that clonal deletion operated in the thymus to maintain tolerance (Table 1). In the thymus of $Tg^{b/d}$ mice, Tg^+ cells expressed the TCR at a ten-fold lower level when compared to Tg^+ TCR expression in $Tg^{d/d}$ mice. This population of TCR^{low} thymocytes may have been immature precursors that had not yet undergone deletion. In any event, these T cells did not efficiently populate the secondary *lymphoid* organs such as the lymph nodes and spleen.

In the intestine, an extrathymic pathway of development has been demonstrated for intraepithelial lymphocytes (2,3,7,27,30) and for some $\alpha\beta$ TCR lamina propria

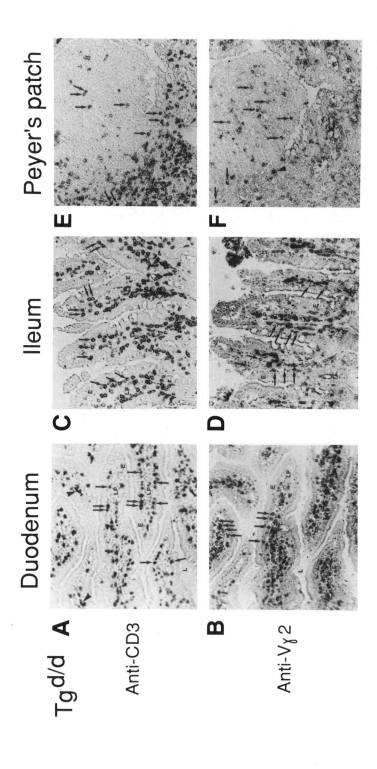

Duodenum   Ileum   Peyer's patch

Tg^d/d

A   C   E

Anti-CD3

B   D   F

Anti-Vγ2

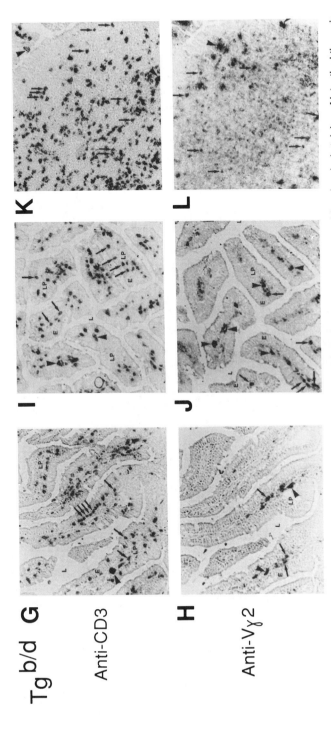

FIG. 2. Self-reactive γδ TCR transgenic cells are present in intestinal epithelial compartment. Immunohistochemical staining of intestinal tissue is shown after serial sections were stained with anti-CD3 (all T cells) and anti-Vγ2 (identifying Tg⁺ cells) mAbs. *Arrows* denote some of the positively stained cells. *Arrowheads* indicate endogenous or nonspecific peroxidase activity. E, epithelium; L, lumen or exterior; LP, lamina propria.

lymphocytes (2). As discussed in the previous section, γδ TCR Tg$^+$ cells were capable of populating all three compartments of the intestine of syngeneic mice. By introducing alloantigen, we were able to examine the mechanisms of tolerance for γδ TCR cells localized to the intestine. In Ag-bearing, Tg$^{b/d}$ mice, Tg$^+$ cells were not detected in lamina propria (Fig. 2I, K). The absence of potentially self-reactive Tg$^+$ cells in this compartment correlated with the absence of these cells from peripheral lymphoid organs. These results parallel other αβ TCR models in that deletion of self-reactive cells was the predominant mechanism for maintaining tolerance (2,28). Tg$^+$ cells were detected in non-T cell dependent areas of Tg$^{b/d}$ Peyer's patches (Fig. 2M). This observation is currently being investigated further. These results may be explained by an extrathymic pathway of development for γδ TCR cells homing to Peyer's patches. Alternatively, these cells may represent Tg$^+$ cells in the process of migrating to the epithelial compartment.

Although alloreactive Tg$^+$ γδ TCR cells were deleted from the thymus, Tg$^+$ IELs were clearly present in significant numbers in the intestinal epithelial compartment of Tg$^{b/d}$ mice (Fig. 2H, J). In order to examine Tg$^+$ γδ TCR cells in Ag-bearing animals in detail, IELs were purified and analyzed by flow cytometry. Analysis of isolated IELs correlated with the immunohistochemistry results and, furthermore, demonstrated that surface density of TCR molecules was equal in Tg$^{d/d}$, Tg$^{b/d}$, and nontransgenic mice (1). In Tg$^{b/d}$ mice a minority of Tg$^+$ IELs were CD8$^+$ (Table 1), whereas the remainder exhibited the same CD4$^-$CD8$^-$ phenotype observed in peripheral *lymphoid* tissue. This demonstrated that CD8α expression was not necessary for homing or localization for γδ TCR IELs.

One difference between Tg$^{d/d}$ and Tg$^{b/d}$ mice was the observation that the percentage of Tg$^+$ γδ TCR IELs in Ag-bearing Tg$^{b/d}$ mice decreased over time compared to Tg$^{d/d}$ mice (Table 1). At 6 weeks of age the percentage of Tg$^+$ IELs in Tg$^{b/d}$ mice was 20% less than in Tg$^{d/d}$ mice. However, in 20-week-old Tg$^{b/d}$ mice the percentage of Tg$^+$ IELs was less than half that observed in Tg$^{d/d}$ mice. These data suggested that deletion or turnover was occurring in epithelial tissues of Ag-bearing animals.

THE PHENOTYPE OF γδ TCR TRANSGENIC IELs

Although histologic data suggested that Tg$^{b/d}$ IELs were not autoaggressive, the question remained: Were IELs from Tg$^{b/d}$ mice functionally immature or had they encountered self-Ag and become tolerant? Our initial approach to this question was to examine the surface phenotype of Tg$^{b/d}$ and Tg$^{d/d}$ IELs. Previous reports from germ-free and nude mice have suggested that Thy-1$^-$ IELs represent a functionally immature subset and that Thy-1 expression may upregulate with antigenic stimulation (reviewed by Lefrançois in this text). It has also been suggested that Thy-1$^-$ T cells in Peyer's patches are terminally differentiated cells that are refractory to stimulation and unable to upregulate Thy-1 (29). The data summarized in Table 2 show that Tg$^+$ IELs from Tg$^{b/d}$ mice were largely Thy-1$^-$. In addition, a small subset

TABLE 2. *IEL from Ag-bearing Tg⁺ mice are largely Thy-1⁻ and express surface activation markers. Cells were gated on the basis of staining with anti-Vγ2 mAb, and percentages of IELs staining with FITC and PE-conjugated mAbs are shown.*

Markers	$Tg^{d/d}$	$Tg^{b/d}$
Thy-1	74%	15%
CD5	21%	7%
CD45R	29%	90%
IL2R	1%	2%
CD44	15%	80%

expressed low levels of Thy-1 (Thy-1^{dul}) with virtually no IELs expressing high levels of Thy-1 as seen on peripheral T cells and $Tg^{d/d}$ IELs. In contrast, the majority of $Tg^{d/d}$ IELs were clearly Thy-1$^+$ with some detectable Thy-1^{dul} expression (30). We also examined CD5 and CD45R/B220 expression, as these markers had previously been observed on Thy-1$^+$ and Thy-1$^-$ IELs respectively, in normal mice (23). In Table 2, expression of CD5 can be seen on greater numbers of $Tg^{d/d}$ IELs, whereas CD45R/B220 is preferentially expressed on $Tg^{b/d}$ IELs. The possibility that these markers identify subsets of IELs derived in the thymic rather than extrathymic pathways is being investigated. Without further data these correlations remain speculative.

It has been suggested that the induction of peripheral tolerance may involve an activation event. Therefore, we examined $Tg^{b/d}$ IELs for surface markers suggestive of an activation event. Specifically, we examined expression of IL-2 receptor (IL-2R) as an early activation marker and CD44 (Pgp-1) as a more stable marker observed on memory T cells (31). Staining of $Tg^{b/d}$ IELs with anti-IL-2Rα mAb was not different from that seen in $Tg^{d/d}$ mice. However, Tg$^+$ IELs from $Tg^{b/d}$ mice expressed greater levels of the activation marker, CD44, as compared to $Tg^{d/d}$ IELs. The increased CD44 expression on $Tg^{b/d}$ IELs suggested that these cells had been previously activated, possibly by alloantigen.

THE FUNCTION OF γδ TCR IELs IN SYNGENEIC AND AG-BEARING MICE

Our initial approach to examine the function of Tg$^+$ γδ TCR cells was to assess the proliferative responses of isolated IELs from $Tg^{d/d}$, $Tg^{b/d}$, and non-Tg mice. The IELs in these experiments were sorted for purity on the basis of expression of the transgenic TCR alone. Intraepithelial lymphocytes from $Tg^{b/d}$ mice were unresponsive when compared to $Tg^{d/d}$ IELs cocultured with Ag$^+$ splenic APCs (Fig. 3A). The nonresponsiveness of the $Tg^{b/d}$ IELs was also demonstrated using anti-Vγ2 mAb-coated plates (1). Since the anti-Vγ2 mAb activates independently of δ usage, the nonresponsiveness of the $Tg^{b/d}$ IELs was not due to their inability to recognize antigen. Furthermore, the lack of proliferation of $Tg^{b/d}$ IELs could not be recon-

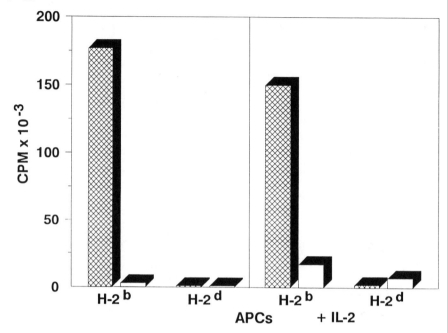

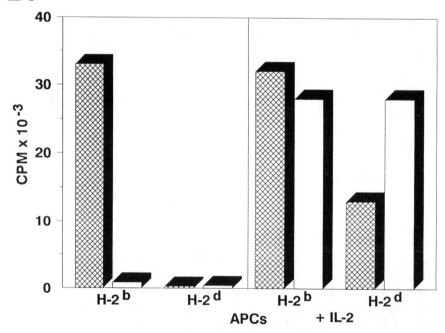

FIG. 3. IELs from Tg$^{d/d}$ but not Tg$^{b/d}$ mice proliferate in response to allogeneic splenocytes. Responder IEL were sorted on the basis ot Tg$^+$ expression **(A)** and for Thy-1^{dul} Tg$^+$ expression **(B)** from Tg$^{d/d}$ (*hatched bars*) and Tg$^{b/d}$ mice (*open bars*). Wells were pulsed for 18 hours with ^{3}H-thymidine after 2 days of culture with H-2^d and H-^{2b} splenocytes, with and without rIL-2.

stituted with exogenous rIL-2. We also demonstrated that $Tg^{b/d}$ IELs did not release detectable levels of IL-2, IL-3, or interferon-γ, whereas $Tg^{d/d}$ IELs were able to release significant levels of all three of these lymphokines (1). Taken together, these initial studies suggested that IELs from $Tg^{b/d}$ mice were unresponsive to TCR-mediated stimulation.

As discussed in the previous section, IELs from $Tg^{d/d}$ and $Tg^{b/d}$ mice expressed distinct levels of Thy-1. We and others have shown that Thy-1$^-$ IELs are functionally inactive as compared to Thy-1$^+$ IELs with regard to cytolytic activity (32), lymphokine production, and proliferation (24). Thus, it was possible that the lack of proliferation observed for $Tg^{b/d}$ IELs was related to the relative inability of Thy-1$^-$ IELs to be activated or proliferate even in the presence of rIL-2. IELs from both $Tg^{d/d}$ and $Tg^{b/d}$ mice had a small population of Thy-1^{dul} cells. In $Tg^{b/d}$ mice these cells may represent cells undergoing clonal inactivation in the Ag$^+$ environment. To examine the proliferative response of Tg$^+$ IELs that express lower levels of Thy-1, Thy-1^{dul} IELs from both $Tg^{d/d}$ and $Tg^{b/d}$ mice were purified and stimulated. As seen in Fig. 3B, Thy-1^{dul} $Tg^{d/d}$ IELs proliferated vigorously. In contrast, purified Thy-1^{dul} IELs from $Tg^{b/d}$ mice proliferated less well to Ag$^+$ splenic APCs, indicative of an unresponsive or anergic state (33). Thus, Tg$^+$ IELs expressing equivalently low levels of Thy-1 were unresponsive in $Tg^{b/d}$ but not $Tg^{d/d}$ mice. Furthermore, addition of rIL-2 reconstituted the proliferative response of Thy-1^{dul} $Tg^{b/d}$ IELs. In fact, the enhanced proliferative response was independent of the presence of allogeneic H-2^b spleen cells. These results suggested that Thy-1^{dul} $Tg^{b/d}$ IELs had failed to proliferate due to a lack of IL-2 secretion. The proliferation of $Tg^{b/d}$ IELs with exogenous rIL-2 and syngeneic spleen suggested that Thy-1^{dul} $Tg^{b/d}$ IELs had previously encountered Ag, which led to upregulation of high-affinity IL-2R. This level of IL-2R may have been undetectable by anti-IL-2R staining (Table 2). Taken together, these data suggested that at least the Thy-1^{dul} IELs from $Tg^{b/d}$ mice had undergone an activation event but had been rendered unresponsive to further TCR-mediated stimulation.

DOWNREGULATION OF THY-1

The previous results suggested that the lower level of Thy-1 expression was correlated with the induction of tolerance. One mechanism that could explain this finding was that Thy-1 was downregulated when IELs encountered self-Ag. Alternatively, Thy-1$^+$ IELs may be deleted resulting in the enrichment of immature Thy-1$^-$ IELs. In order to distinguish these two possibilities, a direct relationship between Ag exposure and Thy-1 downregulation was established. Freshly isolated IELs from $Tg^{d/d}$ mice were sorted on the basis of Thy-1 expression and 10^7 Tg$^+$ Thy-1$^+$ IELs injected into C.B-17, H-2^d and C3H, H-2^k (Ag-bearing) severe combined immunodeficient (SCID) mice. At 6 weeks, IELs were isolated and analyzed by flow cytometry. As shown in Fig. 4A, Thy-1 was expressed by a greater percentage of Tg$^+$ IELs in syngeneic C.B-17 SCID compared to C3H SCID mice. Further-

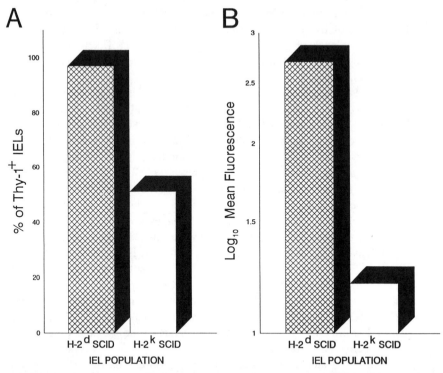

FIG. 4. Thy-1$^+$ IELs from Tg$^{d/d}$ mice downregulate Thy-1 when transferred into Ag-bearing SCID mice. Transgenic IELs from Tg$^{d/d}$ mice were sorted for Thy-1 expression and injected into syngeneic C.B-17 (H-2^d) and Ag-bearing C3H (H-2^k) SCID mice. After 6 weeks IELs were isolated from recipient SCID and analyzed by flow cytometry. **A,** The percentages of Thy-1$^+$, Tg$^+$ IELs isolated from syngeneic (*hatched bars*) and Ag-bearing (*open bars*) SCID. **B,** The mean fluorescence of anti-Thy-1 staining is shown for Tg$^+$ IEL isolated from SCID recipients. Cells were gated on the basis of staining with FITC conjugated anti-V$_\gamma$2 mAb, and results are shown for staining with PE-conjugated anti-Thy-1.

more, the level of Thy-1 expressed by Tg$^+$ IELs in C3H SCIDs was less than 3% of that observed in C.B-17 SCIDs (Fig. 4B). Therefore, a direct relationship between downregulation of Thy-1 and Ag-exposure was demonstrated for Tg$^+$ IELs.

TOLERANCE OF γδ TCR IELs IN BONE MARROW CHIMERAS

We constructed radiation bone marrow (BM) chimeras to examine the role of APC populations in mediating tolerance induction for IELs. The phenotype of Tg$^+$ IELs analyzed 8 weeks after reconstitution is shown in Table 3. In these chimeras, Tg$^+$ IELs developed in the absence of Ag (d/d → d/d), in the presence of Ag restricted to BM-derived APCs (b/d → d/d), in the presence of Ag restricted to radioresistant APCs (d/d → b/d), and when Ag was expressed by both BM-derived and radioresistant APCs (b/d → b/d). The total yields of IEL preparations did not differ significantly among individual euthymic chimeras. Functional analysis revealed that Tg$^+$ IELs that developed in the presence of antigen were unresponsive to Ag (1). These results show that Tg$^+$ IELs could be detected in all four chimera combinations but that significantly fewer Tg$^+$ IELs were present in BM chimeras that expressed Ag. These data correlate with findings from intact Tg$^{b/d}$ mice, where deletion was observed during tolerance induction for IELs (Table 1). Further analysis revealed that the smallest amount of deletion occurred in those chimeras where Ag was restricted to radioresistant APCs (d/d → b/d). In comparison, the percentage of Tg$^+$ IELs was lowest when AG expression was restricted to BM-derived APCs (b/d → d/d). This degree of deletion was greater than that observed when Ag was expressed on both APC populations (b/d → b/d). One interpretation of these data (in b/d → b/d chimeras) is that the induction of clonal energy occurred for IELs that encountered Ag on radioresistant APCs. The induction of clonal anergy may have allowed IELs to "escape" deletion and persist in a nonfunctional state in the epithelial compartment. It should also be noted that in b/d → d/d chimeras, Thy-1 downregulation may have occurred during IEL development outside the intraepithelial compartment. Because there are few BM-derived APCs in the epithelial compartment, it would appear that in b/d → d/d chimeras tolerance occurred prior to localization. These data further suggest that Thy-1 downregulation was a predominant mechanism involved in tolerance induction for γδ TCR IELs.

To examine whether IEL tolerance induction was thymic-dependent, euthymic and thymectomized BM chimeras were constructed. Transgenic IELs isolated from thymectomized BM chimeras resembled euthymic BM chimeras (Table 3) and intact Tg$^{b/d}$ mice (Table 1) by several criteria. First, Tg$^+$ IELs were present in Ag-bearing, thymectomized BM chimeras despite their absence in peripheral *lymphoid* tissue. Second, Tg$^+$ IELs in Ag-bearing mice were largely Thy-1$^-$, whereas

TABLE 3. *Development of transgenic IEL in euthymic and thymectomized radiation chimeras. Chimeras were generated by injecting 10^7 isolated bone marrow (BM) into irradiated euthymic and thymectomized (ATx) recipients as follows: Tg$^{d/d}$ BM into BALB/c (H-2^d) mice (d/d → d/d), Tg$^{b/d}$ BM into BALB/c mice (b/d → d/d), Tg$^{d/d}$ BM into CB6 F1 (H-2$^{b/d}$) mice (d/d → b/d), and Tg$^{b/d}$ BM into CB6 F1 mice (b/d → b/d). Flow- cytometric analysis of IEL isolated from chimeras 8 weeks after reconstitution is shown. The percentage of lymphoid cells that expressed the transgenic TCR was determined using an anti-V$_\gamma$2 mAb (% Tg$^+$). the percentage of Thy-1$^+$ and CD8$^+$ IELs was then calculated for cells that were positive for anti-V$_\gamma$2 staining. The percent of IEL staining positive is based on control staining with irrelevant mAb.*

		Phenotype of Tg$^+$ IELs	
Chimeras	% Tg$^+$	% Thy1$^+$	% CD8$^+$
d/d → d/d	84	90	23
b/d → d/d	19	28	16
d/d → b/d	57	3	78
b/d → b/d	48	14	61
ATx b/d → b/d	72	44	94

Thy-1$^+$ Tg$^+$ IELs predominated in syngeneic Tg$^{d/d}$ mice. Third, Tg$^+$ IELs in thymectomized and euthymic b/d→b/d BM chimeras (Table 3) were largely CD8$^+$, whereas Tg$^+$ IELs in d/d→d/d chimeras and Tg$^{d/d}$ mice (Table 1) were predominantly CD8$^-$. In either case, the persistence of Tg$^+$ IELs in Ag-bearing mice is likely the result of extrathymic development.

SUMMARY

The models of tolerance for αβ TCR and γδ TCR IELs have several features in common. In each model, potentially self-reactive IELs were detected despite deletion of thymic T cells expressing self-reactive TCRs. The explanation for this apparent "escape" from thymic deletion was that IELs were extrathymically-derived. Furthermore, the potentially self-reactive IELs in these models were unresponsive to TCR-mediated activation. This suggests that the IELs had undergone tolerance induction or were unable to be activated by TCR-mediated stimuli, perhaps because of immaturity. Deletion was observed for both αβ TCR and γδ TCR IELs. Populations of αβ TCR IELs known to be functional (CD4$^+$ or CD8αβ$^+$) were deleted in the extrathymic pathway (2). The absence of Thy-1$^+$ γδ TCR Tg$^+$ IELs in Ag-bearing mice suggests that this functionally active subset may have been deleted. Another mechanism for tolerance we suggested was apparent for Tg$^{b/d}$ γδ TCR IELs. These IELs had likely become anergic following an activation event. The induction of clonal anergy among these cells may also have led to clonal deletion. Whether this mechanism accounts for clonal inactivation and deletion of αβ TCR IELs is not known. However, we have observed that in DBA/2 mice potentially self-reactive IELs were predominantly Thy-1$^-$, whereas other Vβ-expressing subsets were largely Thy-1$^+$ (unpublished observations). Thus the induction of tolerance to self-Ag may involve developmental events common for both αβ TCR and γδ TCR cells that shape IEL phenotype and function.

The examination of potentially self-reactive IELs in αβ TCR and γδ TCR models of tolerance has highlighted areas of development that are not well understood. We have repeatedly alluded to the importance of defining the phenotypic and functional properties of IELs. It has been difficult to distinguish between immature IEL precursors and IELs that have been functionally inactivated following encounter with self-Ag. Furthermore, distinct lineages of IELs exist. The variable expression of Thy-1, CD4, CD8αβ, CD8αα, CD5, and CD45R suggests that both thymic and extrathymically derived IELs may express multiple phenotypes in response to distinct developmental pressures. These issues highlight the complexity of IEL development and underscore the need for further examination of well-defined models.

REFERENCES

1. Barrett TA, Delvy M, Kennedy D, et al. Mechanism of self-tolerance of γδ T cells in epithelial tissues. *J Exp Med* 1992;175:65–70.

2. Poussier P, Edouard P, Lee C, Binnie M, Julius M. Thymus-independent development and negative selection of T cells expressing T cell receptor αβ in the intestinal epithelium: evidence for distinct circulation patterns of gut- and thymus-derived T lymphocytes. *J Exp Med* 1992;176:187–199.
3. Rocha B, Vassalli P, Guy-Grand D. The Vβ repertoire of mouse homodimeric α CD8[+] intraepithelial lymphocytes reveals a major extrathymic pathway of T cell differentiation. *J Exp Med* 1991;173:483–486.
4. Rocha B. von Boehmer HP, Guy-Grand D. Selection of intraepithelial lymphocytes with CD8 α/α co-receptors by self-antigen in the murine gut. *Proc Natl Acad Sci USA* 1992;89:5336–5340.
5. Carding SR, Hayday AC, Bottomly K. Cytokines in T-cell development. *Immunol Today* 1991; 12:239–245.
6. Nikolic-Zugic J, Bevan MJ. Role of self-peptides in positively selecting the T-cell repertoire. *Nature* 1990;344:65–67.
7. Mayerhofer G. Thymus-dependent and thymus-independent subpopulations of intestinal intraepithelial lymphocytes: a granular subpopulation of probable bone marrow origin and relationship to mucosal mast cells. *Blood* 1980;55:532–535.
8. Kisielow P, Bluthmann H, Staerz UD, Steinmetz M, von Boehmer H. Tolerance in T-cell-receptor transgenic mice involves deletion of nonmature CD4[+]8[+] thymocytes. *Nature* 1988;333:742–748.
9. Kappler JW, Staerz U, White J, Marrack PC. Self-tolerance eliminates T cell specific for Mls-modified products of the major histocompatibility complex. *Nature* 1988;332:35–40.
10. Pircher H, Burki K, Lang R, Hengartner H, Zinkernagel RM. Tolerance induction in double specific T-cell receptor transgenic mice varies with antigen. *Nature* 1989;342:559–561.
11. MacDonald HR, Schneider R, Lees RK, et al. T-cell receptor Vβ predicts reactivity and tolerance to Mls[a]-encoded antigens. *Nature* 1988;332:40–45.
12. Kappler JW, Roehm N, Marrack P. T cell tolerance by clonal elimination in the thymus. *Cell* 1987;49:273–280.
13. Bill J, Kanagawa O, Woodland DL, Palmer E. The MHC Molecule I-E is necessary but not sufficient for the clonal deletion of Vβ11-bearing T cells. *J Exp Med* 1989;169:1405–1419.
14. Sha WC, Nelson CA, Newberry RD, Kranz DM, Russell JH, Loh DY. Positive and negative selection receptor on T cells in transgenic mice. *Nature* 1988;336:73–76.
15. Rammensee H, Kroschewski R, Frangoulis B. Clonal anergy induced in mature Vβ6 T lymphocytes on immunizing Mls-1[a] expressing cells. *Nature* 1989;339:541–543.
16. Ramsdell F, Lantz T, Fowlkes BJ. A nondeletional mechanism of thymic self-tolerance. *Science* 1989;246:1038–1041.
17. Blackman MA, Gerhard-Burgert H, Woodland DL, Palmer E, Kappler JW, Marrack P. A role for clonal inactivation in T cell tolerance to Mls-1[a]. *Nature* 1988;345:540–544.
18. Houlden BA, Matis LA, Cron RQ, et al. A TCRγδ cell recognizing a novel TL-encoded gene product. *Cold Spring Harbor Symp Quant Biol* 1989; Vol. LIV:45.
19. Dent AL, Matis LA, Hooshmand F, Widacki SM, Bluestone JA, Hedrick SM. Self-reactive γδ T cells are eliminated in the thymus. *Nature* 1990;343:714–719.
20. Bluestone JA, Cron RQ, Cotterman M, Houlden BA, Matis LA. Structure and specificity of T cell receptor on major histocompatibility complex antigen-specific CD3[+], CD4[-], CD8 T lymphocytes. *J Exp Med* 1988;168:1899–1916.
21. Goodman T, Lefrançois L. Intraepithelial lymphocytes: anatomical site, not T cell receptor form, dictates phenotype and function. *J Exp Med* 1989;170:1569–1581.
22. Bluestone JA, Cron RC, Barrett TA, et al. Repertoire development and ligand specificity of murine TCRγδ cells. *Immunol Rev* 1991;120:5–33.
23. Bucy RP, Chen C-LH, Cooper MD. Tissue localization and CD8 accessory molecule expression of TCRγδ cells in human. *J Immunol* 1989;142:3045–3049.
24. Barrett TA, Gajewski T, Chang EB, Beagley K, Bluestone JA. Differential function of intestinal intraepithelial lymphocyte subsets. *J Immunol* 1992;149:1124–1130.
25. Coffman RL, Lebman DA, Shrader B. Transforming growth factor β specifically enhances IgA production by lipopolysaccharide-stimulated murine B lymphocytes. *J Exp Med* 1989;170:1039–1044.
26. Itohara S, Farr AG, Lafaillek JJ. Bonneville M, Takagaki Y, Haas W, Tonegawa S. Homing of a γδ thymocyte subset with homogeneous T-cell receptors to mucosal epithelia. *Nature* 1990;343:754–757.
27. Lefrançois L, LeCorre R, Mayo J, Bluestone JA, Goodman T. Extrathymic selection of TCRγδ T cells by class II major histocompatibility complex molecules. *Cell* 1990;63:333–340.

28. Blackman M, Kappler J, Marrack P. The role of the T-cell receptor in positive and negative selection of developing T-cells. *Science* 1990;248:1335–1341.
29. Harriman GR, Lycke NY, Elwood LJ, Strober W. Lymphocytes that express CD4 and the αβ-T cell receptor but lack Thy-1: preferential localization in Peyer's patches. *J Immunol* 1990;145:2406–2414.
30. Barrett TA, Tatsumi Y, Bluestone JA. Tolerance of TCRγδ cells in the intestine. *J Exp Med* 1993;177:1755–1762.
31. Ernst DN, Hobbs MV, Torbett BE, et al. Differences in the expression profiles of CD45RB, Pgp-1, and 3G11 membrane antigens and in the patterns of lymphokine secretion by splenic CD4[+] T cells from young and aged mice. *J Immunol* 1990;145:1295–1302.
32. Lefrançois L, Goodman T. *In vivo* modulation of cytolytic activity and Thy-1 expression of TCRγδ[+] intraepithelial lymphocytes. *Science* 1989;243:1716–1718.
33. Schwartz RH. A cell culture model for T lymphocyte clonal anergy. *Science* 1990;248:1349–1356.

Mucosal Immunology: Intraepithelial Lymphocytes,
edited by H. Kiyono and J. R. McGhee.
Raven Press, Ltd., New York © 1993.

9

Effector Functions of Human Intraepithelial Lymphocytes

Ellen C. Ebert

Department of Medicine, University of Medicine and Dentistry of New Jersey,
Robert Wood Johnson Medical School, One Robert Wood Johnson Place,
New Brunswick, NJ.

Intraepithelial lymphocytes (IEL) are in a unique location, singly interspersed between intestinal epithelial cells (EC) and next to a basement membrane composed of myofibroblasts. There, the IEL are exposed to antigens presented or released at the basolateral surfaces of EC (1). If the tight junctions between the EC are "loosened," as with interferon-γ (2), the flow of antigens into the intraepithelial space is greater and less selective. Lymphocytes in such a location are likely to function independently of macrophages and other lymphocytes and may instead depend on EC, myofibroblasts, or soluble factors from the lamina propria.

This laboratory has focused on the functions of human IEL, using *in vitro* assays. The most studied of the human intestinal lymphocytes are the lamina propria lymphocytes (LPL) from the colon because of the availability of colonic surgical specimens, which are often resected from elderly patients with cancer. The IEL, a distinct compartment of lymphocytes with phenotypes and functions that differ from LPL, have been studied infrequently because they are difficult to isolate in large numbers from colonic mucosa, and because surgical specimens of jejunum, from which IEL can be isolated in abundance, are scarce. The advantages of using jejunal mucosa obtained from gastric bypass operations for morbid obesity are that the patients are young and healthy and that IEL and LPL can be isolated together and compared. Using this uniform, abundant source of IEL, the phenotype and functions of this unusual compartment of lymphocytes have been investigated.

ISOLATION OF IEL

In order to isolate IEL (3,4), the jejunal mucosa is first treated with dithiothreitol to dissociate the superficial mucus layer, which interferes with subsequent cell separations. The IEL and EC are then separated from the lamina propria by vigorous shaking in a solution of ethylenediamine tetraacetic acid in a medium without calcium and magnesium ions. The cells collected in the supernates contain IEL and EC. All of the IEL are viable, whereas the majority of EC from jejunal villi, which are terminally differentiated, die during the isolation. Crypt EC from colon, in contrast, are predominantly undifferentiated, proliferating cells that maintain their viability for a short time after separation. The IEL are separated from EC using a discontinuous density gradient of Percoll. This procedure results in a cell preparation containing over 90% lymphocytes, with a phenotype expected of IEL (see below). In order to isolate LPL, the remaining tissue is partially digested with collagenase for 4 hours. The tissue is then pressed through a wire mesh to release the remaining cells. The LPL are also purified by a density gradient. This method yields 100 to 300 million IEL and 40 to 80 million LPL from a 40 cm^2 piece of jejunal mucosa.

The effect of this isolation procedure on the IEL was determined by treating PBL in the same manner. Of the many functions tested, only the detection of vasoactive intestinal peptide (VIP) receptors on PBL was altered (5). But, because the IEL are protected by being embedded in tissue, they are probably less exposed to the treatments than are PBL in suspension.

PHENOTYPE OF IEL

Flow cytometric analysis reveals that the majority of IEL have the same size and granularity as PBL (Fig. 1), indicating that most are *not* large, granular lymphocytes. They are $93 \pm 5\%$ CD2$^+$, $83 \pm 8\%$ CD3$^+$, $6 \pm 6\%$ CD4$^+$, $83 \pm 7\%$ CD5$^+$, and $89 \pm 2\%$ CD8$^+$. The mean densities of CD2, CD3, and CD8 antigens are the same on IEL and PBL. Only CD5 expression is lower on IEL (4). Immunohistochemical studies show a large fraction of IEL to be CD5$^-$ (6), perhaps because this less sensitive technique does not identify lymphocytes with a low density of CD5.

The majority of CD3$^+$ IEL have a T cell receptor (TCR) of the α/β type. This contrasts with murine intestinal IEL, which mainly express $\gamma\delta$ TCR. Single-sided polymerase chain reaction (PCR) amplification cloning and quantitative PCR amplification of the TCR chains from fresh IEL demonstrate that IEL are oligoclonal in their TCR expression, although the predominant V-α and V-β types differ from one individual to the next (7). Oligoclonal TCR expression also occurs in LPL, with most V-α and V-β chains being different from those in autologous IEL (8).

PROLIFERATION AND LYMPHOKINE PRODUCTION BY IEL

IEL proliferate only minimally in response to mitogens, such as phytohemagglutinin (PHA); to superantigens, such as staphylococcal enterotoxin B (SEB); and to antibody to CD3 (4,9). This low proliferative response is only minimally increased by the addition of recombinant interleukin-2 (IL-2) or by autologous irradiated peripheral blood (PB) monocytes, and is unaffected by the addition of recombinant IL-1β, IL-4, or IL-6.

In contrast, IEL proliferate vigorously to stimuli of the CD2 molecule, such as

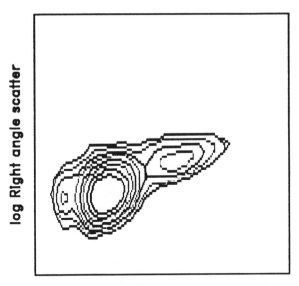

Forward angle scatter

FIG. 1. Flow cytometry plot depicting subpopulations of IEL according to relative size (forward angle scatter) and granularity (right angle scatter). There are two predominant lymphocyte populations: the smaller, less granular one (Map 1) and the larger, more granular one (Map 2).

the mitogenic antibodies, $T11_2$ and $T11_3$, or the combination of PHA and sheep red blood cells (SRBC). The minimal proliferative response of IEL to PHA is accompanied by low IL-2 production and receptor generation. These events of activation are markedly augmented, however, when IEL are cultured with SRBC in addition to PHA. The production of the cytokines, IL-2 and interferon-γ (IFNγ), by IEL is also markedly increased by stimulation through CD2 rather than CD3 (10). A similar preferential activation through the CD2 molecule has been shown using LPL (11), suggesting that this is a property of all lymphocytes in the intestinal mucosa.

CYTOTOXIC ACTIVITY BY IEL

The location of IEL, adjacent to EC, suggests that they may play a role in the destruction of dysplastic or frankly malignant EC. Several mechanisms may be involved: spontaneous cytotoxicity (SC), lymphokine-activated killer (LAK) activity, and cytotoxic T lymphocyte (CTL) activity.

In the circulation, SC activity, the lysis of target cells by freshly isolated unprimed lymphocytes, is due to natural killer (NK) cells. But the SC activity of IEL is different from such NK activity (12; Table 1). The effector cells in IEL are

TABLE 1. *Comparison of the SC Activity by IEL to the NK Activity by PBL*

	SC activity by IEL	NK activity by PBL
Effector cell		
Phenotype	$CD2^+CD3^+CD4^-CD8^+$ $CD16^-NKH1^-$	$CD2^+CD3^-CD4^-CD8^-$ $CD16^+NKH1^+$
Response to IFN-γ	None	Increased lytic activity
Target cell susceptibility	EC tumors	EC tumors and K-562 cells

$CD2^+CD3^+CD4^-CD8^+CD16^-NKH1^-$, whereas NK cells in peripheral blood lymphocytes (PBL) are $CD2^+CD3^-CD4^-CD8^-CD16^+NKH1^+$. Preincubation of effector cells with IFNγ has no effect on the lytic activity of IEL, but markedly increases the lytic activity of PBL. IEL will spontaneously kill EC tumors, but not the highly NK-sensitive K-562 cells, whereas NK cells in peripheral blood lyse both target cell types. These findings suggest that IEL specifically destroy EC tumors using a mechanism that differs from that of circulating lymphocytes.

IEL are capable of LAK activity that is *not* target cell restricted (10). The precursor LAK IEL and LPL are mainly of the $CD4^-CD8^-$ phenotype, as opposed to the $CD8^+$ IEL responsible for SC activity (13). The target cell restriction of one, but not the other, activity is probably due to differences in the phenotypes of the cytotoxic cells and mechanisms of action. Also, LAK activity is not enhanced by the addition of SRBC to the culture, as is the proliferative response of IEL. This, too, is a consequence of the different phenotypes involved, since proliferation is carried out predominantly by the $CD8^+$ IEL.

CTL activity, an important host defense against malignancies and infections, is manifested by murine IEL (14) but not human LPL (15). When lymphocytes were cultured with irradiated allogeneic PBL for 5 days (stimulator cells), peripheral blood $CD8^+$ T lymphocytes lysed fresh PBL, whereas IEL and LPL did not (16). Since the irradiated stimulator PBL are still intact after 7 days in culture (which is not true for murine splenocytes), they may reduce apparent cytotoxicity by acting as unlabeled targets in the cytotoxicity assay. To avoid this problem, the sensitizing culture was extended. That is, intestinal lymphocytes were cultured with allogeneic PBL and IL-2 for 17 days; fresh medium and IL-2 were added on days 7 and 14. Cytotoxic activity of the effector cells was then tested against the same PBL used as stimulator cells and against novel PBL, so that CTL activity could be differentiated from background LAK activity. The difference in cytotoxicity was defined as CTL activity. In this system, IEL and LPL *did* demonstrate CTL activity, although the cytotoxic activity by IEL was significantly less than that by PB $CD8^+$ T lymphocytes. This difference may be due, in part, to the rapid growth in this system of $CD4^+$ IEL, which, after 17 days, represented 15 to 30% of the IEL.

BINDING OF IEL TO COLON CANCER CELLS

IEL demonstrate SC and LAK activities against EC tumors; therefore the binding of effector to target was evaluated because this is an initial event in cytotoxicity

Proposed mechanism:

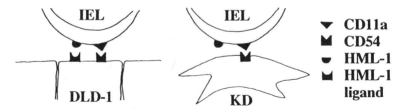

FIG. 2. Proposed mechanism of IEL binding to DLD-1 (colonic adenocarcinoma) and KD (fibroblast) cell lines. The binding to DLD-1 cells occurs by the adhesion of CD11a and HML-1 surface receptors on IEL to their complementary ligands, CD54 and an undefined molecule, respectively, on DLD-1 cells. In contrast, IEL bind to KD by the CD11a/CD54 interaction, but not HML-1. (Illustration by Arthur I. Roberts.)

(17). When a monolayer of DLD-1 cells (colonic adenocarcinoma) was incubated with radiolabeled lymphocytes at 37°C, it bound a larger fraction of IEL than PBL. IEL also adhered to other EC tumor lines, such as HT-29 (colonic adenocarcinoma) and 5637 (bladder epidermoid carcinoma), as well as to the nonepithelial tumor A375 (malignant melanoma); all cell lines were obtained from American Type Culture Collection, Rockville, MD. Binding to EC tumors was totally inhibited by antibody to HML-1 in combination with antibody to either CD11a or CD54. IEL also bound, but to a much lesser extent, to the nonmalignant monolayers of KD (lip fibroblast) and HISM (jejunal smooth muscle). This binding, however, was inhibited by antibodies to CD11a and CD54, but not by antibody to HML-1 (Fig. 2).

ENVIRONMENTAL FACTORS

The IEL may be influenced by their surroundings: epithelial cells, myofibroblasts, and factors secreted by the lamina propria. The neuropeptides, VIP and substance P (SP), were evaluated in depth, since both are found in high concentrations in the intestinal mucosa and modulate immune responses in other systems (18). VIP receptors were found on PBL (both CD4$^+$ and CD8$^+$ T lymphocytes) but not on IEL or LPL, although treating PBL in the same manner as IEL resulted in some decrease in VIP receptor expression (5). SP receptors were not found on IEL or LPL (19). Furthermore, SP receptors were not detected on PBL, despite reports to the contrary (20). In addition, these neuropeptides did not alter the proliferation or SC activity of IEL.

SUMMARY

The study of jejunal IEL from patients undergoing gastric bypass operations for morbid obesity has several advantages: (a) the large number and purity of IEL isolated from jejunal mucosa, (b) the uniformity of the intestinal specimens resected, and (c) the health and youth of the individuals studied.

Jejunal IEL have many unique features. These lymphocytes, predominantly CD8[+] T cells, have oligoclonal $\alpha\beta$ TCR expression. This may dictate their reactivity to a limited range of stimuli, perhaps resulting in tolerance to food antigens and commensal bacteria. The proliferative responses and production of IL-2 or IFN-γ by IEL are much greater after stimulation through the CD2 molecule than through CD3. The CD8[+] IEL are responsible for SC selectively directed against EC tumors, but not the highly NK-susceptible K-562 cells. In contrast, the CD4[-]CD8[-] IEL are responsible for LAK activity against both target types. IEL bind to colon cancer cells by the interaction of HML-1 and CD11a on IEL to an undefined ligand and CD54 on the cancer cell. Binding of IEL to mesenchymal cells involves the CD11a/CD54 interaction, but not HML-1. The specificity of SC against EC tumors and the phenotypic resemblance of IEL to lymphocytes infiltrating colon cancer (21) suggest that IEL may contribute to the initial immune defense against dysplastic EC or *in situ* colonic adenocarcinomas. IEL may also be involved in the development of an immune response to deleterious agents. Studies of their functions *in vitro* will provide clues to their role in the human intestine.

ACKNOWLEDGMENTS

This work was supported by a grant from the National Institutes of Health (DK 42166). The author would like to thank Arthur I. Roberts for his technical expertise and advice and Robert E. Brolin, M.D., for providing jejunal tissue.

REFERENCES

1. Russell GJ, Walker WA. Role of the intestinal mucosal barrier and antigen uptake. In: Targan SR, Shanahan F, eds. *Immunology and immunopathology of the liver and gastrointestinal tract*. New York: Igaku-Shoin Medical Publishers; 1990:15–31.
2. Madara JL, Stafford J. Interferon-gamma directly affects barrier function of cultured intestinal epithelial monolayers. *J Clin Invest* 1989;83:724–727.
3. Ebert EC, Roberts AI, Brolin RE, Raska K. Examination of the low proliferative capacity of human jejunal intraepithelial lymphocytes. *Clin Exp Immunol* 1986;65:148–157.
4. Ebert EC. Proliferative responses of human intraepithelial lymphocytes to various T-cell stimuli. *Gastroenterology* 1989;97:1372–1381.
5. Roberts AI, Panja A, Brolin RE, Ebert EC. Human intraepithelial lymphocytes: immunomodulation and receptor binding of vasoactive intestinal peptide. *Dig Dis Sci* 1991;36:341–346.
6. Selby WS, Janossy G, Bofill M, Jewell DP. Intestinal lymphocyte subpopulations in inflammatory bowel disease: an analysis by immunohistological cell isolation techniques. *Gut* 1984;25:32–40.
7. Balk SP, Ebert EC, Blumenthal RL, McDermott FV, Wucherpfennig K, Landau SB, Blumberg RS. Oligoclonal expansion and CD1 recognition by human intestinal intraepithelial lymphocytes. *Science* 1991;253:1411–1415.
8. Blumberg RS, Yockey C, Gross GG, Ebert EC, Balk SP. Human intestinal intraepithelial lymphocytes are derived from a limited number of T cell clones that utilize multiple VβF cell receptor genes. *J Immunol* 1993;150:5144–5153.
9. O'Connell SM, Roberts AI, Ebert EC. The CD2 receptor regulates the proliferation of intraepithelial lymphocytes in response to phytohemagglutinin but not to staphylococcal enterotoxin B. *Gastroenterology* 1992;102(4):A673(abst).

10. Ebert EC. Intra-epithelial lymphocytes: interferon-gamma production and suppressor/cytotoxic activities. *Clin Exp Immunol* 1990;82:81–85.
11. Qiao L, Schurmann G, Betzler M, Meuer SC. Activation and signaling status of human lamina propria T lymphocytes. *Gastroenterology* 1991;101:1529–1536.
12. Taunk J, Roberts AI, Ebert EC. Spontaneous cytotoxicity of human intraepithelial lymphocytes against epithelial cell tumors. *Gastroenterology* 1992;102:69–75.
13. Ebert EC, Roberts AI. Lymphokine-activated killing by human intestinal lymphocytes. *Cell Immuno* 1993;146:107–116.
14. Ernst PB, Clark DA, Rosenthal KL, Befus AD, Bienenstock J. Detection and characterization of cytotoxic T lymphocyte precursors in the murine intestinal intraepithelial leukocyte population. *J Immunol* 1986;136:2121–2126.
15. MacDermott RP, Bragdon MJ, Jenkins KM, Franklin GO, Shedlofsky S, Kodner IJ. Human intestinal mononuclear cells. II: Demonstration of a naturally occurring subclass of T cells which respond in the allogeneic mixed leukocyte reaction but do not affect cell-mediated lympholysis. *Gastroenterology* 1981;80:748–757.
16. Ebert EC. Do the CD45RO⁺CD8⁺ intestinal intraepithelial T lymphocytes have the characteristics of memory cells? *Cell Immunol* 1993;147:331–340.
17. Roberts AI. O'Connell SM, Ebert EC. Intestinal intraepithelial lymphocytes bind to colon cancer cells by HML1 and CD11a. *Cancer Res* 1993;53:1608–1611.
18. Payan DG, Goetzl EJ. Modulation of lymphocyte function by sensory neuropeptides. *J Immunol* 1985;135:783–786.
19. Roberts AI, Taunk J, Ebert EC. Human lymphocytes lack substance P receptors. *Cell Immunol* 1992;141:457–465.
20. Payan DG, Brewster DR, Missirian-Bastian A, Goetzl EJ. Substance P recognition by a subset of human T lymphocytes. *J Clin Invest* 1984;74:1532–1539.
21. Jarry A, Cerf-Bensussan, N, Brousse N, Guy-Grand D, Muzeau F, Potet F. Same peculiar subset of HML1⁺ lymphocytes present within normal intestinal epithelium is associated with tumoral epithelium of gastrointestinal carcinomas. *Gut* 1988;29:1632–1638.

Mucosal Immunology: Intraepithelial Lymphocytes,
edited by H. Kiyono and J. R. McGhee.
Raven Press, Ltd., New York © 1993.

10

Development and Function of Human Intraepithelial Lymphocytes

Jo Spencer* and Thomas T. MacDonald†

*Department of Histopathology, University College and Middlesex School of Medicine,
University St., London, England, and †Department of Paediatric Gastroenterology,
St Bartholomew's Hospital, West Smithfield, London, England.*

Our knowledge of the origin, diversity and function of intraepithelial lymphocytes (IEL) in experimental animals is increasing rapidly, although many fundamental questions remain unanswered. Studies of human tissue so far have concluded that IEL in humans and experimental animals differ in many of their most fundamental characteristics, and it is important therefore that they are considered independently. In this chapter, we discuss the ontogenic development of IEL in humans, their origin, and their function.

ONTOGENY OF HUMAN IEL

In humans, IEL can be identified between the intestinal epithelial cells around the time of development of villus and crypt structures, at 10 to 11 weeks gestation (1,2). In an electron micrographic study, 3 IEL/1000 enterocytes were identified at 11 weeks gestation, increasing to 28 IEL/1000 epithelial cells by 16 weeks. Occasional clusters of cells were observed, but most cells were single and situated basally in the epithelium at both proximal and distal ends of the fetal intestine (2).

More recent immunohistochemical studies have shown that most of the IEL in the fetus are $CD3^+$ (Fig. 1) (3). A non-T cell ($CD7^+$, $CD3^-$), non-NK cell population, present in the tips of the villi in human postnatal intestine (4), is absent in the fetus (5), suggesting that this population matures later or accumulates postnatally in response to food or intestinal bacteria. This cell type may be a precursor of a subgroup of T cells, since in long-term cultures blood $CD7^+$, $CD3^-$ lymphocytes have been shown to give rise to $\alpha\beta$ TCR^+ and $\gamma\delta$ TCR^+ T cells (6). Densely granulated IEL have not been identified in the fetus, but all IEL from fetal tissue have been shown to contain one or more lysosomal granules (2).

The T cell subpopulations present in fetal intestine differ from those in postnatal intestine. As in postnatal intestine, fetal IEL are different from the T cells that

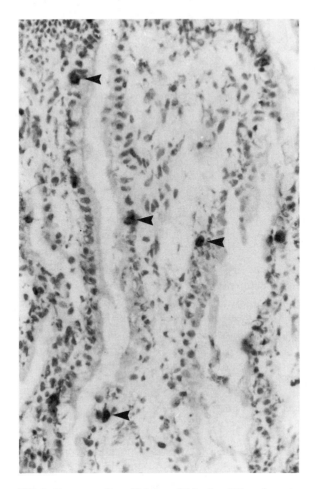

FIG. 1. Frozen section of fetal small intestine (17 weeks gestation) stained using anti-CD3. T cells are clearly indentifiable between the epithelial cells (*arrow- heads*). Immunoperoxidase, original magnification × 125.

develop in other lymphoid tissues (3). T cells in tissues such as fetal lymph node, Peyer's patch, and spleen, and in the intestinal lamina propria are mostly CD4$^+$, whereas CD4$^+$ T cells are rare in fetal intestinal epithelium (3,7,8). A graph showing the appearance of CD3$^+$, CD5$^+$, CD8$^+$, and CD4$^+$ IEL in the fetus with increasing age is shown in Fig. 2, and a comparison of subpopulations present in the fetus at 20 weeks compared with postnatal IEL subpopulations is shown in Table 1.

In adult intestine, the majority of CD3$^+$ IEL co-express CD8 (9), whereas in the fetus only approximately one-half of the CD3$^+$ IEL co-express CD8. The CD5$^+$ IEL population is also reduced in the fetus (3). The double negative (CD4$^-$, CD8$^-$)

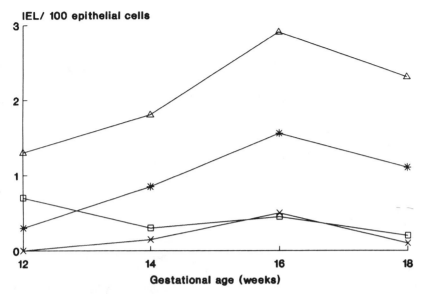

FIG. 2. Intraepithelial lymphocytes expressing CD3 (*triangles*) and CD8 (*asterisks*) increase in density in the epithelium between 12 and 18 weeks gestation. Relatively few fetal IEL express CD4 (*squares*) or CD5 (*X*).

IEL population, which comprises approximately 6% of adult CD3$^+$ IEL (4), is expanded as a proportion of the T cells in the fetus (5). The double negative cells have been shown in adults to express the $\gamma\delta$ TCR rather than the more commonly expressed $\alpha\beta$ form of the TCR (10,11). In adults, the $\gamma\delta$ TCR expressed by T cells from peripheral blood differs from that expressed by IEL. Whereas the Vδ2 gene

TABLE 1. *IEL subpopulations in the fetal small intestine at 20 weeks in comparison with the populations present in adult tissues*

IEL phenotype	20-week fetus	Adult
CD3$^+$, CD4$^-$, CD8$^+$ (%CD3)	45	80
CD3$^+$, CD4$^-$, CD8$^-$ (%CD3)	50	6
CD7$^+$, CD3$^-$ (%CD7)	0	15
CD5$^+$ (%CD3)	17	53
$\gamma\delta$ TCR (%CD3)	25	12
Vδ1$^+$ (%CD3)	0	4
Vδ2$^+$ (%CD3)	25	1

segment is preferentially expressed by peripheral blood T cells, the Vδ1 segment is preferentially expressed by IEL (12,13). This is not the case in the fetus. The Vδ1-expressing IEL are not detectable in fetal intestinal epithelium despite ardent searching in many immunoperoxidase stained specimens (12). This result is particularly surprising considering that Vδ1[+] cells account for 50% of the γδ TCR[+] T cells in cord blood (14). The Vδ2-expressing IEL and the total γδ TCR[+] T cell population detected by antibodies to the constant region of the delta chain are approximately the same percentage of the total CD3[+] population in the fetus (12). The number of IEL expressing Vδ2 in the fetus as a percentage of the total cells in the epithelium (including the epithelial cells) is approximately equivalent to the number of IEL expressing Vδ2 as a percentage of the total cells in the epithelium in adult life (12). This suggests that the intraepithelial Vδ2 population remains stable throughout life and that the increase in Vδ1 cells postnatally may be environmentally driven, as is thought to occur in the blood. A similar situation with γδ TCR[+] T cells occurs in mice, where the number of γδ TCR[+] IEL is the same in germ-free and conventional mice, the increase in IEL in the latter being due to an expansion of αβ TCR[+] T cells (15).

Like adult IEL, fetal IEL express the mucosal lymphocyte antigen HML1, which is a novel α chain, disulphide linked to a β7 integrin molecule (16,17). HML1 has been shown to be inducible on peripheral T cells by prolonged mitogenic stimulation (18). In the human fetus, it is unlikely that there is sufficient exogenous antigenic stimulation to induce HML1 expression, and, in addition, no CD25[+] cells are present in normal fetal intestinal lamina propria or Peyer's patches (19). It is more likely that HML1 is induced locally on T cells in the gut, probably by TGF-β (20).

There is a gap in our knowledge of the number of IEL in the last 20 weeks of gestation. The number of CD3[+] IEL has not been determined in newborn infants. There clearly must be an increase in number between the fetus and the infant, where the IEL density is approximately the same as in normal adults (5,9,21). The relative degree of expansion in the antigen-free gut preterm and after birth is still unknown. In a single 1-day-old newborn, there were very few CD3[+] IEL in the small bowel (22).

ORIGIN OF HUMAN IEL

Several observations have clearly illustrated the origin of IEL from cells in the lamina propria. Morphologically, IEL can be observed to have trailing cytoplasmic pseudopods in a direction that suggests that they can migrate back and forth between the epithelium and the lamina propria. The epithelial basement membrane has been shown to be punctured around the sites of IEL, which is thought to reflect migration through the basement membrane from the lamina propria (2,23). In a dynamic study in isolated explants of human fetal intestine in which lamina propria T cells were stimulated with mitogenic concentrations of anti-CD3 antibody, the origin of HML1[+] IEL from activated lamina propria cells was demonstrated (16).

It is not known whether any human IEL, like γδ TCR⁺ T cells in mice, mature independently of the thymus. Extrathymic changes in the ratio of Vδ1:Vδ2 in the γδ TCR⁺ T cell population have been reported to occur after birth, with a gradual expansion of the Vδ1-expressing population (14). The appearance of IEL in humans at 10 to 11 weeks corresponds with the appearance of the first thymic emigrants. Thymus tissue with epithelial and stromal cells is identifiable in the fetus at around 6 weeks gestation (24). CD3⁺ cells with αβ TCR are present by 10 weeks gestation, by which time cortical and medullary zones are identifiable (25). γδ TCR⁺ T cells are rare in the thymus at this time (0.02% total thymocytes), but they undergo a substantial 35-fold increase in number at 14 weeks gestation. Most of the γδ TCR⁺ T cells in the thymus express the Vδ1 gene segment. Cells expressing the Vδ2 segment are rare (26). This suggests that if either of these populations matures extrathymically, it would be more likely to be the Vδ2-expressing population. Supporting this idea in adult tissues, no change in peripheral T cells expressing Vδ2 was observed in a study of a patient with thymic atresia (27). The early appearance of Vδ2⁺ IEL in the fetus may be due to lack of need for thymic selection. In adult tissues, however, T cells expressing Vδ2 are a minority population of γδ TCR⁺ T cells in the gut.

A reduction in the total number of IEL in the elderly has been observed, although the particular subsets of IEL that change have not yet been determined (28).

Studies in rats have suggested that epithelial class II antigens and the presence of IEL are associated, and that epithelial class II is induced by factors derived from IEL (29). In humans these are clearly unrelated because IEL are observed from 14 weeks gestation, but the earliest time at which epithelial class II expression has been observed is 19 weeks gestation (30).

FUNCTION OF HUMAN IEL

One of the first studies of isolated human IEL showed that they are capable of cytotoxic activity in a mitogen-induced system, but that they differ in the targets they are able to kill when compared to cells isolated from the lamina propria or blood (31). More recent studies have shown that IEL do not kill the K562 cell line, which is highly sensitive to NK activity, but that they do kill targets of epithelial origin (32,33), suggesting that IEL or a subpopulation of IEL may function as a surveillance system to detect and kill infected or defective epithelial cells. The effector cells that kill epithelial cells are CD8⁺ T cells, and the activity cannot be increased by IFN-γ, indicating that these cells are fully activated *in vivo*.

The recognition element for IEL on target/presenting cells is not known. It has recently been shown that CD1d of the CD1 a-d group of nonpolymorphic MHC class I-like glycoproteins is expressed by intestinal epithelial cells. IEL lines have been shown to have cytolytic activity against class I negative cell lines transfected with CD1a-d. This activity was greatest against the CD1c transfectants, and it was shown to be mediated by the TCR/CD3 complex (34). Although CD1c is not expressed by intestinal epithelium, it is possible that it could be induced in inflammation, in which case it could be a ligand involved in the selection of cytotoxic IEL populations. Since CD1d is constitutively expressed (35), it has been proposed that it may be involved in IEL selection, if indeed this occurs in the epithelium in humans.

Suppression of lamina propria and peripheral blood cell proliferation by activated IEL has also been observed, and this has led to speculation that these cells may be involved in oral tolerance (36). However, since IEL are granulated, it is difficult to exclude the possibility that the suppression is due to the cytotoxic effect of proteases in the IEL granules.

Human IEL rarely proliferate *in situ*, but the rate of division is increased in enteropathies such as coeliac disease (37). However, isolated IEL have poor proliferative responses to most T cell mitogens, although they produce cytokines in response to the same stimuli (38,39,40). Recent attempts to define the stimuli that induce IEL proliferation have shown that cytokines can enhance mitogen-induced proliferation, but that stimulation indexed by CD25 expression is low nevertheless. Maximal proliferation of IEL has been achieved through the stimulation of the CD2 molecule. This has been shown in IEL to be more efficient than crosslinking the TCR complex using antibodies to CD3 (41).

SUMMARY

IELs are present in human fetal intestine from 10-11 weeeks gestation. They are predominantly CD3$^+$. Approximately 45% of CD$^+$ IELs express CD8 and 50% are double negative. In postnatal tissues, double negative T cells predominantly express the $\gamma\delta$ TCR, the majority of which in the intestine use Vδ 1. In the fetus $\gamma\delta$ T cells expressing Vδ 1 are absent and T cells using Vδ 2 are present with the same frequency per 100 cells in the epithelium as in the adult. If, as in mice, a sub-population of $\gamma\delta$ intraepithelial T cells matures extrathymically, it is likely to be that using Vδ 2.

Functionally, IELs have cytotoxic activity against epithelial rather than NK sensitive target cells. Although the restriction element for IEL function is not known, the potential of CD1 to fulfill this role is currently being explored.

REFERENCES

1. Moxey PC, Trier JS. Specialized cell types in the fetal human intestine. *Anat Rec* 1978;191:269–286.
2. Orlic D, Lev R. An electron microscopic study of intraepithelial lymphocytes in human fetal small intestine. *Lab Invest* 1977;37:554–561.
3. Spencer J, Dillon SB, Isaacson PG, MacDonald TT. T cell subclasses in fetal small intestine. *Clin Exp Immunol* 1986;65:553–558.
4. Spencer J, MacDonald TT, Diss TC, Walker-Smith JA, Ciclitira PJ, Isaacson PG. Changes in intraepithelial lymphocyte sub-populations in coeliac disease and enteropathy associated T cell lymphoma (malignant histiocytosis of the intestine). *Gut* 1989;30:339–346.

5. Spencer J, Isaacson PG, Walker-Smith JA, MacDonald TT. Heterogeneity of intraepithelial sub-populations in fetal and postnatal intestine. *J Pediatr Gastroenterol Nutr* 1989;9:173–177.
6. Preffer FI, Kim CW, Fischer KH, Sabga EM, Kradin RL, Colvin RB. Identification of pre-T cells in human peripheral blood: extrathymic differentiation of CD7$^+$, CD3$^-$ cells into CD3$^+$ γ/δ$^+$ or α/β$^+$ T cells. *J Exp Med* 1989;170:177–190.
7. Spencer J, MacDonald TT, Finn T, Isaacson PG. Development of gut associated lymphoid tissue in the terminal ileum of fetal human intestine. *Clin Exp Immunol* 1986;64:536–43.
8. Namikawa R, Mizuno T, Matsuoka, et al. Ontogenetic development of T and B cells and non-lymphoid cells in the white pulp of the human spleen. *Immunology* 1986;57:61–69.
9. Selby WS, Janossy G, Bofill M, Jewell DP. Intestinal lymphocyte sub-populations in inflammatory bowel disease: an analysis by immunohistological and cell isolation techniques. *Gut* 1984;25:32–40.
10. Brenner MB, McLean J, Dialynas DP, et al. Identification of a putative second T-cell receptor. *Nature* 1986;322:145–149.
11. Groh V, Porcelli S, Fabbi M, et al. Human lymphocytes bearing T cell receptor γ/δ are phe-notypically diverse and evenly distributed throughout the lymphoid system. *J Exp Med* 1989;169:1277–1294.
12. Spencer J, Isaacson PG, Diss TC, MacDonald TT. Expression of disulphide linked and non-di-sulphide linked forms of the T cell receptor gamma/ delta heterodimer in human intestinal intra-epithelial lymphocytes. *Eur J Immunol* 1989;19:1335–1338.
13. Halstensen TS, Scott H, Brandtzaeg P. Intraepithelial T cells of the TcRγ/δ$^+$CD8$^+$ and Vδ1/Jδ1$^+$ phenotypes are increased in coeliac disease. *Scand J Immunol* 1989;30:665–672.
14. Parker CM, Groh V, Band H, et al. Evidence for extrathymic changes in the T cell receptor γ/δ repertoire. *J Exp Med* 1990;171:1597–1612.
15. Bandeira A, Mota-Santos T, Itohara S, Degermann S, Heusser C, Tonegawa S, Coutinho A. Local-ization of γ/δ T cells to the intestinal epithelium is independent of normal bacterial colonization. *J Exp Med* 1990;172:239–244.
16. Monk T, Spencer J, Cerf-Bensussan N, MacDonald TT. Activation of mucosal T cells *in situ* with anti-CD3 antibody: phenotype of the activated T cells and their distribution within the mucosal micro-environment. *Clin Exp Immunol* 1988;74:212–22.
17. Cerf-Bensussan N, Jarry A, Brousse N, Lisowska-Grospierre B, Guy Grand D, Griscelli C. A monoclonal antibody (HML1) defining a novel membrane molecule present on human intestinal lymphocytes. *Eur J Immunol* 1987;17:1279–1283.
18. Schieferdecker HL, Ullrich R, Weiss-Breckwoldt AN. The HML1 antigen is an activation antigen. *J Immunol* 1990;144:2541–2549.
19. MacDonald TT, Spencer J. Evidence that activated mucosal T cells play a role in the pathogenesis of enteropathy in the human small intestine. *J Exp Med* 1988;167:1341–1349.
20. Parker CM, Cepek KL, Russell GJ. A family of β7 integrins on human mucosal lymphocytes. *Proc Natl Acad Sci USA* 1992;89:1924–1928.
21. Spencer J, Isaacson PG, MacDonald TT, Thomas AJ, Walker-Smith JA. Gamma/delta T cells and the diagnosis of coeliac disease. *Clin Exp Immunol* 1991;85:109–113.
22. Russell GJ, Bhan AK, Winter HS. The distribution of T and B lymphocyte populations and MHC class II expression in human fetal and post-natal intestine. *Pediatr Res* 1990;27:239–244.
23. Toner PG, Ferguson A. Intraepithelial cells in the human intestinal mucosa. *J Ultrastruct Res* 1971;34:329–344.
24. Goldstein G, MacKay IR. *The human thymus.* Glasgow: Glasgow University Press; 1969.
25. Campana D, Janossy G, Coustan-Smith E, Amlot PL, Tian W-T, Ip S, Wong L. The expression of the T cell receptor associated proteins during T cell ontogeny in man. *J Immunol* 1989;142:57–66.
26. Bottino C, Tambussi G, Ferrini S, et al. Two subsets of human T lymphocytes expressing the γ/δ antigen receptor are identifiable by monoclonal antibodies directed to two distinct molecular forms of the receptor. *J Exp Med* 1988;168:491–505.
27. Geisler C, Pallesen G, Platz P, et al. Novel primary thymic defect with T lymphocytes expressing γ/δ T cell receptor. *J Clin Pathol* 1989;42:705–711.
28. Arranz E, O'Mahony S, Barton JR, Ferguson A. Immunosenescence and mucosal immunity: signif-icant effects of old age on secretory IgA concentration and intraepithelial lymphocyte counts. *Gut* 1992;882–886.
29. Cerf-Bensussan N, Quaroni A, Kurnick JT, Bhan AK. Intraepithelial lymphocytes modulate Ia expression by intestinal epithelial cells. *J Immunol* 1984;132:2244–2252.

30. MacDonald TT, Weinel A, Spencer J. HLA-DR expression in human fetal intestinal epithelium. *Gut* 1988;29:1324–1348.
31. Chiba M, Bartnik W, ReMine SG, Thayer WR, Shorter RG. Human colonic intraepithelial and lamina proprial lymphocytes: cytotoxicity *in vitro* and the potential effects of the isolation method on their functional properties. *Gut* 1981;22:177–186.
32. Taunk J, Roberts AI, Ebert EC. Spontaneous cytotoxicity of human intraepithelial lymphocytes against epithelial cell tumors. *Gastroenterology* 1992;102:69–75.
33. Cerf-Bensussan N, Guy-Grand D, Griscelli C. Intraepithelial lymphocytes of human gut: isolation, characterisation and study of natural killer activity. *Gut* 1985;26:81–88.
34. Balk SP, Ebert EC, Blumenthal RL, McDermott FV, Wucherpfennig KW, Landau SB, Blumberg RS. Oligoclonal expansion and CD1 recognition by human intestinal intraepithelial lymphocytes. *Science* 1991;1411–1415.
35. Blumberg RS, Terhorst C, Bleicher P, et al. Expression of a nonpolymorphic MHC class I-like molecule, CD1D, by human intestinal epithelial cells. *J Immunol* 1991;147:2518–2524.
36. Hoang P, Dalton HR, Jewell DP. Human colonic intraepithelial lymphocytes are suppressor cells. *Clin Exp Immunol* 1991;85:498–503.
37. Halstensen TS, Brandzaeg P. Activated T cells in the coeliac lesion: non-proliferative activation (CD25) of CD4$^+$ α/β cells in the laminapropria but proliferation of α/β and γ/δ cells in the epithelium. *Eur J Immunol* 1993;23:505–510.
38. Greenwood JH, Austin LL, Dobbins WO. *In vitro* characterization of human intraepithelial lymphocytes. *Gastroenterology* 1983;85:1023–1035.
39. Ebert EC, Roberts AI, Raska RE, Raska K. Examination of the low proliferative capacity of human jejunal intraepithelial lymphocytes. *Clin Exp Immunol* 1986;65:148–157.
40. Ebert EC. Intraepithelial lymphocytes: interferon-gamma production and suppressor cytotoxic activities. *Clin Exp Immunol* 1990;82:81–85.
41. Ebert EC. Proliferative responses of human intraepithelial lymphocytes to various T cell stimuli. *Gastroenterology* 1989;97:1372–1381.

Mucosal Immunology: Intraepithelial Lymphocytes,
edited by H. Kiyono and J. R. McGhee.
Raven Press, Ltd., New York © 1993.

11

Phenotypic Characteristics of Human Intraepithelial Lymphocytes

Trond S. Halstensen and Per Brandtzaeg

*Laboratory for Immunohistochemistry and Immunopathology (LIIPAT),
Institute of Pathology, University of Oslo, The National Hospital,
Rikshospitalet, Oslo, Norway.*

Human CD8[+] T cells are, for reasons as yet unknown, preferentially located in the gut epithelium (reviewed in refs. 1,2). Such intraepithelial lymphocytes (IEL) are relatively numerous in the small intestine but less so in colonic mucosa, gastric mucosa (4), and airways; and they are quite rare in the epidermis (3–6). This review will focus on the phenotypic characteristics of human intestinal IEL and discuss some of their functional implications.

T CELL RECEPTOR (TCR) USAGE OF HUMAN IEL

Human IEL share many features with murine IEL but show some important differences. While a high proportion (50 to 90%) of murine small intestinal and skin IEL express γ/δ TCR (7–9), rat (10) and human (11–12) small intestinal IEL are mainly $\alpha\beta$ TCR[+] and human IEL express both the α and β chain of CD8 (13). Moreover, only a small fraction (2 to 8%) of human IEL normally express $\gamma\delta$ TCR (11–20), and these are mainly (75%) negative for CD8α and CD4 (16). This is in contrast to murine $\gamma\delta$ TCR[+] IEL that express the CD8α homodimer (21–22). The large intestine has a lower density of IEL, and its proportion of $\gamma\delta$ TCR[+] cells is higher (23).

Immunohistochemical examination of small (16) and large (23) intestinal IEL has revealed that the $\gamma\delta$ TCR[+] cells are only 25 to 50% or less positive for CD8α *in situ* and that none expresses CD4. However, flow-cytometric analysis of isolated IEL has suggested that all of the small intestinal (24) and 58% of the large intestinal (25) $\gamma\delta$ TCR[+] cells express CD8α. Methodological differences might partly account for this discrepancy, and one possibility is that the isolation procedure could induce CD8α expression. Nevertheless, both *in situ* (16) and flow-cytometric two-color immunofluorescence (26) examinations of IEL in the celiac lesion showed that less than 10% of the $\gamma\delta$ TCR[+] IEL co-expressed CD8α.

Most $\gamma\delta$ TCR[+] IEL (50 to 70%) in the normal human intestine use the Vδ1 chain as detected by mAb A13 (27), usually (about 67%) in conjunction with the joining segment Jδ1 detected by mAb δTSC1 (16,17). This is in contrast to peripheral blood, where the same phenotypic subset accounts for only 30% of the γδ TCR$^+$ cells; the remaining circulating fraction uses Vδ2 (mAb BB3$^+$, ref. 27) in conjunction with Vγ9 (28). This subset is predominantly found in the lamina propria (23), especially in celiac disease (17, Halstensen unpublished). By flow-cytometric analysis, however, isolated IEL from normal small intestinal mucosa have been reported to contain an equal proportion of Vδ1$^+$ and V δ2$^+$ IEL (13), contrasting the immunohistochemical findings mentioned above. Although isolated IEL may become contaminated with Vδ2$^+$ T cells from the lamina propria, individual variations are also often large *in situ*.

The restricted usage of Vδ segments suggests that human IEL are oligoclonal. Although murine γδ TCR$^+$ IEL use predominately Vγ7/Vδ4 or Vγ6 TCR gene products (8), they show an extensive junctional diversity (29,30). The predominant αβ TCR$^+$ CD8$^+$ human IEL subset has recently been shown to be oligoclonal with individual skewing of TCR β-chain usage (31–33). Whether this expression pattern is a general phenomenon throughout the intestinal tract, perhaps being influenced by an individual's HLA-class I or II phenotype, or whether the oligoclonality is topical and influenced by the local microenvironment, is currently unknown. However, colonic mucosa contain significantly fewer IEL than the small intestine, despite a much higher microbial load. Luminal bacterial products (superantigens?) might therefore be of less importance for human IEL density and TCR usage than food antigens.

HUMAN IEL ARE PHENOTYPICALLY MEMORY CELLS

The CD45 complex comprises high-molecular-weight (180 to 220 kDa) membrane glycoproteins expressed on cells of hematopoietic origin (Fig. 1). Variable expression of three alternatively splicing exons (A, B, and C) gives rise to five identified CD45 isoforms preferentially on different subsets of lymphocytes (34). Various mAbs reacting selectively with some CD45 isoforms are referred to as CD45R (restricted) antibodies. CD45RA mAb (restricted to an exon A-encoded epitope) recognizes the larger 220-kDa and 205-kDa forms of CD45 that use exons ABC and AB, respectively; mAb PD/7/a26 recognizes an exon B-encoded epitope (CD45RB) and reacts therefore with the same CD45 isoforms as CD45RA mAb in addition to the 205-kDa and 190-kDa exon BC- and B-encoded isoforms, respectively; and mAb UCHL1 recognizes only the shortest 180-kDa isoform that lacks exon A-, B-, and C-encoded parts (35), giving rise to its designation CD45R0 (36).

CD4$^+$ T cells have been divided into functional subsets on the basis of their reactivity with mAbs specific for CD45RA and CD45R0 (36). Naive or unprimed T cells express the 220-kDa CD45RA isoform, whereas T cells responding to recall antigens ("memory" cells) express high levels of the 180-kDa isoform CD45R0 (reviewed in 37). Intermediate-sized CD45 isoforms encoded either by exon A and B (205 kDa), exon B and C (205 kDa), or exon B only (190 kDa) are, in addition, variably expressed on both functional T cell subsets.

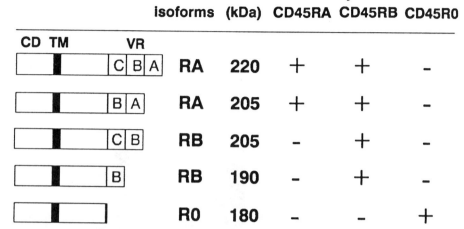

FIG. 1. Schematic depiction of the five identified human CD45 isoforms, variably expressed on subsets of lymphocytes by alternative splicing of exons A, B, and C: mAb to CD45RA recognizes the 220-kDa and 205-kDa products encoded by exons ABC and AB, respectively; mAb PD/7/26/16 to CD45RB recognizes, in addition, the 205-kDa and 190-kDa products encoded by exons BC and B; and mAb to CD45R0 (UCHL1) recognizes the 180-kDa isoform that lacks exon A, B, and C products. CD, cytoplasmic domain; TM, transmembrane part; VR, variable region. (Modified from ref. 40.)

Very few IEL express CD45RA in the normal human intestine; and by *in situ* immunohistochemical examination only 35 to 60% of normal small intestinal CD3$^+$ IEL express high enough levels of CD45R0 to be regarded as positive (38–40). These CD8$^+$, $\alpha\beta$ TCR and $\gamma\delta$ TCR$^+$ IEL subsets that are CD45RA$^-$CD45R0^{low} express preferentially the CD45RB isoform (Fig. 2) (40,41). This pattern is similar to that of murine IEL, which preferentially use exon 5 alone (comparable to human 190-kDa CD45RB), or together with exon 4 (comparable to human 205-kDa CD45RBC) or exon 6 (comparable to human 205-kDa CD45RBA) (42). Low levels of the 180-kDa CD45R0 were also noted on the murine IEL (42). This agrees with the low levels of CD45R0 observed on IEL *in situ* (38–41). However, flow-cytometric analysis of isolated human CD3$^+$ IEL has revealed that the majority express CD45R0 (13, Halstensen et al. unpublished). Perhaps IEL rapidly increase their CD45R0 expression as a result of activation induced by the isolation procedure.

HUMAN IEL EXPRESS SPECIFIC ADHESION MOLECULES

The mechanisms for entry of IEL into the epithelium have recently been explored. Cerf-Bensussan and colleagues (43) first showed that IEL express the epitope for mAb HML-1. This mAb identifies an adhesion molecule belonging to the integrin family consisting of a $\beta7$ chain associated with a new α chain designated α^E

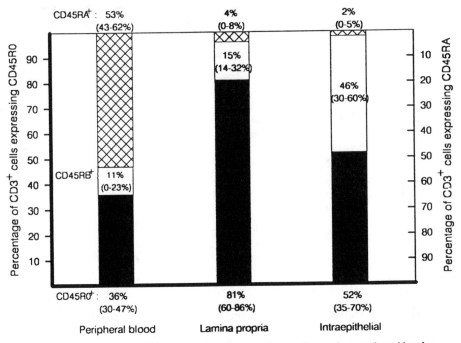

FIG. 2. Percentage of CD3[+] T lymphocytes (median and range) scored positive for CD45RA (*cross-hatched*), CD45R0 (*solid*), or solely for CD45RB (*open*) in peripherial blood, small intestinal mucosa, and jejunal villous epithelium in healthy controls. (Modified from ref. 40.)

(44–47). Other mAbs, such as BP6 (47), B-ly7 (48,49), and Ber-ACT8 (50), also react with this integrin. Almost all (about 90%) IEL, as well as approximately 40% of the lamina propria lymphocytes (LPL), express this molecule according to flow-cytometric analyses (13). Immunofluorescence staining *in situ* suggests that IEL in celiac disease express $\alpha^E\beta7$ at a considerably higher level than T cells in the lamina propria (Halstensen, unpublished). The murine homologue to human integrin $\beta7$ has recently been cloned, and the integrin $\alpha^4\beta7$ was suggested to be a Peyer's patch (PP) adhesion molecule (51,52). It is of interest that human CD3[+] LPL express integrin $\alpha4$ but has little or no detectable $\beta1$ (53), perhaps reflecting that human T cells also use $\alpha^4\beta7$ to enter gut mucosa. Migration from the lamina propria into the epithelium might, therefore, involve a shift in expression of the integrin α chain only (from $\alpha4$ to α^E).

ARE IEL SUPPRESSOR OR CYTOTOXIC CELLS?

Whether human CD8[+] IEL are involved in "oral tolerance" (anergy/suppression?) or mediate cytotoxicity is a question of continuing debate. The functional phenomenon oral tolerance to nonadherent food antigens appears generally accepted, but the putative T cell subset inducing or contributing to such immunological downregulation remains unknown. Although mitogen-activated IEL do not suppress mitogen-induced antibody production (54) or proliferation of peripherial blood lymphocytes (PBL) (55,56) to the same extent as CD8$^+$ PBL do (55), they suppress PHA-induced proliferation of autologous LPL *in vitro* (56).

A high proportion of human IEL contain granules (57,58) and have staining characteristics compatible with the large granular lymphocytes observed in rodent epithelium (59). However, human $\alpha\beta$ TCR$^+$ IEL do not appear to have classical natural killer cell (NK) activity and few IEL express traditional NK cells markers (CD16, CD56) (60,61). Unstimulated IEL are unable to lyse the NK-sensitive cell lines K562 and Daudi. Although interleukin 2 (IL-2)-activated IEL induced some lysis of the former, the latter cell line remains unlysed (55,60). These results suggest target cell specificity, and it has recently been shown that human CD3$^+$, CD8$^+$ IEL preferentially lyse cell lines of epithelial origin (62).

Isolated murine IEL express perforin and granzyme transcript and show strong cytotoxicity in CD3-stimulated "redirected" lysis assays, regardless of TCR phenotype (63–65). However, granulated metrial gland cells in pregnant murine uterus is the only IEL type that has been reported to bind monoclonal or polyclonal antibodies to perforin (66). Both murine (63,65,67) and human (59–60) IEL are phenotypically heterogeneous, suggesting that various subsets might have different functions. Human peripheral blood $\gamma\delta$ TCR T cells contain perforin and serine esterase (68), and $\gamma\delta$ TCR T cell clones from the celiac lesion lyse NK-sensitive targets such as K562, Molt 4, and Daudi cell lines (69). These result suggest that $\gamma\delta$ TCR$^+$ IEL have NK-like cytotoxic potential.

MHC-restricted cytotoxic CD8$^+$ T cells express the accessory molecule CD28 (reviewed in ref. 70). Flow-cytometric examination (mAb 9.3) has shown that most normal human CD3$^+$ IEL are negative for CD28 (71) in contrast to CD3$^+$ LPL, which express this marker *in situ* (mAb Kolt-2; Halstensen, unpublished). Of interest in this context is the finding that human "suppressor" T-cell clones lack CD28 (72).

Stimulated human IEL produce IFN-γ (55), and 10 to 15% of IEL in normal small intestine contain immunohistochemically detectable IFN-γ (73). IFN-γ is toxic to many of the target cells used in cytotoxic assays. These assays may, therefore, to some extent reflect both cytokine-induced and cell to cell contact dependent, perforin-mediated lyses of target cells. Production of IFN-γ by IEL may, however, have a more fundamental role in mucosal immune regulation *in vivo*. Murine $\gamma\delta$ TCR$^+$ IEL have been shown to abrogate oral tolerance (74) and may produce both IFN-γ and IL-5 after activation (75), whereas $\gamma\delta$ TCR$^+$ IEL provide antigen specific B cell help (76). Others have found that stimulated murine IEL produce an array of cytokines such as IL-2, IL-3, IL6, TNF-α, TGF-β1, and IFN-γ, but not IL-5 or IL-4 (77). The IEL are most presumably a heterogeneous population with different functional properties. The immunoregulatory result may depend on the relative proportion and antigen specificity of the various IEL subsets.

EXTRATHYMIC MATURATION OF IEL

Leukocyte stem cells in the bone marrow express CD34 a marker that is not present on IEL (Halstensen, unpublished). However, IEL show a high level of the Fcμ receptor CD7 but less CD5 (78,79). CD7 is also expressed on CD3⁻ pre-T cells in the thymus. Most intense expression of CD7 is observed on the few CD3⁻ IEL (1 to 5% of IEL). This subset differs from peripheral CD7⁺ NK cells by lacking NK markers such as CD56, CD16, or CD8 (59).

Experiments in mice have suggested that IEL expressing only the CD8α homodimer bypass thymic selection and mature within the intestinal epithelium (80,81). Moreover, murine IEL have been shown to contain the recombination activation gene RAG-1, supporting local TCR rearrangment and extrathymic maturation (82). In humans 10 to 20% of IEL have been reported to express the CD8α homodimer only (13). Moreover, flow-cytometric analyses have suggested that approximately 8% of IEL in normal human small intestine coexpress CD4 and CD8 (24), a population that abounds in the thymus. Two-color immunofluorescence examination of IEL *in situ*, however, has revealed few such "double positive" T cells, which were mainly observed in celiac disease (Halstensen, unpublished). Nevertheless, the interesting possibility exists that the CD3⁻ CD7⁺ IEL represent pre-T cells that undergo extrathymic maturation in the intestinal epithelium.

PHENOTYPIC ALTERATIONS OF IEL IN CELIAC DISEASE (GLUTEN-SENSITIVE ENTEROPATHY)

The pathogenic mechanism by which gluten causes jejunal crypt hyperplasia and villous atrophy in celiac disease is unclear, but the strikingly increased density of IEL (reviewed in refs. 1,2) has suggested that this T-cell subset participates significantly in the development of the intestinal lesion. We (16) and others (11,17,83,84) have shown that there is a remarkably increased fraction of γδ TCR⁺ IEL in both untreated and treated (gluten-free diet) celiac disease [Fig. 3; and see Color plate (A) between pages 154 and 155]. By *in situ* two-color immunohistochemical examination we found that the median percentage of CD3⁺ IEL expressing γδ TCR increased from 2% in controls to 20% in untreated celiac disease (range 11 to 53%). The increased percentage persisted after gluten restriction even when the jejunal morphology improved (median 23%, range 16 to 55%). Most γδ TCR⁺ IEL (80 to 90%) were CD4⁻ CD8α⁻ *in situ*, and 67% (58 to 94%) used TCR Vδ1/Jδ1 as revealed by mAb δTCS1. This increase in γδ TCR⁺ IEL appears rather specific for celiac disease (85) as it is generally not observed in tropical sprue (17), cows milk intolerance (17), inflammatory bowel disease (IBD) (86), gastritis (84), or lymphocytic colitis (87, Halstensen et al., unpublished).

Whether jejunal IEL in general, and the γδ TCR⁺ subset in particular, are activated in celiac disease has been explored by several groups. IEL do not express classical T-cell activation markers such as the α chain of the IL-2 receptor (CD25) (88–90) or the human leukocyte class II antigen HLA-DR, either normally or in the

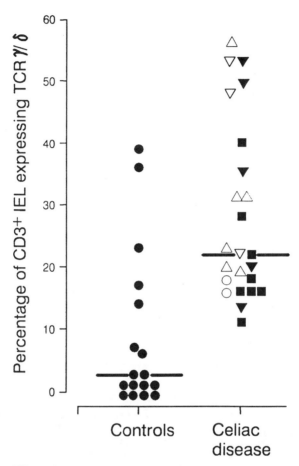

FIG. 3. Scatter diagram of γδ TCR$^+$ IEL distribution in controls with normal jejunal mucosa (*solid circles*) and patients with celiac disease showing various degrees of villous atrophy: total (*squares*); subtotal (*triangles with points down*); partial (*triangles with points up*); or none (*circles*). Closed symbols represent subjects on normal diet, open symbols subjects on gluten-free diet. Median indicated by horizontal lines. (Modified from ref. 16.)

celiac lesion. We recently observed a significantly increased expression of CD45R0 on CD3$^+$ IEL in untreated disease (Fig. 4). However, the expanded γδ TCR$^+$ IEL subset was not more often positive for CD45R0 (59%) than their αβ TCR$^+$ counterparts (75%), and CD45R0 was not particularly expressed by the predominant γδ TCR$^+$ subset (67%) that used the Vδ1/Jδ1-gene segment (mAb δTCS1$^+$) or by the

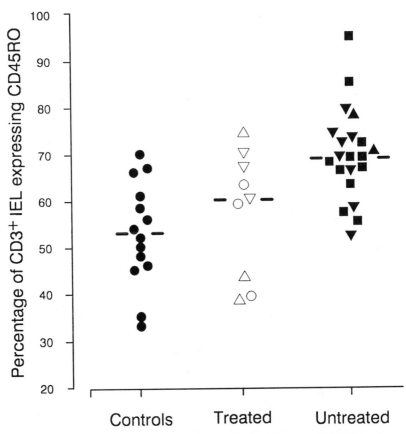

FIG. 4. Scatter diagram of the percentage of CD3$^+$ IEL expressing CD45R0 in controls with normal jejunal mucosa and in patients with treated (gluten-free diet) or untreated celiac disease showing various degrees of villous atrophy (symbols as in Fig. 3). Medians indicated by horizontal lines. (Modified from ref. 40.)

CD8$^+$ IEL subset (62%) (40,41). Conversely, all $\alpha\beta$ TCR CD4$^+$ IEL expressed high levels of CD45R0, comparable to $\alpha\beta$ TCR$^+$ CD4$^+$ T cells in lamina propria. IEL (both $\alpha\beta$ TCR$^+$ CD8$^+$ and $\gamma\delta$ TCR$^+$) expressed instead preferentially the 190/205-kDa CD45RB isoform (41).

Intake of gluten in patients with celiac disease thus leads to intraepithelial accumulation of putative antigen-primed (CD45RA$^-$) memory T cells of both TCR phenotypes, with an expression of CD45RB^{high} rather than CD45R0^{high} also within the expanded $\gamma\delta$ TCR$^+$ subset. This might be of importance in the immunopathology of celiac disease, because various CD45 isoforms are probably involved in the regulation of different activation pathways (8).

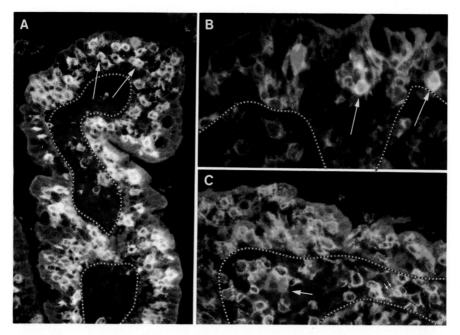

Color plate. Three-color immunofluorescence staining for T cell subsets and activation markers in celiac disease lesion, including both lamina propria and epithelium (*blue*). Tipple exposures of cryosections from jejunal biopsies. **(A)** There is a marked increase in CD3$^+$ IEL (*green*), and a high percentage express the γ/δ TCR (*yellow, arrows*). **(B)** IEL (*CD3, green*) express the nuclear proliferation marker revealed by mAb Ki-67 (*red, arrows*). **(C)** Both macrophages (*arrow*) and T cells (*CD3, green, small arrows*) in the lamina propria express the α-chain of the interleukin-2-receptor (*CD25, red*). Gluten apparently induces a nonproliferative activation of CD4$^+$ T cells in the lamina propria, but a proliferative activation of both γδ TCR$^+$ and αβ TCR$^+$ CD8$^+$ IEL in celiac disease.

PROLIFERATION OF IEL IN THE CELIAC LESION

It has been a matter of controversy whether the raised density of IEL in the celiac lesion represents an absolute numerical increase or is secondary to villous atrophy with reduced extension of the surface epithelium (91). Previous examination of celiac disease specimens revealed an increased fraction of mitotic IEL, which by some authors was considered specific for celiac disease (92) and by others related to the density of IEL regardless of the underlying disorder (93). We recently examined the phenotype of these proliferative IEL in celiac disease. Various CD3$^+$ T-cell subsets (CD4$^+$, CD8$^+$, $\gamma\delta$ TCR$^+$) were examined for expression of the nuclear proliferation marker revealed by mAb Ki-67 (90). Its expression was absent in controls, but a median of 4.5% of CD3$^+$ IEL were positive in partly treated (range 0 to 19%) and 12.8% in untreated celiac disease (range 4.0 to 30.7%; p<0.005 (Fig. 5). Disease controls were regrettably not available.

Direct sequential and two- or three-color *in situ* immunofluorescence staining suggested that both $\gamma\delta$ TCR$^+$ and $\alpha\beta$ TCR CD8$^+$ (but not $\alpha\beta$ TCR CD4$^+$) IEL proliferated in the celiac lesion [see Color plate (B) between pages 154 and 155]. The $\alpha\beta$ TCR$^+$ CD8$^+$ subset was considerably more often positive with mAb Ki-67 (21.5%) than the $\gamma\delta$ TCR$^+$ subset (5.9%; range 0 to 9%; calculated in 12 untreated patients). This might be related to the proportion of $\gamma\delta$ TCR IEL, as both TCR subsets were equally often positive in a patient with almost 40% $\gamma\delta$ TCR$^+$ IEL. Few IEL (0-1 cell per section) expressed CD25 [see Color plate (C) between pages 154 and 155], contrasting the strong expression of this marker predominantly on lamina propria CD4$^+$ T cells in untreated disease (90). Thus, it appeared that gluten induces a nonproliferative activation of CD4$^+$ lamina propria T cells but a proliferative activation of $\alpha\beta$ TCR$^+$ CD8$^+$ and $\gamma\delta$ TCR$^+$ IEL. The mechanism for this is unknown, but "normal" human IEL proliferate poorly after CD3/TCR-mediated activation alone; additional signal as CD2 crosslinking is needed (94). Although the increased density of $\alpha\beta$ TCR$^+$ CD8$^+$ and $\gamma\delta$ TCR$^+$ IEL in the celiac lesion could be secondary to T cell-mediated immune activation in the lamina propria (95,96), a direct primary antigen-driven proliferation of IEL (perhaps CD1-dependent) should not be excluded (30,97).

SUMMARY

Human intestinal IEL show a unique phenotype compared with peripheral and lamina propria T cells. Some of the surface molecules they express might be involved in migration into the epithelium, like the adhesion molecule integrin $\alpha^E\beta7$. Other surface molecules have been implicated as activation markers, e.g., CD7. However, the functional significance of most surface molecules preferentially expressed by IEL remains unknown. Even the simplest and most important difference, the remarkable predominance of $\alpha\beta$ TCR CD8$^+$ IEL, remains an enigma awaiting elucidation. Are IEL simply cytotoxic effector cells controlled by CD4$^+$ T cells in the lamina propria and directed against luminal infectious agents? Or are

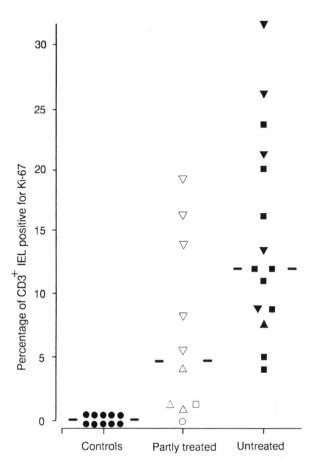

FIG. 5. Scatter diagram of the percentage of CD3 [+] IEL positive for Ki-67 (median indicated) in controls with normal jejunal mucosa (*solid circles*) and patients with celiac disease showing various degrees of villous atrophy (symbols as in Fig. 3). (Modified from ref. 90.)

they suppressor cells involved in mucosal immune regulation, perhaps contributing to the phenomenon of oral tolerance? Only further research may provide the answer. But identifying molecules with differential expression on IEL is a necessary approach to the performance of rational functional studies.

ACKNOWLEDGMENTS

The studies in the authors' laboratory have been supported by the Norwegian Research Council (NAVF/RMF), the Norwegian Cancer Society, and Rakel and Otto Kr. Bruun's Legacy.

REFERENCES

1. Dobbins WO. Human intestinal intraepithelial lymphocytes. *Gut* 1986;27:972–985.
2. Brandtzaeg P, Halstensen TS, Kett K, et al. Immunobiology and immunopathology of human gut mucosa: humoral immunity and intraepithelial lymphocytes. *Gastroenterology* 1989;97:1562–1584.
3. Selby WS, Janossy G, Jewell DP. Immunohistochemical characterization of intraepithelial lymphocytes of the human gastrointestinal tract. *Gut* 1981;22:169–176.
4. Hirata I, Berrebi G, Austin LL, Keren DF, Dobbins WO III. Immunohistological characterization of intraepithelial and lamina propria lymphocytes in control ileum and colon and inflammatory bowel disease. *Dig Dis Sci* 1986;6:593–603.
5. Fournier M, Lebargy F, Ladurie FLR, Lenormand E, Pariente R. Intraepithelial T-lymphocyte subsets in the airway of normal subjects and of patients with chronic bronchitis. *Am Rev Respir Dis* 1989;140:737–742.
6. Foster CA, Yokozeki H, Rappersberger, et al. *J Exp Med* 1990;171:997–1013.
7. Goodman T, Lefrançois L. Expression of the γ-δ T cell receptor on intestinal CD8⁺ intraepithelial lymphocytes in the small intestine of mice. *Nature* 1988;333:855–858.
8. Boneville M, Janeway CA, Ito K, et al. Intestinal intraepithelial lymphocytes are distinct set of γ-δ T cells. *Nature* 1988;336:479–481.
9. Viney JL, MacDonald TT, Kilshaw PJ. T-cell receptor expression in intestinal intraepithelial lymphocyte subpopulation of normal and athymic mice. *Immunology* 1989;66:583–587.
10. Vaage JT, Dissen E, Ager A, Roberts I, Fossum S, Rolstad B. T cell receptor-bearing cells among rat intestinal intraepithelial lymphocytes are mainly alpha/beta+ and are thymus dependent. *Eur J Immunol* 1990;20:1193–1196.
11. Spencer J, Isaacson PG. Human T-cell receptor expression. *Nature* 1989;337:416.
12. Brandtzaeg P, Bosnes V, Halstensen TS, Scott H, Sollid LM, Valnes KN. T lymphocytes in the human gut epithelium preferentially express the α/β antigen receptor and are often CD45R0/UCHL1 positive. *Scand J Immunol* 1989;30:123–128.
13. Jarry A, Cerf-Bensussan N, Brousse N, Selz F, Guy-Grand D. Subset of CD3⁺ (T cell receptor α/β or γ/δ) and CD3⁻ lymphocytes isolated from the normal human gut epithelium display phenotypical features different from their counterparts in peripheral blood. *Eur J Immunol* 1990;20:1097–1103.
14. Groh V, Porcelli S, Fabbi M, et al. Human lymphocytes bearing T cell receptor δ are phenotypically diverse and evenly distributed throughout the lymphoid system. *J Exp Med* 1989;169:1277–1289.
15. Bucy RP, Chen C-LH, Cooper MD. Tissue localization and CD8 accessory molecule expression of Tγδ cells in humans. *J Immunol* 1989;142:3045–3051.
16. Halstensen TS, Scott H, Brandtzaeg P. Intraepithelial T cells of the TcRγ/δ⁺CD8⁻ and V$_\delta$1/J$_\delta$1⁺ phenotype are increased in coeliac disease. *Scand J Immunol* 1989;30:665–672.
17. Spencer J, Isaacson PG, Diss TC, et al. Expression of disulphide-linked and non-disulphide-linked forms of the T cell receptor γ/δ heterodimer in human intestinal intraepithelial lymphocytes. *Eur J Immunol* 1989;19:1335–1338.
18. Trejdosiewicz LK, Smart CJ, Oakes DJ, Howdle PD, Malizia G, Campana D, Boylston AW. Expression of T-cell receptor TcR1 (γ/δ) and TcR2 (α/β) in the human intestinal mucosa. *Immunology* 1989;68:7–12.
19. Vroom TM, Scholte G, Ossendorp F, Borst J. Tissue distribution of human γ/δ T cells: no evidence for general epithelial tropism. *J Clin Pathol* 1991;44:1012–1017.
20. Trejdosiewicz LK. Intestinal intraepithelial lymphocytes and lymphoepithelial interactions in the human gastrointestinal mucosa. *Immunol Let* 1992;32:13–20.
21. Parrott DMV, Tait C, MacKenzie S, Mowat AM, Davies MDJ, Micklem HS. Analysis of the effector functions of different populations of mucosal lymphocytes. *Ann NY Acad Sci* 1983;403:307–319.
22. Guy-Grand D, Cerf-Bensussan N, Malissen B, Malassis-Seris M, Briottet C, Vassalli P. Two gut intraepithelial CD8⁺ lymphocytes populations with different T cell receptors: a role for the gut epithelium in T cell differentiation. *J Exp Med* 1991;173:471–481.
23. Fukushima K, Masuda T, Ohtani H, Sasaki I, Funayama Y, Matsumo S, Nagura H. Immunohistochemical characterization, distribution and ultrastructure of lymphocytes bearing the gamma/delta T-cell receptor in the human gut. *Virchows Arch [Cell Pathol]* 1991;60:7–13.
24. Lynch S, Feighery C, Weir DG, Kelleher D, Farrelly CO. Flow cytometric analysis of human IEL from small intestinal biopsies: evidence of extra-thymic T cell differentiation. Abstract # 32, International coeliac symposium, Dublin, Ireland, 1992.
25. Deusch K, Lüling F, Reich K, Classen M, Wagner H, Pfeffer K. A. major fraction of human

intraepithelial lymphocytes simultaneously express the γ/δ T cell receptor, the CD8 accessory molecule and preferentially uses the V$_δ$1 gene segment. *Eur J Immunol* 1991;21:1053–1059.

26. Lynch S, Kelleher D, Feighery C, Weir DG, Farrelly CO. Double negative γ/δ lymphocytes: a novel population in coeliac gut epithelium. Abstract # 31, International coeliac symposium, Dublin, Ireland, 1992.

27. Bottino C, Tambussi G, Ferrini S, et al. Two subsets of human T lymphocytes expressing γ/δ antigen receptor are identifiable by monoclonal antibodies directed to two distinct molecular forms of the receptor. *J Exp Med* 1989;168:491–505.

28. Faure F, Jitsukawa S, Triebel F, Hercend T. CD3/TiγA: a functional γ-receptor complex expressed on human peripheral lymphocytes. *J Immunol* 1988;140:1372–1379.

29. Takagaki Y, Decloux A, Bonneville M, Tonegawa S. Diversity of γ/δ T-cell receptors on murine intestinal intraepithelial lymphocytes. *Nature* 1989;339:712–715.

30. Asarnow DM, Goodman T, LeFrançois L, Allison JP. Distinct antigen receptor repertoires of two classes of murine epithelium-associated T cells. *Nature* 1989;341:60–62.

31. Balk SP, Ebert EE, Blumenthal RL, McDermott FV, Wucherpfenning K, Landau SB, Blumberg RS. Oligoclonal expansion and CD1 recognition of cluster of differentiation 1 antigens by human intestinal intraepithelial lymphocytes. *Science* 1991;253:1411–1415.

32. Kerckove Van C, Russell GJ, Deusch K, Reich K, Bhan AK, DerSimonian H, Brenner MB. Oligoclonality of human intraepithelial T cells. *J Exp Med* 1992;175:57–63.

33. Pluschke G, Taube H, Krawinkel U, Pfeffer K, Hermann W, Classen M, Deusch K. Oligoclonality and skewed T cell receptor Vβ gene segment expression in *in vitro* activated human intestinal intraepithelial lymphocytes. *Int Immunol* 1993; in press.

34. Streuli M, Morimoto C, Schreiber M, Schlossman SF, Saito H. Characterization of CD45 and CD45R monoclonal antibodies using transfected mouse cell line that express individual human leukocyte common antigens. *J Immunol* 1988;141:3910–3919.

35. Terry LA, Brown MH, Beverley PCL. The monoclonal antibody UCHL1, recognizes a 180,000 MW component of the human leucocyte-common antigen, CD45. *Immunology* 1988;64:331–336.

36. Smith SH, Brown MH, Rowe D, Callard RE, Beverley PCL. Functional subsets of human helper-inducer cells defined by a new monoclonal antibody. UCHL1. *Immunology* 1988;58:63–68.

37. Clement LT. Isoforms of the CD45 common leukocyte antigen family: markers for human T-cell differentiation. *J Clin Immunol* 1992;12:1–10.

38. Harvey J, Jones DB, Wright DH. Leucocyte common antigen expression of T cells in normal and inflamed human gut. *Immunology* 1989;68:13–17.

39. Janossy G, Bofill M, Muir J, Beverley PCL. The tissue distribution of T lymphocytes expressing different polypeptides. *Immunology* 1989;66:517–525.

40. Halstensen TS, Scott H, Brandtzaeg P. Human intraepithelial T lymphocytes are mainly CD45RA$^-$RB$^+$ and show increased co-expression of CD45RO in celiac disease. *Eur J Immunol* 1990;20: 1825–1830.

41. Halstensen TS, Farstad IN, Scott H, Fausa O, Brandtzaeg P. Intraepithelial TCRα/β$^+$ lymphocytes express CD45RO more often than the TCR γ/δ$^+$ counterparts in coeliac disease. *Immunology* 1990;71:460–466.

42. Goodman TG, Chang H-L, Esselman WJ, LeCorre R, Lefrancois L. Characterization of the CD45 molecule on murine intestinal intraepithelial lymphocytes. *J Immunol* 1990;145:2959–2966.

43. Cerf-Bensussan N, Jarry A, Brousse N, Lisowska-Grospierre B, Guy-Grand D, Griscelli C. A monoclonal antibody (HML-1) defining a novel membrane molecule present on human intestinal lymphocytes. *Eur J Immunol* 1987;17:1279–1285.

44. Cerf-Bensussan N, Bègue B, Gagnon J, Meo T. The human intraepithelial lymphocyte marker HML-1 is an integrin consisting of a β7 subunit associated with a distinct α chain. *Eur J Immunol* 1992;22:273–277.

45. Parker CM, Cepek KL, Russel GJ, Shaw SK, Posnett DN, Schwarting R, Brenner MB. A family of β$_7$ integrins on human mucosal lymphocytes. *Proc Natl Acad Sci USA* 1992;89:1924–1928.

46. Krissansen GW, Print CG, Prestidge RL, et al. Immunologic and structural relatedness of the integrin beta 7 complex and the human intraepithelial antigen HML-1. *FEBS Lett* 1992;296:25–28.

47. Micklem KJ, Dong Y, Willis A, et al. HML-1 antigen on mucosa-associated T cells, activated cells, and hairy leukemic cells is a new integrin containing the beta 7 subunit. *Am J Pathol* 1992;139: 1297–1301.

48. Visser L, Shaw A, Slupsky J, Vos H, Poppema S. Monoclonal antibodies reactive with hairy cell leukemia. *Blood* 1989;74:320–325.

49. Schwarting R, Dienemann D, Kruschwitz M, Fritsche G, Stein H. Specificities of monoclonal antibodies B-ly7 and HML-1 are identical. *Blood* 1990;75:320–321.
50. Kruschwitz M, Fritzsche G, Schwarting R, et al. Ber-ACT8: new monoclonal antibody to the mucosa lymphocyte antigen. *J Clin Pathol* 1991;44:636–645.
51. Yuan Q, Jiang WM, Leung E, Hollander D, Watson JD, Krissansen GW. Molecular cloning of the mouse integrin beta 7 subunit. *J Biol Chem* 1992;267:7352–7358.
52. Hu MC-T, Crowe DT, Weissman IL, Holzmann B. Cloning and expression of mouse integrin $\beta_p(\beta_7)$: a functional role in Peyer's patch-specific lymphocyte homing. *Proc Natl Acad Sci USA* 1992;89:8254–8258.
53. Schieferdecker HL, Ullrich R, Hirseland H, Zeitz M. T cell differentiation antigens on lymphocytes in the human intestinal lamina propria. *J Immunol* 1992;149:2816–2822.
54. Greenwood JH, Austin LL, Dobbins WO. In vitro characterization of human intestinal intra-epithelial lymphocytes. *Gastroenterology* 1983;85:1023–1034.
55. Ebert EC. Intra-epithelial lymphocytes: interferon-gamma production and suppressor/cytotoxic activities. *Clin Exp Immunol* 1990;82:81–85.
56. Hoang P, Dalton HR, Jewell DP. Human colonic intra-epithelial lymphocytes are suppressor cells. *Clin Exp Immunol* 1991;85:498–503.
57. Meader RD, Landers DF. Electron and light microscopic observation on relationships between lymphocytes and intestinal epithelium. *Am J Anat* 1967;121:763–774.
58. Toner PG, Ferguson A. Intraepithelial cells in the human intestinal mucosa. *J Ultrastruct Res* 1971; 34:329–344.
59. Cerf-Bensussan N, Schneeberger EE, Bhan AK. Immunohistologic and immunoelectron microscopic characterization of the mucosal lymphocytes of human small intestine by the use of monoclonal antibodies. *J Immunol* 1983;130:2615–2622.
60. Cerf-Bensussan N, Guy-Grand D, Griscelli C. Intraepithelial lymphocytes of human gut: isolation, characterization and study of natural killer activity. *Gut* 1985;26:81–88.
61. Chiba M, Bartnik W, ReMine SG, Thayer WR, Shorter RG. Human colonic intraepithelial and lamina propria lymphocytes: cytotoxicity *in vitro* and potential effects of the isolation method on their functional properties. *Gut* 1981;22:177–186.
62. Taunk J, Roberts AI, Ebert EC. Spontaneous cytotoxicity of human intraepithelial lymphocytes against epithelial cell tumors. *Gastroenterology* 1992;102:69–75.
63. Goodman T, Lefrancois L. *In vivo* modulation of cytolytic activity and Thy-1 expression in TCR γ/δ^+ intraepithelial lymphocytes. *Science* 1989;243:1716–1718.
64. Viney JL, Kilshaw PJ, MacDonald TT. Cytotoxic α/β^+ and γ/δ^+ T cells in murine intestinal epithelium. *Eur J Immunol* 1990;20:1623–1626.
65. Guy-Grand D, Malassis-Seris M, Briottet C, Vassalli P. Cytotoxic differentiation of mouse intraepithelial T lymphocytes is induced locally. Correlation between functional assays, presence of perforin and granzyme transcripts and cytoplasmic granules. *J Exp Med* 1991;173:1549–1552.
66. Joag SV, Zheng L-M, Persechini P, Michl J, Parr E, Young JD-E. The distribution of perforin in normal tissue. *Immunol Let* 1991;28:195–200.
67. Lefrançois L. Phenotypic complexity of intraepithelial lymphocytes of the small intestine. *J Immunol* 1991;147:1746–1751.
68. Koizumi H, Liu C-C, Zheng LM, Joag SV, Bayne NK, Holoshitz J, Young JD-E. Expression of perforin and serine esterase by human γ/δ T cells. *J Exp Med* 1991;173:499–502.
69. Rust C, Kooy Y, Peña S, Mearins M-L, Kluiin P, Koning F. Phenotypical and functional characterization of small intestinal TcRγδ$^+$ T cells in coeliac disease. *Scand J Immunol* 1992;35:459–468.
70. June CH, Ledbetter JA, Linsley PS, Thomson CB. Role of the CD28 receptor in T cell activation. *Immunol Today* 1990;11:211–216.
71. Mayer L, Shlien R. Evidence for function of Ia molecules on gut epithelial cells in man. *J Exp Med* 1987;166:1471–1483.
72. Li SG, Ottenhoff THM, van den Elsen P, Koning F, Zhang L, Mak T, De Vries RRP. Human suppressor T cell clones lack CD28. *Eur J Immunol* 1990;20:1281–1288.
73. Al-Dawoud A, Nakshabendi I, Foulis A, Mowat AM. Immunohistochemical analysis of mucosal gamma-interferon production in coeliac disease. *Gut* 1992;23:1482–1486.
74. Fujihashi K, Kiyono H, Aicher WK, Green DR, Singh B, Eldridge JH, McGhee JR. Immunoregulatory function of CD3$^+$, CD4$^-$, and CD8$^-$ T cells. γδ T cell receptor-positive T cells from nude mice abrogate oral tolerance. *J Immunol* 1989;143:3415–3422.

75. Taguchi T, McGhee JR, Coffman RL, Beagley KW, Eldridge JH, Takatsu K, Kiyono H. Analysis of Th1 and Th2 cells in murine gut-associated tissues. Frequencies of CD4$^+$ and CD8$^+$ T cells that secrete IFN-gamma and IL-5. *J Immunol* 1990;145:68–77.
76. Fujihashi K, Taguchi T, Aicher WK, McGhee JR, Bluestone JA, Eldridge JH, Kiyono H. Immunoregulatory functions for murine intraepithelial lymphocytes: γ/δ T cell receptor-positive (TCR$^+$) T cells abrogate oral tolerance, while α/β TCR$^+$ T cells provide B cell help. *J Exp Med* 1992;175:695–707.
77. Barret TA, Gajewski TF, Danielpour D, Chang EB, Beagley KW, Bluestone JA. Differential function of intestinal intraepithelial lymphocyte subsets. *J Immunol* 1992;149:1124–1130.
78. Malizia G, Trejdosiewicz LK, Wood GM, Howdle PD, Janossy G, Losowsky MS. The microenvironment of coeliac disease: T cell phenotype and expression of the T2 "T blast" antigen by small bowel lymphocytes. *Clin Exp Immunol* 1985;60:437–446.
79. Trejdosiewicz LK, Malizia G, Badr-el-Din S, et al. T cell and mononuclear phagocyte populations of the human small and large intestine. *Adv Exp Med Biol* 1987;216A:463–473.
80. Rocha B, Vassalli P, Guy-Grand D. The Vβ repertoire of mouse gut homodimer α CD8$^+$ intraepithelial T cell receptor α/β$^+$ lymphocytes reveals a major extrathymic pathway of T cell differentiation. *J Exp Med* 1991;173:483–486.
81. Rocha B, von Boehmer H, Guy-Grand D. Selection of intraepithelial lymphocytes with CD8 α/α coreceptors by self antigen in the murine gut. *Proc Natl Acad Sci USA* 1992;89:5336–5340.
82. Guy-Grand D, Broecke CV, Briottet C, Malassis-Seris M, Selz F, Vassalli P. Different expression of the recombination activity gene RAG-1 in various populations of thymus, peripheral T cells and gut thymus-independent intraepithelial lymphocytes suggests two pathways of T cell receptor rearrangement. *Eur J Immunol* 1992;22:505–510.
83. Savilahti E, Arato A, Verkasalo M. Intestinal γ/δ receptor-bearing T lymphocytes in celiac disease and inflammatory bowel diseases in children. Constant increase in celiac disease. *Pediatr Res* 1990;28:579–581.
84. Trejdosiewicz LK, Calabrese A, Smart CJ, et al. γδ T cell receptor-cells of the human gastrointestinal mucosa: occurrence and V region gene expression in *Helicobacter pylori*-associated gastritis, coeliac disease and inflammatory bowel disease. *Clin Exp Immunol* 1991;84:440–444.
85. Spencer J, Isaacson P, Macdonald TT, et al. Gamma/delta T cells and the diagnosis of coeliac disease. *Clin Exp Immunol* 1991;85:109–113.
86. Fukushima K, Masuda T, Ohtani H, Sasaki I, Funayama Y, Matsuno S, Nagura H. Immunohistochemical characterization, distribution, and ultrastructure of lymphocytes bearing T-cell receptor gamma/delta in inflammatory bowel disease. *Gastroenterology* 1991;101:670–678.
87. Armes J, Gee DC, Macrae FA, Shroeder W, Bhathal PS. Collagenous colitis jejunal and colorectal pathology. *J Clin Pathol* 1992;45:784–787.
88. Selby WS, Janossy G, Bofill M, et al. Lymphocyte subpopulations in the human small intestine. The findings in normal mucosa and in the mucosa of patients with adult coeliac disease. *Clin Exp Immunol* 1983;52:219–228.
89. Kelly J, O'Farrelly CO, O'Mahony DG, et al. Immunoperoxidase demonstration of the cellular composition of the normal and coeliac small bowel. *Clin Exp Immunol* 1987;68:177–188.
90. Halstensen TS, Brandtzaeg P. Activated T lymphocytes in the celiac lesion: nonproliferative activation (CD25) of CD4$^+$ αβ cells in the lamina propria but proliferation (Ki-67) of αβ and γδ cells in the epithelium. *Eur J Immunol* 1993;23:505–510.
91. Marsh MN. Studies of intestinal lymphoid tissue. III: Quantitative analyses of epithelial lymphocytes in the small intestine of human control subjects and of patients with celiac sprue. *Gastroenterology* 1980;79:481–492.
92. Marsh MN, Haeney MR. Studies of intestinal lymphoid tissue. VI: Proliferative response of small intestinal lymphocytes distinguishes gluten- from non-gluten-induced enteropathy. *J Clin Pathol* 1993;36:149–160.
93. Ferguson A, Ziegler K. Intraepithelial lymphocyte mitosis in a jejunal biopsy correlates with intraepithelial lymphocyte count, irrespective of diagnosis. *Gut* 1986;27:675–679.
94. Ebert EC. Proliferative responses of human intraepithelial lymphocytes to various T-cell stimuli. *Gastroenterology* 1989;97:1372–1381.
95. MacDonald TT, Spencer J. Evidence that activated mucosal T cells play a role in the pathogenesis of enteropathy in human small intestine. *J Exp Med* 1988;167:1341–1349.
96. Monk T, Spencer J, Cerf-Bensussan N, MacDonald TT. Stimulation of mucosal T cells *in situ* with

anti-CD3 antibody: location of the activated T cell and their distribution within the mucosal microenvironment. *Clin Exp Immunol* 1988;74:216–222.

97. Porcelli S, Morita CT, Brenner MB. CD1b restricted the response of human CD4$^-$8$^-$ T lymphocytes to a microbial antigen. *Nature* 1992;360:593–597.
98. Janossy G, Tidman N, Selby WS, Thomas JA, Granger S. Human T lymphocytes of inducer and suppressor type occupy different microenvironment. *Nature* 1980;228:81–84.

Mucosal Immunology: Intraepithelial Lymphocytes,
edited by H. Kiyono and J. R. McGhee.
Raven Press, Ltd., New York © 1993.

12

Intraepithelial Lymphocytes in Birds

Yoshihito Kasahara, Chen-lo H. Chen, Thomas W. F. Göbel,
R. Pat Bucy, and Max D. Cooper

*Division of Developmental and Clinical Immunology, Departments of Medicine,
Pediatrics, Microbiology, and Pathology, and the Howard Hughes
Medical Institute, University of Alabama at Birmingham, Birmingham, AL.*

Intraepithelial lymphocytes (IEL) represent a unique population of lymphoid cells. T cells in this location may differ from the bulk of T cells in other tissues in their pattern of receptor expression, functional activities, and developmental origin. We have examined the IEL in chickens, since comparative studies in birds and mammals may provide significant insight into lymphocyte development pathways. For example, the separate developmental pathways of T and B cells and their origin from multipotential stem cells was initially revealed in the avian model (1,2). Identification of avian immunoglobulin and T cell receptor (TCR) genes (3–6) and the generation of monoclonal antibodies (mAb) identifying T and B cell receptors (reviewed in 7) have renewed interest in the avian model for study of the immune system. Comparative analysis of avian lymphocyte development and function reveals striking conservation of the major T and B cell features defined in mammals (8,9). Analysis of the avian IEL may reveal conserved features that lead to a better understanding of the vertebrate mucosal immune system.

ANATOMICAL DEFINITION OF THE GUT-ASSOCIATED LYMPHOID TISSUE IN BIRDS

The gut-associated lymphoid tissue (GALT) is one of the major afferent portals of entry for many pathogens. Collectively, it contains more lymphocytes than any other lymphoid tissue (10). The avian intestinal tract displays both similarities to and differences from the mammalian intestinal tract. Besides the overall physiologic function, the avian intestinal tract shares similar histologic structure, having an abundance of lymphoid cells distributed throughout the epithelium and in the lamina propria. Major differences in the avian gut include presence of the gizzard and duodenal bulb in the upper intestinal tract, cecal tonsils, a unique cloaca that receives the ureters as well as the fecal stream, and the bursa of Fabricius at the outlet of the intestinal tract. Intestinal lymphocytes are scattered throughout the lamina propria and epithelium, and occasional submucosal lymphoid aggregates are seen. The organized lymphoid structures include Peyer's patches (PP), cecal tonsils, and Meckel's diverticulum (11). Up to five or six PP can be found in the intestine of young chickens, while only one or two are found in adult chickens (12). The chicken PP are roughly comparable to the mammalian counterpart, containing mostly CD4[+] T cells, B cells, and their plasma cell progeny (12–14).

The cecal tonsils are paired blind loops of bowel that are connected to the intestine at the ileocecal junction. The cecal tonsils have multiple small plicae and numerous mucous-containing goblet cells, the mucosal histology resembling that of the rodent cecum. At the base of each cecal tonsil is a discrete lymphoid nodule resembling a mammalian PP. These lymphoid nodules contain central crypts, diffuse lymphoid tissues, and germinal centers (15). Both T and B cells are present in the germinal centers; and plasma cells, which produce IgM, IgG, and IgA, are found in the cecal tonsils (14). The function of cecal tonsils is unknown, but active pinocytosis of orally administrated carbon particles has been demonstrated, suggesting functional similarity with the mammalian PP (12).

Meckel's diverticulum is a remnant of the yolk sac attachment to the small intestine that usually persists as a discrete structure for the lifetime of the chicken. Germinal centers and B cells have been detected in the Meckel's diverticulum (12), but no clear immunological role has been demonstrated for this tissue.

Located at the end of the intestine is the bursa of Fabricius, a unique structure consisting of a hollow tissue pouch containing hundreds of lymphoid follicles, which are highly pinocytotic. Maintaining direct communication with the lumen of the cloaca via the bursal duct, the bursa serves as the primary lymphoid organ for B lymphocyte development in birds (2,8). The bursal duct directly connects the lumen of the bursa to the cloacal lumen and the fecal stream (16). This unique anatomical relationship could suggest an effector functional role, but whether the bursa plays a role as a secondary lymphoid organ is still a controversial issue.

PHENOTYPIC CHARACTERISTICS OF INTESTINAL EPITHELIAL LYMPHOCYTES

A distinctive population of epithelial lymphocytes forms a key element of the GALT. Besides their particular localization, there are several indications that this population of IEL represents a functionally distinctive lymphocyte subset. First, frequencies of the T cell subsets are quite different in the epithelium than in the lamina propria (13). In the chicken three subpopulations of T cells are defined by the mAb reactive with T cell receptors: TCR1[+] cells express γδ TCR (17); and TCR2[+] and TCR3[+] cells express Vβ1 and Vβ2 αβ TCR, respectively (18–21). TCR1[+] cells comprise the most abundant subpopulation of T cells in the epithelium, while TCR2[+] cells predominate in the lamina propria. The TCR3[+] cells are relatively infrequent in the intestine. In addition to this distinctive pattern of T cell distribution in the epithelium, the chicken IEL population contains a unique population of cytoplasmic $CD3^+$ cells that express neither $\alpha\beta$ nor $\gamma\delta$ TCR. We have termed these TCR0 cells (22,23) to denote their lack of T cell receptors despite their resemblance to T cells. The TCR0 subset forms between 15 and 40% of the IEL compartment (22). These cells, which appear to be the homologues of mammalian NK cells, are described below. The vast majority of the intraepithelial TCR0 cells express the CD8 coreceptor, but both they and the TCR1 IEL population may express the $CD8\alpha\alpha$ homodimer, rather than the $CD8\alpha\beta$ heterodimer found on most $\alpha\beta$ TCR cells.

INTRAEPITHELIAL $\gamma\delta$ T CELLS

Developmental Origin

While the thymus is known to be the major source of T cells, experiments in mice have suggested that many of the $\gamma\delta$ TCR^+ IEL are generated extrathymically (24). The IEL in nude mice with an atrophic thymus are predominantly $\gamma\delta$ TCR^+ T cells, and bone marrow or fetal liver transplants into irradiated, thymectomized mice give rise to $\gamma\delta$ IEL (25,26). Thymectomized mice acquire $CD8^+$ $\gamma\delta$ TCR^+ IEL in significant numbers, and transcripts of the recombinase activating gene (RAG-1) have been detected in IEL (27). These data suggest that TCR rearrangement occurs in IEL and that $\gamma\delta$ TCR^+ cells may be derived *in situ* from extrathymic precursors.

Studies of chick-quail chimeras suggest instead that embryonic $\gamma\delta$ TCR^+ and $\alpha\beta$ TCR^+ T cells are generated exclusively in the avian thymus (23,28). In the chicken, early thymectomy effectively aborts development of $\gamma\delta$ TCR^+ T cells in the circulation, indicating that sustained thymic seeding is essential for normal development of the peripheral $\gamma\delta$ TCR^+ T cell pool (29,30).

To examine further the origin and kinetics of avian $\gamma\delta$ TCR^+ T cells, Dunon and coworkers (31) analyzed the intestinal colonization by $\gamma\delta$ TCR^+ T cells using transplants between congenic ov^+ and ov^- chick strains (H.B19ov^+ and H.B19ov^-). The ov alloantigen is expressed on most hemopoietic precursors during embryonic life, and by T lineage cells, peripheral B cells and some bursal B cells, after hatching (32). When embryonic day 14 (E14) thymocytes, 25% of which are $\gamma\delta$ TCR^+ T cells, were obtained from H.B19 ov^+ chickens and injected into E15–16 ov^- recipients, the donor ov^+ $\gamma\delta$ TCR^+ cells homed to the recipient small intestine within 2 days after injection. The percentage of donor $\gamma\delta$ TCR^+ T cells in the intestine remained relatively constant until hatching, when a dramatic decrease in frequency occurred as a consequence of dilution by influx of the host $\gamma\delta$ TCR^+ T cells. When the donor E14 ov^+ cells were injected into thymectomized recipients 2 days after hatching, 20% of the $\gamma\delta$ TCR population were of donor origin over the first month of life, whereas only a low percent of donor ov^+ cells persisted in the intestine of nonthymectomized recipients. These results indicate a thymic origin for a long-lived population of $\gamma\delta$ TCR^+ cells in the intraepithelial compartment. The progeny of stem cells belonging to the second wave of thymus colonization begin to mature around the time of hatching (33), and data obtained in the thymocyte chimeric model suggests that γδ TCR$^+$ T cells in this and subsequent waves home to the intestine, beginning immediately after hatching.

To examine the possibility that precursor thymocytes might differentiate into γδ TCR$^+$ T cells extrathymically, γδ TCR$^-$ thymocytes of the E14 ov$^+$ chickens were injected into E16 ov$^-$ recipients, but progeny γδ TCR$^+$ cells were not found in the recipients even 2 months after hatching. Similarly, E13 splenocytes or bone marrow cells as a source of donor stem cells rarely yield intestinal γδ TCR$^+$ cells of donor origin in E16 recipients (31).

These results indicate that the thymus is the prime source of γδ TCR$^+$ IEL, at least early in chicken development. A similar conclusion has been reached in sheep, where early thymectomy results in a life-long deficit of γδ TCR$^+$ T cells (34). γδ TCR$^+$ T cells are the predominant IEL cell type in both chicken and sheep, whereas they represent 50% of the IEL in mice and 5 to 10% of IEL in humans (35,36). Although unlikely in our view, it is theoretically possible that these differences in frequency reflect species differences in the proportion of thymus-derived γδ TCR$^+$ T cells.

Intestinal γδ TCR$^+$ T Cells Express the CD8 Coreceptor

Unlike the γδ TCR$^+$ T cells in blood, which usually express neither CD4 nor CD8, two-thirds of the γδ TCR$^+$ T cells in the chicken intestine and spleen express CD8 (13,19). The CD8 structure is a heterodimer composed of two glycosylated polypeptides designated α (Lyt2 in mice) and β (Lyt3 in mice) (37,38). In mice, the α and β chains have different sizes, whereas the α and β chains of the human CD8 appear to be of the same size. The CT8 anti-chicken CD8 mAb precipitates a 64-kDa dimer of 34-kDa chains (39). Another anti-chicken CD8 mAb, EP42, has now been identified which may recognize the CD8β chain (M. J. H. Ratcliffe, unpublished). Assuming this specificity assignment is correct, analysis of γδ TCR$^+$ IEL suggests that approximately 15% are CD8$^-$, 40% express CD8αβ, and 45% express CD8αα. In contrast, the vast majority of the CD8$^+$ γδ TCR$^+$ T cells in other tissues express the CD8αβ heterodimer (F. K. Kong et al., unpublished). Murine T cells bearing the CD8αα coreceptor are thought to be thymus-independent in their development (40). It would be interesting to analyze the frequency of CD8αα$^+$ IEL in thymectomized chickens, since chicken γδ TCR$^+$ IEL are derived predominantly, if not exclusively, from the thymus.

INTRAEPITHELIAL NK CELLS

Chicken NK cells have been identified by their ability to mediate MHC-unrestricted cytotoxicity, and the highest NK activity has been observed for the IEL population (41,42). IEL along the intestinal tract may exhibit different levels of NK activity, being higher in the jejunum and ileum and lower in the duodenum and caecum (43). Specific markers for avian NK cells do not yet exist, but the NK activity is unaffected by treatment with anti-thymocyte, anti-B cell sera, and irradiation (44). Anti-asialo GM sera that react with NK cells in several mammalian species may crossreact with some of the chicken IEL (45). Recently two mAb have been described that inhibit the NK activity of chicken spleen cells (46), but the nature of the antigens and the cells identified by these antibodies is not yet defined.

Avian TCR0 cells resemble mammalian NK cells in their expression of cytoplasmic CD3 and lack of a cell surface TCR/CD3 complex (22,47). In adult chickens, TCR0 cells are detected mainly in the intestinal epithelium, where most express the CD8 antigen (22). Less than 1% of the CD3$^+$ cells identifiable in tissue sections of the adult spleen are TCR0 cells, although splenocytes capable of spontaneous cytotoxicity can be readily detected in the adult spleen (41).

TCR0 cells can be obtained from the E14 spleen before the appearance of T cells, and these can be grown in conditioned medium prepared by concanavalin A (Con A) stimulation of adult spleen cells (T. W. F. Göbel et al., manuscript submitted). Most of these cells express cytoplasmic CD3 and surface CD8. These CD8$^+$ cells can kill NK-susceptible target cells, and share many features with mammalian NK cells, including the expression of IL-2 receptors, CD8, and Fcγ receptors (Table 1). As for mammalian NK cells (48), CD8 molecules on the TCR0 cells appear to be CD8$\alpha\alpha$ homodimers (C. H. Chen et al., unpublished observation).

TCR0 cells are large granular lymphocytes (T. W. F. Göbel et al., manuscript submitted) that ultrastructurally resemble mammalian NK cells (49). They also resemble chicken spleen cells with NK activity (50). Classical morphologic criteria can be used to divide chicken IEL into subpopulations of lymphocytes (77%), "globule" leukocytes (22%), and eosinophils (1%) (51). The globule lymphocytes contain azidophilic granules of variable sizes, are slightly larger than the average lymphocyte, and may represent NK effector cells (52). These globule cells are probably synonymous with the TCR0 cells that we have defined as NK cells.

The cultured TCR0 cells contain at least two of the three CD3 γ, δ and ϵ chains

TABLE 1. *Comparison of avian and mammalian NK cells*

	Avian	Mammalian
Independent lymphoid lineage	Yes	Yes
Morphology	LGL	LGL
Molecular markers:		
CD2	?	+
CD3 (cytoplasmic)	+	+
CD8$\alpha\alpha$	+	+
CD25	+	+
CD45	+	+
FcγR	+	+
Receptor molecules	?	60–90 kD
Distribution	Blood, lymphoid tissues, and intestinal epithelium	
Function	Spontaneous cytotoxicity	

(T. W. F. Göbel et al., manuscript submitted). In this way they resemble NK cells in the human fetus, which may express all of the CD3 components, albeit very low levels of partially glycosylated CD3 γ chains. NK cells in human adults, on the other hand, express CD3 ε chains only after activation (53). The majority of the cultured TCR0 cells and of those among the IEL population are CD8$^+$ (13; T. W. F. Göbel et al., manuscript submitted), which may suggest that these cells are activated either by the cytokines added to the cultures or by intestinal antigen stimulation.

The developmental origin of TCR0 cells was examined in chick-quail chimeras (23) because the lineage history of NK cells has been controversial. When E6 chick spleens were transplanted into E3 quails, TCR0 cells of donor origin were detected in the recipients. The development of these TCR0 cells in the donor E6 spleen is clearly thymus-independent, since the first wave of thymocyte precursors does not enter the chick thymus before E6.5. Moreover, chick TCR0 cells do not differentiate into conventional T cells even when they migrate into the quail thymus. The avian NK cells thus represent a thymus-independent lineage, the development of which is unaffected by early thymectomy (our unpublished observations). Similarly, the development of "globule leukocytes" with NK activity is unaffected by either bursectomy or thymectomy (54,55).

The shared expression of CD3 proteins in NK cells and T cells may imply that they are derived from the same progenitor cells. In this regard, it has been suggested that commitment for differentiation along T cell versus NK cell lineages depends on the microenvironment (47,56). FcγRII/RIII are expressed by most mouse thymocytes prior to the expression of T cell markers. These cells can become mature T cells in the thymus, but retain the NK cell phenotype when allowed to continue their development in an extrathymic site (56).

INTESTINAL T CELLS MAY EXPRESS AN ADHESION/RETENTION MOLECULE

Homing and retention of lymphocytes to specific tissues may be controlled by integrins (57). Chicken intestinal lymphocytes selectively express a cell surface molecule that is identified by the A19 mouse mAb (58). The A19 antigen is expressed infrequently by cells in the lamina propria, while 50% of IEL express it at relatively high levels. Of the intestinal T cells, approximately 80% express A19, whereas non-T cells in the intestine do not express the A19 antigen. Thymocytes, splenocytes, blood lymphocytes, and bone marrow mononuclear cells rarely express the A19 antigen in detectable levels, nor is it detected in nonlymphoid tissues.

The A19 antigen is a heterodimeric glycoprotein consisting of 145-kDa (α) and 75-kDa (β) chains. Reduction releases a fragment of 26 kDa from the α chain, which then migrates as a 120-kDa protein. Reduced β chains display a higher apparent molecular weight, suggesting the presence of intrachain disulfide bonds. The biochemical characteristics and tissue distribution of A19 are thus similar to those of the M290 or RGL-1 integrin molecules in rodents (59,60) and MLA in humans (61). MLA has been identified as a novel integrin molecule containing the α^E and β_{71} chains (62,63). The murine M290 antigen also belongs to the integrin family, utilizing α^{M290} and β_7 subunits (64,65). Although both molecules are not normally expressed by blood lymphocytes, late expression can be induced by mitogens (59,63,66). Similarly, A19 expression by chicken T cells can be induced by Con A in the presence of culture supernatants derived from Con A stimulated splenocytes, and this induction is enhanced by treatment with the human TGF-β1 (58).

The A19 complex thus appears to be the avian homologue of the mammalian $\alpha^E\beta_7$ integrins, which are thought to be involved in intestinal lymphocyte homing, retention, or adhesion (Table 2). A19$^+$ cells appear first in the intestine on the day after hatching, although T cells lacking the A19 antigen arrive in the intestine several days before hatching. Treatment of newly hatched chicks with the A19 mAb does not inhibit development of A19$^+$ T cells in the intestinal epithelium. For these reasons, A19 is unlikely to be a homing molecule for intestinal T cells. A19$^+$ cells can bind specifically to the intestinal epithelium, and the A19 mAb may inhibit this binding in a dose-dependent manner (H. Grenz et al., unpublished observations), making the A19 integrin an excellent candidate molecule for the retention of T cells in the intestine.

IEL FUNCTION

The anatomical separation of intraepithelial and lamina proprial compartments may have important functional implications for intestinal lymphocytes. To explore the meaning of this compartmentalization, the functions of IEL have been examined by *in vitro* assays in both birds and mammals. Plant mitogen stimulation or CD3

TABLE 2. *Conserved intestinal T-cell integrin*

Species	Human	Mouse	Rat	Chicken
Antigens defined by mAb	HML-1 B-ly7 Ber-ACT8	M290	RGL-1	A19
Molecular weights (kDa)				
α chain	175 (α^E, α^{MLA})	135 (α^{M290})	125	145
β chain	105 (β_7)	100 (β_7)	100	75
Tissue distribution				
intestinal epithelium	94%[a]	90%	84%	53%
intestinal lamina propria	40%	30%	51%	10–25%
other	Hairy cell leukemia	Lung IEL		
Late T-cell activation antigen	+		+	
TGF$^-$β1 enhancement	+	+		+

[a]Percentage of total lymphocyte population.

crosslinking induces proliferation of chicken and mouse IEL, but the proliferative response is less vigorous than that observed for blood or splenic T cells (67–69). Human IEL, on the other hand, respond well to CD3 crosslinkage (70,71). We have observed that avian $\gamma\delta$ TCR$^+$ T cells are highly dependent on growth factors that are produced by $\alpha\beta$ TCR$^+$ T cells (Y. Kasahara et al., manuscript in preparation). The predominance of $\gamma\delta$ TCR$^+$ T cells in chicken and mouse IEL populations may figure in the relatively poor responses of IEL to mitogens.

Many investigators have demonstrated cytolytic activity by freshly isolated IEL. In the case of cytotoxicity by avian TCR1 cells, the target cell killing can be triggered via the $\gamma\delta$ TCR complex (M. Chan et al., unpublished observations). Murine CD8$^+$ $\gamma\delta$ TCR$^+$ cells have been shown to display cytolytic activity, suggesting *in vivo* activation of these cells (35,72). Spontaneous cytotoxicity against tumor target cells by IEL, but not by lamina proprial lymphocytes, has been reported in chickens (41,42). The phenotype of these natural killer cells has not been determined, and they could be either TCR0 or $\gamma\delta$ TCR$^+$ T cells.

The response to intestinal infections may uniquely invoke the IEL populations. Immune defense to coccidiosis, an important avian intestinal disease caused by Eimeria parasites, appears to be cell-mediated (73,74). Cyclosporine A treatment of chickens enhances their susceptibility to primary Eimeria infection and abrogates the development of resistance to secondary challenge (75). NK cell activity by IEL decreases after primary Eimerian infection, and then increases following secondary infection, a functional activity that correlates with an increase in the numbers of asialo GM-positive IEL (45). NK cells capable of killing rotavirus-infected target cells have been demonstrated among the IEL population during intestinal rotavirus infection (42).

SUMMARY

Avian IEL constitute a distinctive lymphocyte population made up of two T-cell subpopulations ($\gamma\delta$ TCR$^+$ and $\alpha\beta$ TCR$^+$ T cells), a large third population of lymphoid cells with constitutive NK cell activity, and a relatively minor population of B lymphocytes. All of the IEL are derived from multipotent hemopoietic stem cells. The two T-cell subpopulations are seeded from the thymus, and express an intestine-specific integrin that may retain them in the epithelial compartment. The IEL population differs from the lymphocyte population in the underlying intestinal lamina propria in that $\gamma\delta$ TCR$^+$ T cells and NK cells predominate in the epithelial population, whereas higher frequencies of $\alpha\beta$ TCR$^+$ T cells and B cells are found in the lamina propria. It is unclear whether the epithelial populations represent primary effector cells involved in defense against intestinal pathogens, whether the IEL serve to modulate potentially destructive hypersensitivity reactions to intestinal antigens, or whether they serve a clean-up function to repair the ravages of intestinal inflammation. Until these questions can be answered precisely, study of IEL will remain an active field of research.

ACKNOWLEDGMENTS

Studies performed in this laboratory were supported in part by USPHS grants AI 30879, CA 13148 and AR 03555, awarded by the National Institutes of Health. TWFG is supported by Deutsche Forschungsgemeinshaft. MDC is an investigator of the Howard Hughes Medical Institute. We thank Mrs. Ann Brookshire for help in preparation of the manuscript.

REFERENCES

1. Moore MAS, Owen JJT. Chromosome marker studies on the development of the haemopoietic system in the chick embryo. *Nature* 1965;208:956–990.
2. Cooper MD, Peterson DA, Good RA. Delineation of the thymic and bursal lymphoid systems in the chicken. *Nature* 1965;205:143–146.
3. Weill J-C, Reynaud C-A. The chicken B cell compartment. *Science* 1987;238:1094–1098.
4. Parvari R, Avivi A, Lentner F, Ziv E, Tel-Or S, Burstein Y, Schechter I. Chicken immunoglobulin γ-heavy chains: limited V_H gene repertoire, combinatorial diversification by D gene segments and evolution of the heavy chain locus. *EMBO J* 1988;7:739–744.
5. Mansikka A. The chicken IgA heavy chains: implications to the evolution of heavy chain isotypes. *J Immunol* 1992;149:855–861.
6. Tjoelker LW, Carlson LM, Lee K, et al. Evolutionary conservation of antigen recognition: the chicken T-cell receptor β-chain. *Proc Natl Acad Sci USA* 1990;87:7856–7860.
7. Chen CH, Pickel JM, Lahti JM, Cooper MD. Surface markers on avian immune cells. In: Sharma JM, ed. *Avian cellular immunology*. Boca Raton: CRC Press;1991:1–22.
8. Ratcliffe MJH. Development of the avian B lymphocyte lineage. *Crit Rev Poult Biol* 1989;2:207–234.
9. Cooper MD, Chen CH, Bucy RP, Thompson CB. Avian T cell ontogeny. *Adv Immunol* 1991;50:87–117.
10. Mestecky J, McGhee JR. Immunoglobulin A (IgA): molecular and cellular interactions involved in IgA biosynthesis and immune response. *Adv Immunol* 1987;40:153–245.
11. Schat KA, Myers TJ. Avian intestinal immunity. *Crit Rev Poult Biol* 1991;3:19–34.
12. Befus AD, Johnston N, Leslie GA, Bienenstock J. Gut-associated lymphoid tissue in the chicken. I. Morphology, ontogeny, and some functional characteristics of Peyer's patches. *J Immunol* 1980;125:2626–2632.
13. Bucy RP, Chen CH, Cihak J, Lösch U, Cooper MD. Avian T cells expressing γδ receptors localize in the splenic sinusoids and the intestinal epithelium. *J Immunol* 1988;141:2200–2205.
14. Jeurissen SH, Janse EM, Koch G, de Boer GF. Postnatal development of mucosa-associated lymphoid tissues in chickens. *Cell Tissue Res* 1989;258:119–124.
15. Glick B, Holbrook KA, Olah I, Perkins WD, Stinson R. An electron and light microscope study of the caecal tonsil, the basic unit of the caecal tonsil. *Dev Comp Immunol* 1981;5:95–104.
16. Bockman DE, Cooper MD. Pinocytosis by epithelium associated with lymphoid follicles in the bursa of Fabricius, appendix and Peyer's patches. An electron microscopic study. *Am J Anat* 1973;136:455–477.
17. Sowder JT, Chen CH, Ager LL, Chan MM, Cooper MD. A large subpopulation of avian T cells express a homologue of the mammalian T γδ receptor. *J Exp Med* 1988;167:315–322.
18. Cihak J, Ziegler-Heitbrock HWL, Trainer H, Schranner I, Merkenschlager M, Lösch U. Characterization and functional properties of a novel monoclonal antibody which identifies a T cell receptor in chickens. *Eur J Immunol* 1988;18:533–537.
19. Chen CH, Cihak J, Lösch U, Cooper MD. Differential expression of two T cell receptors, TCR1 and TCR2, on chicken lymphocytes. *Eur J Immunol* 1988;18:539–543.
20. Char D, Sanchez P, Chen CH, Bucy RP, Cooper MD. A third sublineage of avian T cells can be identified with a T cell receptor-3-specific antibody. *J Immunol* 1990;145:3547–3555.
21. Lahti JM, Chen CH, Tjoelker LW, et al. Two distinct αβ T-cell lineages can be distinguished by the differential usuage of T-cell receptor Vβ gene segments. *Proc Natl Acad Sci USA* 1991;88:10956–10960.

22. Bucy RP, Chen CH, Cooper MD. Development of cytoplasmic CD3$^+$/T cell receptor-negative cells in the peripheral lymphoid tissues of chickens. *Eur J Immunol* 1990;20:1345–1350.
23. Bucy RP, Coltey M, Chen CH, Char D, Le Douarin NM, Cooper MD. Cytoplasmic CD3$^+$ surface CD8$^+$ lymphocytes develop as a thymus-independent lineage in chick-quail chimeras. *Eur J Immunol* 1989;19:1449–1455.
24. Lefrançois L. Extrathymic differentiation of intraepithelial lymphocytes: generation of a separate and unequal T-cell repertoire? *Immunol Today* 1991;12:436–438.
25. Guy-Grand D, Cerf-Bensussan N, Malissen B, Malassis-Seris M, Briottet C, Vassalli P. Two gut intraepithelial CD8$^+$ lymphocyte populations with different T cell receptors: a role for the gut epithelium in T cell differentiation. *J Exp Med* 1991;173:471–481.
26. Bandeira A, Itohara S, Bonneville M, Burlen-Defranons O, Mota-Santos T, Coutinho A, Tonegawa S. Extrathymic origin of intestinal intraepithelial lymphocytes bearing T-cell antigen receptor γδ. *Proc Natl Acad Sci USA* 1991;88:43–47.
27. Guy-Grand D, Broecke CV, Briottet C, Malassis-Seris M, Selz F, Vassalli P. Different expression of the recombination activity gene RAG-1 in various populations of thymocytes, peripheral T cells and gut thymus-independent intraepithelial lymphocytes suggests two pathways of T cell receptor rearrangement. *Eur J Immunol* 1992;22:505–510.
28. Coltey M, Bucy RP, Chen CH, et al. Analysis of the first two waves of thymus homing stem cells and their T cell progeny in chick-quail chimeras. *J Exp Med* 1989; 170:543–557.
29. Chen CH, Sowder JT, Lahti JM, Cihak J, Lösch U, Cooper MD. TCR3: a third T-cell receptor in the chicken. *Proc Natl Acad Sci USA* 1989;86:2351–2355.
30. Cihak J. Hoffmann-Fezer G, Ziegler-Heibrock HWL, et al. T cells expressing the Vβ1 T-cell receptor are required for IgA production in the chicken. *Proc Natl Acad Sci USA* 1991;88:10951–10955.
31. Dunon D, Cooper MD, Imhof BA. Thymic origin and migration patterns of intestinal γδ T cells. *J Exp Med* 1993;177:257–263.
32. Vainio O, Veromaa TV, Eerola E, Toivanen P. Characterization of two monoclonal antibodies against chicken T lymphocyte surface antigens. In: Weber WT, Ewert DL, eds. *Avian immunology*. New York: Alan R Liss; 1987:99–108.
33. Coltey M, Jotereau FV, Le Douarin NM. Evidence for a cyclic renewal of lymphocyte precursor cells in the embryonic chick thymus. *Cell Differ* 1987;22:71–82.
34. Hein WR, Dudler L, Morris B. Differential peripheral expansion and *in vivo* antigen reactivity of α/β and γ/δ T cells emigrating from the early fetal lamb thymus. *Eur J Immunol* 1990;20:1805–1813.
35. Goodman T, LeFrançois L. Expression of the γ/δ T-cell receptor on intestinal CD8$^+$ intraepithelial lymphocytes. *Nature* 1988;333:855–858.
36. Bucy RP, Chen CH, Cooper MD. Tissue localization and CD8 accessory molecule expression of T γδ cells in humans. *J Immunol* 1989;142:3045–3049.
37. Littman DR. The structure of the CD4 and CD8 genes. *Ann Rev Immunol* 1987;5:561–584.
38. Norment AM, Littman DR. A second subunit of CD8 is expressed in human T cells. *EMBO J* 1988;7:3433–3439.
39. Chan MM, Chen CH, Ager LL, Cooper MD. Identification of the avian homologues of mammalian CD4 and CD8 antigens. *J Immunol* 1988;140:2133–2138.
40. Rocha B, Vassalli P, Guy-Grand D. The Vβ repertoire of mouse gut homodimeric α CD8$^+$ intraepithelial T cell receptor α/β$^+$ lymphocytes reveals a major extrathymic pathway of T cell differentiation. *J Exp Med* 1991;173:483–486.
41. Lillehoj HS, Chai J-Y. Comparative natural killer cell activites of thymic bursal, splenic and intestinal intraepithelial lymphocytes of chickens. *Dev Comp Immunol* 1988;12:629–643.
42. Myers TJ, Schat KA. Natural killer cell activity of chicken intraepithelial leukocytes against rotavirus-infected target cells. *Vet Immunol Immunopathol* 1990;26:157–170.
43. Chai J-Y, Lillehoj HS. Isolation and functional characterization of chicken intestinal intra-epithelial lymphocytes showing natural killer activity against tumour target cells. *Immunology* 1988;63:111–117.
44. Lam KM, Linna TJ. Transfer of natural resistance to Marek's disease (JMV) with non-immune spleen cells. I: Studies of cell population transferring resistance. *Int J Cancer* 1979;24:662–667.
45. Lillehoj HS. Intestinal intraepithelial and splenic natural killer cell responses to Eimerian infections in inbred chickens. *Infect Immun* 1989;57:1879–1884.
46. Chung K-S, Lillehoj HS. Development and functional characterization of monoclonal antibodies recognizing chicken lymphocytes with natural killer cell activity. *Vet Immunol Immunopathol* 1991;28:351–363.

47. Lanier LL, Spits H, Phillips JH. The developmental relationship between NK cells and T cells. *Immunol Today* 1992;13:392–395.

48. Terry LA, Disanto JP, Small TN, Flomenberg N. Differential expression of the CD8 and Lyt-3 antigens on a subset of human T-cell receptor γ/δ-bearing lymphocytes. In: Knapp W, Dorken B, Gilks WR, et al., eds. *Leucocyte typing IV. White cell differentiation antigens.* Oxford: Oxford University Press; 1989:345–346.

49. Trinchieri G. Biology of natural killer cells. *Adv Immunol* 1987;47:187–376.

50. Schat KA, Calnek BW, Weinstock D. Cultivation and characterization of avian lymphocytes with natural killer cell activity. *Avian Pathol* 1986;15:539–556.

51. Back O. Studies on the lymphocytes in the intestinal epithelium of the chicken. I: Ontogeny. *Acta Pathol Microbiol Scand* 1972;80:84–90.

52. Kitagawa H, Hashimoto Y, Kon Y, Kudo N. Light and electron microscopic studies on chicken intestinal globule leukocytes. *Jpn J Vet Res* 1988;36:83–117.

53. Lanier LL, Chang C, Spits H, Phillips JH. Expression of cytoplasmic CD3ε proteins in activated human adult natural killer (NK) cells and CD3γ,δ,ε complexes in fetal NK cells. *J Immunol* 1992;149:1876–1880.

54. Back O. Studies on the lymphocytes in the intestinal epithelium of the chicken. III. Effect of thymectomy. *Int Arch Allergy Appl Immunol* 1970;39:192–200.

55. Back O. Studies on the lymphocytes in the intestinal epithelium of the chicken. IV. Effect of bursectomy. *Int Arch Allergy Appl Immunol* 1970;39:342–351.

56. Rodewald H-R, Moingeon P, Lucich JL, Dosiou C, Lopez P, Reinherz EL. A population of early fetal thymocytes expressing FcγRII/III contains precursors of T lymphocytes and natural killer cells. *Cell* 1992;69:139–150.

57. Hynes RO. Integrins: versatility, modulation, and signaling in cell adhesion. *Cell* 1992;69:11–25.

58. Haury M, Kasahara Y, Schaal S, Bucy RP, Cooper MD. Intestinal T lymphocytes in the chicken express an integrin-like antigen. *Eur J Immunol* 1993;23:313–319.

59. Kilshaw PJ, Murant SJ. A new surface antigen on intraepithelial lymphocytes in the intestine. *Eur J Immunol* 1990;20:2201–2207.

60. Cerf-Bensussan N, Guy-Grand D, Lisowska-Grospierre B, Griscelli C, Bhan AK. A monoclonal antibody specific for rat intestinal lymphocytes. *J Immunol* 1986;136:76–82.

61. Cerf-Bensussan N, Jarry A, Brousse N, Lisowska-Grospierre B, Guy-Grand D, Griscelli C. A monoclonal antibody (HML-1) defining a novel membrane molecule present on human intestinal lymphocytes. *Eur J Immunol* 1987;17:1279–1285.

62. Micklem KJ, Dong Y, Willis A, et al. HML-1 antigen on mucosa-associated T cells, activated cells, and hairy leukemic cells is a new integrin containing the β7 subunit. *Am J Pathol* 1991;139:1297–1301.

63. Parker CM, Cepek KL, Russell GJ, Shaw SK, Posnett DN, Schwarting R, Brenner MB. A family of β7 integrins on human mucosal lymphocytes. *Proc Natl Acad Sci USA* 1992;89:1924–1928.

64. Yuan Q, Jiang W-M, Hollander D, Leung E, Watson JD, Drissansen GW. Identity between the novel integrin β7 subunit and an antigen found highly expressed on intraepithelial lymphocytes in the small intestine. *Biochem Biophys Res Commun* 1991;176:1443–1449.

65. Kilshaw PJ, Murant SJ. Expression and regulation of β7(βp) integrins on mouse lymphocytes: relevance to the mucosal immune system. *Eur J Immunol* 1991;21:2591–2597.

66. Schieferdecker HL, Ullrich R, Weiss-Breckwoldt AN, Schwarting R, Stein H, Riecken E-O, Zeitz M. The HML-1 antigen of intestinal lymphocytes is an activation antigen. *J Immunol* 1990;144:2541–2549.

67. Lawn AM, Rose ME, Bradley JWA, Rennie MC. Lymphocytes of the intestinal mucosa of chickens. *Cell Tissue Res* 1988;251:189–195.

68. Mosley L, Whetsell M, Klein JR. Proliferative properties of murine intestinal intraepithelial lymphocytes (IEL): IEL expressing TCRαβ or TCRγδ are largely unresponsive to proliferative signals mediated via conventional stimulation of the CD3-TCR complex. *Int Immunol* 1991;3:563–569.

69. Mowat AM, Tait RC, MacKenzie S, Davies MDJ, Parrott DMV. Analysis of natural killer effector and suppressor activity by intraepithelial lymphocytes from mouse small intestine. *Clin Exp Immunol* 1983;52:191–198.

70. Miyawaki T, Kasahara Y, Taga K, Yachie A, Taniguchi N. Differential expression of CD45R0 (UCHL1) and its functional relevance in two subpopulations of circulating TCR-γ/δ + lymphocytes. *J Exp Med* 1990;171:1833–1838.

71. Sarnacki S, Begue B, Bue H, Le Deist F, Cerf-Bensussan N. Enhancement of CD3-induced activa-

tion of human intestinal intraepithelial lymphocytes by stimulation of the β7-containing integrin defined by HML-1 monoclonal antibody. *Eur J Immunol* 1992;22:2887–2892.

72. Fujihashi K, Taguchi T, Aicher WK, McGhee JR, Bluestone JA, Eldridge JH, Kiyono H. Immunoregulatory functions for murine intraepithelial lymphocytes: γ/δ T cell receptor-positive (TCR⁺) T cells abrogate oral tolerance, while α/β TCR⁺ T cells provide B cell help. *J Exp Med* 1992; 175:695–707.

73. Lillehoj HS, Ruff MD, Bacon LD, Lamont SJ, Jeffers TK. Genetic control of immunity to *Eimeria tenella*. Interaction of MHC genes and non-MHC linked genes influences levels of disease susceptibility in chickens. *Vet Immunol Immunopathol* 1989;20:135–148.

74. Lillehoj HS, Ruff MD. Comparison of disease susceptibility and subclass specific antibody response in SC and FP chickens experimentally inoculated with *E. tenella, E. acervulina,* or *E. maxima. Avian Dis* 1987;31:112–119.

75. Lillehoj HS. Effects of immunosuppression on avian coccidiosis: cyclosporin A but not hormonal bursectomy abrogates host protective immunity. *Infect Immun* 1987;55:1616–1621.

Mucosal Immunology: Intraepithelial Lymphocytes,
edited by H. Kiyono and J. R. McGhee.
Raven Press, Ltd., New York © 1993.

13

The Protection of Epithelial Integrity by Intraepithelial Lymphocyte Populations: γδ T Cell Receptors Constitutively and Inducibly Associated with Epithelia

Adrian C. Hayday, Scott J. Roberts, and Erastus C. Dudley

*Department of Biology and Section of Immunobiology,
Yale University, 219 Prospect St., New Haven, CT.*

Located at the interface of the body with the external environment, intraepithelial lymphocytes (IEL) seem ideally placed to provide a first line of defense against pathogens, such as human immunodeficiency virus, that frequently first encounter the body at an epithelial surface. Moreover, human epithelial surfaces are a major site for the development of malignancy, and if malignant or premalignant cells are to elicit an immune response, again IEL seem ideally situated to provide a first line of surveillance. Thus, in 1988, we presented an hypothesis that IEL might serve both these functions (1). In this chapter, we assess the current validity of this hypothesis, with particular reference to the role of γδ TCR$^+$ IEL. In so doing, we consider recently derived data, pertinent to the hypothesis, that two types of γδ TCR are associated with epithelial sheets—one constitutively, the other inducible upon infection (2).

γδ TCR$^+$ IEL AND THE FIRST LINE OF DEFENSE HYPOTHESIS

Interest in IEL increased in response to the demonstration that in chickens and in mice, the IEL repertoires are disproportionately enriched in γδ TCR$^+$ T cells (3–7). Hence, attempts have been made to understand IEL on the basis of properties that distinguish γδ TCR$^+$ T cells from αβ TCR$^+$ T cells. Possibly the most distinctive property of γδ TCR$^+$ T cells is their limited TCR diversity (8). The relatively small number of functional Vγ genes (six or seven in mice, eight in humans) limits the *combinatorial* diversity theoretically available to the γδ TCR (8). Moreover, combinatorial diversity is *de facto* further limited in specific murine epithelia by the predominant use of only a single Vγ region (e.g., Vγ5 in skin γδ TCR$^+$ T cells; Vγ6 in uterine γδ TCR$^+$ T cells; Vγ7 in gut γδ TCR$^+$ T cells) (9). While it is theoretically true that γδ TCRs can exploit high *junctional* diversity, there has been no formal demonstration that junctional diversity significantly enhances antigen specificity either for γδ TCR⁺ T cells in general, or for epithelial γδ T cells in particular. Moreover, in the murine γδ TCR⁺ T cell repertoires of the skin, uterine, and oral epithelia, junctional diversity is also extremely limited (9–11).

The derivation of epithelial γδ TCR⁺ T cells with limited junctional diversity can be traced back to highly favored gene rearrangements among early fetal thymocytes (11,12). The abundance of these rearrangements cannot be attributed to positive selection on T cells expressing the corresponding TCR, because the same junctions are favored even in cases where the γδ TCR cannot be expressed as protein (13,14). This having been said, it remains plausible that the remarkable homogeneity of γδ TCR sequences in some epithelial repertoires is enhanced by a selective advantage conferred upon cells expressing the corresponding TCRs.

The limited diversity of epithelial γδ TCR⁺ T cells was hypothesized by us to be compatible with putative constraints on antigen presentation unique to epithelia (1). Specifically, if IEL recognize antigen on either epithelial cells or epithelia-associated macrophages/dendritic cells, the restricted mobility of those APCs within epithelial sheets will limit, relative to the systemic circulation, the number of antigen-presenting-cell–T-cell interactions that can occur in a set period of time. Thus, for any IEL to be activated, the antigen surveillance system must forgo the exquisite antigen specificity conferred by high TCR junctional diversity, since this reduces the probability of any one T cell undergoing a successful interaction with an antigen presenting cell. Instead, a high probability of successful interactions must rely on TCRs of reduced diversity, specific for a few (possibly one) antigens. To effect protection of epithelial integrity against a variety of challenges, we argued that the antigen is likely to be a self-antigen, expressed at unusual levels when epithelial cells are infected, transformed, or in other ways "stressed." Candidate antigens include class Ib major histocompatibility complex (MHC) proteins (1), and heat-shock proteins (hsps) (10). The recognition mechanism of the ligand by the γδ TCR maybe akin to that of superantigen (SAG) recognition by αβ TCRs (15). Since hsps in particular are expressed at very high levels even in the uninduced state, it may be that the ligand for the TCR is expressed constitutively, and that upon stress, epithelial cells activate IEL by induction of a second signal. The beneficial effector response of activated γδ TCR⁺ IEL might range from direct cytolysis of infected epithelial cells, to the secretion of cytokines that regulate an effective local immune response (1).

TESTS OF THE FIRST LINE OF DEFENSE HYPOTHESIS

T Cell Specificity for Stress Antigens: γδ TCR⁺ T Cells and Some αβ TCR⁺ T Cells Recognize Stress-Associated Antigens on Unconventional APCs

Studies have identified, from both humans and mice, γδ TCR⁺ T cells that release IL-2 in response to recognition of hsps. The initial such description was by O'Brien et al. (16) for a set of murine thymic γδ TCR⁺ hybridomas that react to mycobacterial hsp63. Moreover, most of the hybridomas spontaneously secrete IL-2 (very rare among αβ TCR⁺ T cell hybridomas), apparently because of a response to highly conserved mouse hsp63 presented by the T cell hybridomas themselves (16). The response is inhibitable with anti-CD3 antibodies, thereby implicating the TCR in the recognition events. The major hsp63 epitope maps to positions 180 to 196 on the protein, and a synthetic peptide of this sequence elicits a response from the hybridomas, suggesting that the cells recognize processed antigen, as do αβ TCR[+] T cells (17). Moreover, injection of this peptide into mice leads to an increased capability to derive hsp-reactive γδ TCR[+] hybridomas *de novo* (18). However, the fact that different γδ TCR[+] T cell hybridomas with different junctional γδ TCR sequences (19) recognize the same hsp peptide raises doubts about the strict parallel of this recognition with αβ TCR[+] T cell recognition of peptides. That hsp63 recognition might be more akin to a V-region specific SAG response is supported by the usage by responding hybridomas of a common Vγ region, Vγ1, and frequently a single Vδ region, Vδ6.3 (18,19). Likewise, numerous Vγ9 Vδ2(+) and human γδ T cells recognize the Burkitts lymphoma, Daudi, in a response that also involves self-hsp63 recognition (20).

Recognition of hsps is also implicated as a property of epithelial γδ TCR[+] T cells. Murine, dendritic, epidermal Vγ5, Vδ1(+) T cells release IL-2 after co-culture with syngeneic keratinocytes, particularly with those that have been heat-shocked (21,22). Hence, taken together, these data support the hypothesis that γδ TCR[+] cells, including those in epithelia, recognize self-stress antigens on the surface of unorthodox APCs.

Class Ib MHC recognition by γδ TCR[+] T cells has also received experimental support. Murine γδ TCR[+] T cell lines have been described that recognize products of the TL locus (23,24). A general relevance of such recognition is suggested by the expression of TL27[b](T22[b]) on the intestinal epithelium, where it may be capable of antigen presentation to IEL (25,26). Moreover, general induction of serine esterase activity in γδ TCR[+] IEL by exposure to TL has been reported (27). Furthermore, the murine γδ TCR[+] T cell response to the synthetic peptide polymer $G^{50}T^{50}$ (glutamic acid, tyrosine) is restricted by Qal, rather than by highly polymorphic class I or class II MHC products (28).

Such properties are not unique to γδ TCR[+] T cells. Some αβ TCR[+] T cells have been described with nonpolymorphic class I MHC recognition specificities (29). Interestingly, such αβ TCR[+] T cells may themselves be disproportionately associated with epithelia, where the αβ TCR repertoire may be of more limited diversity (30,31). For example, gut-associated human αβ TCR[+] T cells have been described that recognize CD1 antigens (30), and CD1 antigen expression is detectable on gut epithelium (32,33). Hence, IEL, whether αβ TCR[+] or γδ TCR[+], may share structural and functional properties that include the recognition of stress-associated antigens and MHC polypeptides on unconventional APCs.

Epithelial γδ TCR T Cell Responses: Epithelium-Associated T Cell Populations Show Conspicuous Changes in Response to Natural, Epithelial-Tropic Pathogens

Although provocative, the capability of γδ TCR[+] T cell lines and hybridomas and epithelial αβ TCR[+] T cells to recognize heat-shocked epithelial cells, hsps, class Ib MHC, and CD1 is insufficient in and of itself to support the first line of defense hypothesis. To test the hypothesis further, we and others have tested the assumption that a first line of defense would presumably show some response to natural agents of epithelial stress.

By day 12 postinfection (D12PI) of mice with influenza virus, the numbers of γδ TCR$^+$ T cells that could be recovered in the lung lavage was significantly increased (34). At this point TCR$^+$ significantly elevated expression of hsp63 RNA was detectable by hybridization *in situ* (34,35). These data strongly suggest that epithelial stress elicits directly or indirectly, responses among lung-associated γδ TCR$^+$ T cells. However, the most dramatic increase in γδ TCR$^+$ cell numbers occurred relatively late (after the significant increase in αβ TCR$^+$ T cells) and not immediately (as might be expected for a first line of defense). Moreover, a problem besetting full interpretation of these data is the difficulty in demonstrating that the γδ TCR$^+$ T cell changes are reflective of a true, epithelium-associated repertoire. To overcome this, we examined the response of intestinal epithelial T cells to stress induced by infection with the naturally occurring, epithelial-tropic, coccidian protozoan, *Eimeria vermiformis*.

After administration by lavage of sublethal doses of *E. vermiformis* to BALB/c mice, the number of IEL (γδ TCR$^+$ and αβ TCR$^+$) increases over four-fold between D10PI and D15PI (36). By cell surface marker analysis, the increased numbers of cells appear to be *bona fide* CD8$^+$ IEL (36). Hence, this clearly demonstrates a capability of gut IEL populations (γδ TCR$^+$ and αβ TCR$^+$) to respond to natural challenges of the epithelium. However, as with the influenza infection of the lung epithelium, the major increase in IEL occurs subsequent to the major increase in numbers of systemic αβ TCR$^+$ T cells (as measured by mesenteric lymph node swelling).

Histological examination of gut tissue from *Eimeria*-infected mice revealed few if any mitoses among IEL. Thus, changes in the IEL populations in infected mice are not easily attributed to IEL proliferation *in situ*. A similar situation exists in human wheat protein sensitive enteropathies, such as coeliac disease, where significant increases in IEL T cell numbers also cannot be correlated with increased mitoses *in situ*. Instead, the increases in IEL T cells may be attributable to infiltration from the systemic circulation and/or to renewed hematopoiesis (see below).

γδ TCR$^+$ IELs and Tumor Surveillance: Immune Surveillance of Tumors Has Not Been Attributable to an IEL T Cell Response to Stress Proteins

Although ideally placed to monitor deleterious cell transformation events within epithelia, IEL in general, and γδ TCR$^+$ IEL in particular, have not been strongly linked to any form of immune tumor surveillance. In cases where immunogenic tumor-associated antigens have been identified, they have comprised alterations in self-protein expression that are recognized by circulating αβ TCR$^+$ T cells (37). In cases where tumor infiltrating "lymphocytes" have been studied, there has been little evidence for a major role for stress antigen reactive $\gamma\delta$ TCR$^+$ cells (38). Furthermore, SCID mice and RAG½ -/- mice that contain no B or T cells show no clear evidence for increased incidences of tumor development.

However, this issue is not fully resolved. The capability of $\gamma\delta$ TCR$^+$ and other IEL T cells to interact *in vitro* with *bona fide* epithelial cells at various stages of cell transformation has not been thoroughly studied, in large part because appropriate culture conditions both for IEL and for a spectrum of epithelial cells have not been fully developed. Moreover, the failure of RAG½ -/- mice to develop tumors at an increased rate relative to immunocompetent mice may not have been assessed under the appropriate conditions of tumor induction. Thus, the potential of IEL of limited diversity to recognize transformed cells by virtue of their expression of stress-related antigens remains to be fully examined.

Dual $\gamma\delta$ TCR Expression in IELs: Intestinal IEL Populations and Hybridomas Show Expression of Productively Rearranged Vγ7 and Vγ1 Genes

Murine $\gamma\delta$ TCR$^+$ T cells that are constitutively associated with different epithelia demonstrate, to a first approximation, a striking tissue-specific pattern of $\gamma\delta$ TCR expression (Vγ5-Vδ1 in the skin; Vγ6-Vδ1 in the tongue; Vγ7-Vδ4 in the gut). However, both in the lungs of influenza-infected mice and in the intestines of *Eimeria*-infected mice, a conspicuous pattern of Vγ1 (and/or Vγ2) expression becomes apparent. By T cell sorting, the induced expression among the IEL of *Eimeria*-infected mice could be attributed to $\gamma\delta$ TCR$^+$ IEL (36). Moreover, by use of a novel PCR population analysis (39), the expression was shown to be of productively rearranged Vγ1 genes (see Fig. 4 in ref. 39). Likewise, in pairs (rather than pools) of mice studied by Kyes and Hayday (2), $\gamma\delta$ TCR$^+$ T cells isolated from several epithelia showed productively rearranged Vγ1 expression that varied dramatically from mouse to mouse. Expression was particularly strong in the intestines of mice adventitiously infected with the enteric form of mouse hepatitis virus (2). As a result, we have postulated the general existence of two distinct types of $\gamma\delta$ TCR$^+$—one type being constitutively associated with an epithelium and the other being inducible within epithelia after infection (2). The potential value to the host of this induced expression is unknown, but it is interesting that the induced Vγ1-gene is commonly associated with recognition of hsps, which are expressed in increased levels in tissues subject to infection or damage.

To further examine this aspect of $\gamma\delta$ TCR usage in intestinal IEL, a series of $\gamma\delta$ TCR$^+$ hybridomas were made using as a fusion partner the TCR deficient variant of BW5147 (40). Two such hybridomas were studied in great detail. They both express productively rearranged Vγ7 genes—ordinarily associated with gut $\gamma\delta$ TCR$^+$ T cells. However, they both additionally express productively rearranged Vγ1 (41). This gene was not expressed in the fusion partner. A similar failure of isotypic exclusion was demonstrated for a $\gamma\delta$ TCR$^+$ T cell hybridoma, studied by Heilig and

Tonegawa (42), that also harbored two productive TCR γ gene rearrangements. Although the surface coexpression of two $\gamma\delta$ TCRs has not been demonstrated for these hybridomas, such was the case for a skin $\gamma\delta$ TCR$^+$ T cell line studied by Koning and colleagues (43).

These observations of multiple productive γ TCR gene rearrangements in cloned $\gamma\delta$ TCR$^+$ T cells may be attributable to an artifact of cell culture, particularly of hybridomas. Alternatively, these observations may be consistent with the increased expression of productively rearranged Vγ1 genes *in vivo* in IEL postinfection with *Eimeria* (36), and in adventitiously infected mice (2). The organization of the murine γ TCR gene locus renders possible coexpression of Vγ1 and Vγ2 with Vγ7 rearrangements (8). Thus, the increased expression of Vγ1 that we detect in $\gamma\delta$ TCR$^+$ cells postinfection of mice may be attributable to induced expression and/or rearrangement of Vγ1 genes in cells already positive for other (Vγ7) rearrangements. This hypothesis could account for the increase in Vγ1 expression in the absence of overt IEL proliferation.

However, the hypothesis cannot be simply accepted without acknowledgment of the significant predictions that it makes in several areas. For example, it suggests that gene rearrangement (RAG½ activity) continues in a cell with a productive γ gene rearrangement. In fact, multiple TCR usage may not be unique to $\gamma\delta$ TCR$^+$ T cells. $\alpha\beta$ TCR$^+$ T cells have been described with more than one productive rearrangement at the α TCR locus (44), and, consistent with this, ongoing rearrangement in certain $\alpha\beta$ TCR$^+$ T cell lines (45) and in thymocytes (46) has been demonstrated. Thus, whether ongoing TCR gene rearrangement is a common physiologic property of IEL warrants investigation.

In addition, the fact that Vγ1 rearrangements in the IEL examined are disproportionately productive suggests that the Vγ1-based product of the rearrangement confers a selective advantage on the cells expressing it. In turn, this suggests that such cells may functionally co-express two TCRs *in vivo*, in apparent violation of the clonal selection hypothesis. Is it possible that $\gamma\delta$ TCR$^+$ T cells and/or epithelial T cells do not "obey" the clonal selection paradigm? Perhaps—if the response of the T cells in question fulfills any of the following criteria: (a) The cells do not circulate, and thus have little likelihood of (potentially harmful) contact with numerous host cells; (b) the cells neither expand extensively nor initiate an expansive immune response, also limiting (potentially harmful) interactions with self; and (c) the TCRs in question do not make a "self–nonself discrimination," because they are primarily reactive to self-stress antigens. Since all of these are plausible for $\gamma\delta$ TCR$^+$ IEL, the capability for ongoing or multiple TCR gene rearrangement in IEL needs to be further examined. This will demand protocols that facilitate IEL cloning and differentiation *in vitro*.

IEL: CELLS AT A CROSSROADS

The dynamic responses of IEL populations to natural epithelial challenge, coupled with the characterized specificities of $\gamma\delta$ TCR$^+$ T cell lines and hybridomas for stress-associated antigens on unconventional APCs, all support the hypothesis that IEL in general, and $\gamma\delta$ TCR$^+$ IEL in particular, respond to potential breaches of epithelial integrity.

Whether this constitutes a first line of defense is a matter for debate. *Defense* implies a contribution to the host's suppression of the pathogen. The effector responses of IEL *in vivo* remain to be characterized before *defense* can be an accepted descriptor. *First line* may seem at variance with the "delayed" kinetics of the major increases in IEL in infected animals. However, this takes a too narrow view of *first line*. Primary infection by an epithelial-tropic pathogen is, in most cases, rapidly followed by replication of the pathogen, thereby creating a massively increased pathogen load capable of secondary infection of the host. For example, after *E. vermiformis* infection of BALB/c mice, oocysts are shed starting at D7PI. After one day's oxygenated sporulation, there will be a huge titer of infectious parasite in the local environment. It is possible that at this time (approximately D8PI through D12PI) $\alpha\beta$ T cell mediated, species-specific immunity has not yet developed. Thus, the large increase in the number of IEL detectable at these time points may be of value in attenuating reinfection (discussed in ref. 36). Possible mechanisms include cytolysis of infected enterocytes or secretion of IFN-γ that inhibits intracellular pathogen replication. It is possible that inhibitory cytokines released by IEL are also effective inhibitors of local lymphocytic infiltrates from the systemic circulation. If this is so, a major function of IEL may be to prevent breaches of epithelial integrity that could result from acute unregulated inflammation.

SUMMARY

The IEL repertoire is dynamic under conditions of natural infection, and stands at an anatomical crossroad where it may preserve epithelial integrity from threats that come both from without (pathogens) and from within (the host's immune system). Whether, by virtue of the latter capacity, IEL constitute suppressor T cells (47), needs to be thoroughly investigated. The creation of "knockout mice," such as the $\alpha\beta$ TCR$^+$ T cell deficient mice that we recently codeveloped (48), should aid greatly in such investigations.

ACKNOWLEDGMENTS

We should like to express our thanks to Drs C. A. Janeway, Jr., R. Tigelaar, and R. C. Findly for their advice, ideas, and enthusiasm for this work, and to the N.I.H. for grant support.

REFERENCES

1. Janeway CA Jr, Jones B, Hayday AC. Specificity and function of cells bearing $\gamma\delta$ T cell receptors. *Immunol Today* 1988;9:73–76.
2. Kyes S, Hayday AC. Disparate types of $\gamma\delta$ T cells. *Res Immunol* 1990;141:582–587.

3. Bucy P, Chen CL, Cihak J, Löaxh U, Cooper M. Avian T cells expressing γδ receptors localize in the splenic sinusoids and the intestinal epithelium. *J Immunol* 1988;141:2200–2205.
4. Kuziel WA, Takashima A, Bonyhadi M, Bergstresser J, Allison P, Tigelaar RE, Tucker PW. Regulation of T cell receptor γ chain RNA expression in murine thy-1(+) dendritic epidermal cells. *Nature* 1987;328:263–266.
5. Stingl G, Koning F, Yamada H, et al. Thy-1$^+$ dendritic epidermal cells express T3 antigen and the T-cell receptor γ chain. *Proc Natl Acad Sci USA* 1987;84:4586–4589.
6. Goodman T, Lefrançois L. Expression of the γδ T cell receptor on intestinal CD8(+) intraepithelial lymphocytes. *Nature* 1988;333:855–858.
7. Kyes S, Carew E, Carding SR, Janeway CA Jr, Hayday AC. Diversity in T cell receptor γ gene usage in intestinal epithelium. *Proc Natl Acad Sci USA* 1989;84:5527–5531.
8. Hayday A. T cell receptor γδ. In: Delves P, Roitt I, eds. *Encyclopedia of Immunology*. London: Academic Press; 1992:1428–1433.
9. Itohara S, Farr A, Lafaille JJ, Bonneville M, Takagaki Y, Haas W, Tonegawa S. Homing of a gamma delta thymocyte subset with homogeneous T-cell receptors to mucosal epithelia. *Nature* 1990;343:754–757.
10. Asarnow DM, Kuziel WA, Bonyhadi M, Tigelaar RE, Tucker PW, Alison JP. Limited diversity of γδ antigen receptor genes of Thy-1(+) dendritic epidemeral cells. *Cell* 1988;55:837–847.
11. Lafaille JJ, DeCloux A, Bonneville M, Takagaki Y, Tonegawa S. Junctional sequences of T cell receptor γδ genes: implications for γδ T cell lineages and for a novel intermediate of V-(D)-J joining. *Cell* 1989;59:859–870.
12. Havran W, Allison JP. Origin of Thy-1$^+$ dendritic epidermal cells of adult mice from fetal thymic precursors. *Nature* 1990;344:68–70.
13. Itohara S, Mombaerts P, Lafaille JJ, Iacomini J, Nelson A, Farr A, Tonegawa S. T cell receptor δ gene mutant mice: independent generation of αβ T cells and programmed rearrangements of γδ T cell receptor genes. *Cell* 1993;72:337–348.
14. Asarnow DM, Cado D, Raulet DH. Selection is not required to produce invariant T cell receptor γ gene junctional sequences. *Nature* 1993;362:158–160.
15. Rust CJJ, Verreck F, Vietor H, Koning F. Specific recognition of staphylococcal enterotoxin A by human T cells bearing receptors with the Vγ9 region. *Nature* 1990;346:572–574.
16. O'Brien RL, Happ MP, Dallas A, Palmer E, Kubo R, Born WK. Stimulation of a major set of lymphocytes expressing T cell receptor γδ by an antigen derived from *Mycobacterium tuberculosis*. *Cell* 1989;57:667–674.
17. Born WK, Hall L, Dallas A, et al. Recognition of a peptide antigen by heat shock reactive γδ T lymphocytes. *Science* 1990;249:67–69.
18. Fu Y-X, Cranfill R, Vollmer M, van der Zee R, O'Brien RL, Born WK. In vivo response of murine γδ T cells to heat shock protein derived peptide. *Proc Natl Acad Sci USA* 1993;90:322–326.
19. Happ MP, Kubo RT, Palmer E, Born WK, O'Brien RL. Limited receptor repertoire in a mycobacteria-reactive subset of γδ lymphocytes. *Nature* 1989;342:696–698.
20. Fisch P, Malkovsky M, Kovats S, et al. Recognition by human Vγ9/Vδ2 T cells of a GroEL homolog on Daudi Burkitts lymphoma cells. *Science* 1990;250:1269–1273.
21. Havran W, Chien Y-H, Allison JP. Recognition of self antigens by skin-derived T cells with invariant γδ antigen receptors. *Science* 1991;252:1430–1432.
22. Tigelaar RE, Lewis. Recognition of heat-stressed autologous murine keratinocytes by skin-derived γδ(+) dendritic epidermal T cell lines. *Personal communication*.
23. Bluestone JA, Cron RQ, Cotterman M, Houlden RA, Matis LA. Structure and specificity of γδ T cell receptor on major histocompatibility complex antigen-specific CD3$^+$, CD4$^-$, CD8 T lymphocytes. *J Exp Med* 1988;168:1899–1916.
24. Ito K, Van Kaer L, Bonneville M, Hsu S, Murphy DB, Tonegawa S. Recognition of the product of a novel MHC TL region gene (27^b) by a mouse γδ T cell receptor. *Cell* 1990;62:549–561.
25. Wu M, Van Kaer L, Itohara S, Tonegawa S. Highly restricted expression of the thymic leukemia antigens on intestinal epithelial cells. *J Exp Med* 1991;174:213–218.
26. Hershberg R, Eghtesady P, Sydora B, Brorson K, Cheroutre H, Modlin R, Kronenberg M. Expression of the thymus leukemia antigen in the intestinal epithelium. *Proc Natl Sci USA* 1990;87:9727–9731.
27. Eghtesady P, Kronenberg M. Intestinal γδ T lymphocytes are autoreactive for stressed intestinal epithelial cells.1992; *unpublished communication*.
28. Vidovic D, Roglic M, McKune K, Guerder S, MacKay C, Dembic Z. Qa-1 restricted recognition of foreign antigen by a γδ T-cell hybridoma. *Nature* 1989;340:646–650.

29. Porcelli S, Brenner MB, Greenstein JL, Balk SP, Terhorst C, Bleicher PA. Recognition of cluster of differentiation 1 antigen by human CD4⁻CD8⁻ cytolytic T lymphocytes. *Nature* 1989;341:447–450.

30. Balk SP, Ebert EC, Blumenthal RL, McDermott FV, Wucherpfennig KW, Landau SB, Blumberg RS. Oligoclonal expansion and CD1 recognition by human intestinal intraepithelial lymphocytes. *Science* 1991;253:1411–1415.

31. Dunn DA, Gadenne A-S, Simha S, Lerner EA, Bigby M, Bleicher PA. T cell receptor Vβ expression in normal human skin. *Proc Natl Acad Sci USA* 1993;90:1267–1271.

32. Blumberg RS, Terhorst C, Bleicher P, et al. Expression of a nonploymorphic MHC class I-like molecule, CDId, by human intestinal epithelial cells. *J Immunol* 1991;147:2518–2524.

33. Bleicher PA, Balk SP, Hagen SJ, Blumberg RS, Flotte TJ, Terhorst C. Expression of murine CD1 on gastrointestinal epithelium. *Science* 1990;250:679–682.

34. Carding SR, Allen W, Kyes S, Hayday A, Bottomly K, Doherty P. Late dominance of the inflammatory process in murine influenza by γδ(+) T cells. *J Exp Med* 1990;172:1225–1231.

35. Kyes S. Ontogeny and tissue specificity of murine γδ T cell receptor gene expression. *Ph.D. thesis*, Yale University; 1990.

36. Findly RC, Roberts SJ, Hayday AC. Dynamics of murine intestinal intraepithelial T cell populations after infection by the coccidian parasite, *Eimeria*. *Eur J Immunol* 1993; *submitted for publication*.

37. van der Bruggen P, Troversari C, Chomez P, et al. A gene encoding an antigen recognised by cytolytic T lymphocytes on a human melanoma. *Science* 1991;254:1643–1647.

38. Fajac I, Tazi A, Hance AJ, Bouchonnet F, Riquet M, Battesti JP, Soler P. Lymphocytes infiltrating normal human lung and lung carcinomas rarely express γδ T cell antigen receptors. *Clin Exp Immunol* 1992;87:127–131.

39. Mallick C, Dudley EC, Viney J, Owen MJ, Hayday AC. Rearrangement and diversity of T cell receptor β chain genes in thymocytes: a critical role for the β chain in development. *Cell* 1993;73:513–519.

40. Sano Y, Dudely EC, Hayday AC, Janeway CA Jr. γδ(+) intraepithelaial T cell hybridomas that recognise the B cell lymphoma line. *Immunol* 1993, *in press*.

41. Dudley EC, Sano Y, Janeway CA Jr, Hayday AC. T cell receptor structure in γδ(+) intraepithelial T cell hybridomas that recognise the B cell lymphoma line; *unpublished data*.

42. Heilig JS, Tonegawa S. T-cell γ gene is allelically but not isotypically excluded and is not required in known functional T-cell subsets. *Proc Natl Acad Sci USA* 1987;84:8070–8074.

43. Koning F, Yokoyama WM, Maloy WL, et al. Expression of Cγ4 T cell receptors and lack of isotype exclusion by dendritic epidermal T cell lines. *J Immunol* 1988;141:2057–2062.

44. Malissen M, Trucy J, Letourneur F, et al. A T cell clone expresses two T cell receptor α genes but uses only one αβ heterodimer for allorecognition and self MHC restricted antigen recognition. *Cell* 1988;55:49–59.

45. Marolleau JP, Fondell J, Malissen M, et al. The joining of germ-line Vα to Jα complexes in a T cell receptor α,β positive T cell line. *Cell* 1988;55:291–300.

46. Petrie H, Livak F, Schatz DG, Strasser A, Crispe IN, Shortman K. Multiple rearrangements in TCR-α chain genes maximize the production of useful thymocytes. *J Exp Med* 1993; *submitted for publication*.

47. McMenamin C, Oliver J, Girn B, Holt BJ, Kees UR, Thomas WR, Holt PG. Regulation of T-cell sensitization at epithelial surfaces in the respiratory tract: suppression of IgE responses to inhaled antigens by CD3⁺ TcR α⁻/β⁻ lymphocytes (putative γ/δ T cells). *Immunology* 1991;74:234–239.

48. Philpott K, Viney JL, Kay G, et al. Lymphoid development in mice congenitally lacking T cell receptor αβ-expressing cells. *Science* 1992;256:1448–1452.

Mucosal Immunology: Intraepithelial Lymphocytes,
edited by H. Kiyono and J. R. McGhee.
Raven Press, Ltd., New York © 1993.

14

Antigen-Specific Cytotoxic T-Lymphocytes in the Intestinal Epithelium

Christopher F. Cuff

*Department of Microbiology and Immunology, West Virginia University School of
Medicine, Health Sciences Center, Morgantown, WV.*

This chapter is devoted to a discussion of cytotoxic T-lymphocytes (CTL) in the intestinal intraepithelial compartment. Although the term CTL can be broadly applied to many types of lymphocytes that mediate cytotoxic activity in *in vitro* assays, we will restrict most of our discussion to studies that describe cytotoxic intraepithelial lymphocytes (IEL) that (a) appear as a result of antigen stimulation, and (b) mediate specific activity against that antigen following challenge. These criteria help us focus our discussion on the adaptive immune response of IEL, which is both inducible and antigen-specific. In addition to discussing the experimental evidence that demonstrates the function of CTL in the IEL compartment, we will consider the developmental relationship between CTL in the IEL and other lymphoid tissue. Finally, we will consider the development of CTL in the context of the concept of the intestinal epithelium as a site of extrathymic T cell differentiation.

CTL IN THE IEL COMPARTMENT

From an immunologist's perspective, a classical definition of CTL is that CTL are thymus-derived, CD8[+], Thy-1[+] T cells that recognize protein antigens in the context of class I major histocompatibility (MHC) antigens via an antigen-specific $\alpha\beta$ T cell receptor for antigen ($\alpha\beta$ TCR). In addition to expressing CD8, Thy-1, and $\alpha\beta$ TCR, several other surface antigens are expressed on activated CTL including CD2 (1), CD28 (2), CD44 (3), CD45 (4) and CD3.5 (germinal center and T cell antigen; GCT) (5).

A second class of antigen-specific CTL has also been described. These are CD4[+] CTL that lyse targets in a Class II MHC restricted manner. The role of CD4[+] CTL in intestinal immunity is not understood. Recent evidence suggests that CD4[+] CTL could be important immune effectors, particularly in the absence of class I MHC-restricted CTL (6–8). The relationship between CD4[+] CTL and CTL in the IEL compartment will also be addressed.

In general, it is thought that the role of CTL in maintaining the integrity of the host is to recognize and destroy aberrant cells, whether these aberrant cells are infected by an intracellular pathogen or have undergone transformation. Two features of the intestinal epithelium and the IEL are consistent with the notion that CTL could play such a role in protecting the host. First, there is now general agreement that a significant proportion of IEL express the phenotype of mature CTL. Second, these IEL are intimately associated with absorptive epithelial cells, which are potential targets for CTL. These epithelial cells provide a delicate boundary between the external environment of the intestinal lumen and the internal environment of the host.

From a teleological perspective, there seems to be a need for a mechanism to survey the epithelium for aberrant cells. Although the epithelial cells at the tips of villi are fully differentiated and destined to be sloughed into the lumen and out of the host, stem cells in the crypts and epithelial cells that are not fully differentiated could serve as target cells for invading microbes to gain entry into the host and escape the protective action of IgA antibodies. In addition, the stem cells in the intestinal crypts are constantly undergoing cell division, rendering these cells more susceptible to DNA damage and resulting transformation. Thus, a mechanism specifically to survey the intestinal epithelium can provide a selective evolutionary advantage to the host. This is not a new idea. Immune surveillance was proposed as a function of $\gamma\delta$ TCR$^+$ IEL shortly after the initial description of these cells (9). However in contrast to the current state of the art for $\gamma\delta$ TCR$^+$ IEL, antigen-specific CTL function can be ascribed to conventional T cells in the IEL compartment.

FUNCTIONAL STUDIES OF CTL IN THE IEL COMPARTMENT

Alloantigen-Specific CTL

Using the criteria of inducibility and specificity to define CTL in the IEL compartment, the first report of CTL in the IEL compartment was made by Davies and Parrott in 1980 (10). These investigators found that CTL activity could be induced in the IEL of mice that were given an intraperitoneal challenge with allogeneic P-815 mastocytoma cells. The CTL activity in the IEL paralleled the response of mesenteric lymph node lymphocytes in that the response was elicited after intraperitoneal but not subcutaneous challenge. In addition, the response was greater at 11 days than at 3 days postchallenge. These studies were extended in 1983 by the same group (11). The investigators reported that the CTL activity was specific for the cell that was used to elicit cytotoxic IEL, and that the effector cell population was depleted with anti-Thy-1 antiserum.

One of the difficulties in studying antigen-specific CTL activity in IEL populations is that IEL also contain populations of nonspecific cytotoxic cells, which can contribute to the observed cytotoxicity. This was clearly demonstrated by Klein and Kagnoff (12), who examined the CTL response of IEL from mice primed with alloantigens. The investigators found that alloimmunization upregulated the natural killer (NK) and spontaneously cytotoxic (SC) activity of IEL as well as inducing a cytotoxic cell response against the alloantigens (13). Nonetheless, these studies demonstrated that there was a cytotoxic cell response that was inducible and had some degree of specificity. Still, little was known about the phenotype(s) of the specific effector cells, the kinetics of the response, and the role of the CTL response of IEL in immunity to enteric infection. Additional communications by this group indicated that two CTL clones of IEL derived from alloimmunized mice expressed either antigen-specific activity or a broad reactivity against allogeneic and syngeneic targets (14). The broadly reactive clones were cytotoxic when cultured with high concentrations of interleukin-2, but proliferated in an antigen-specific manner when they were maintained in low concentrations of cytokines. Both clones were Thy-1$^+$, Lyt-2$^+$ and asialoGm-1$^+$. Long-term *in vitro* culture of alloantigen-specific CTL derived from the intestinal epithelium lost the ability to lyse targets in an antigen-specific manner, but maintained the ability to proliferate in an antigen-specific manner (15). Because these phenomena distinguished IEL from splenic alloantigen-specific CTL clones, the authors speculated that these CTL from the epithelium could be derived from thymus-independent precursors and thus could be distinguished from conventional T cells derived from peripheral lymphoid tissues.

In 1986, Ernst et al. (16) published an extensive study detailing the phenotype and frequency of alloantigen-specific precursor CTL (CTLp) that developed in the epithelium following *in vitro* activation of alloantigen-specific IEL. Their studies conclusively demonstrated that inducible (*in vitro*), antigen-specific CTL could be generated from IEL. In this system, IEL from H-2^k mice were activated in one-way mixed lymphocyte cultures with allogeneic splenocytes of the H-2^d or H-2^b haplotypes. When the resulting CTL were tested against syngeneic tumor cell targets, it was found that cytotoxicity was significantly higher against tumors that expressed the H-2 haplotype that was syngeneic to the stimulator cells. More convincingly, IEL efficiently lysed blast cells from concanavalin A (Con A)-stimulated spleen cells that were syngeneic to the stimulators, but mediated no activity against Con A-stimulated splenocytes that were not of the same haplotype as the stimulator. The investigators also demonstrated that the CTL were Thy-1$^+$ and Lyt-2$^+$ (CD8α). In addition, the CTLp were shown to be Thy-1$^+$ and Lyt-2$^+$ by depletion or cell sorting prior to *in vitro* stimulation. Limiting dilution analyses indicated that the frequency of alloantigen-specific CTLp were 1 to 2 per 10^4, as compared to frequencies of specific CTLp in spleen of 2 to 5 per 10^4. Thus, IEL contained populations of alloantigen-specific CTL or CTLp that appeared to be similar in phenotype and function to conventional CTL in the periphery. The authors conjectured that the IEL could mount an immune response against enteric pathogens. However, it had not yet been shown that IEL could mediate a CTL response against an enteric pathogen.

Virus-Specific Cytotoxic IEL

Two viruses have been shown to induce a classical CTL response by IEL. These closely related enteric viruses are reovirus and rotavirus. Reovirus (respiratory enteric orphan virus) is a nonenveloped, double-stranded, RNA-containing virus that is ubiquitous in nature and naturally infects many mammalian species. It has been demonstrated that reovirus serotype 1/Lang (1/L) specifically binds to membranous (M) cells that cover the Peyer's patches (17). This specific binding to M cells, coupled with the fact that reovirus is a self-replicating antigen in the gastrointestinal tract, probably accounts for the potent cellular and humoral mucosal immune responses that are observed following infection.

London et al. (18) reported that enteric reovirus infection elicited reovirus-specific CTLp in the Peyer's patches, which gave rise to virus-specific CTL following secondary *in vitro* culture with virus-pulsed antigen-presenting cells. The effector CTL were CD8[+] and Thy-1[+]. A secondary report (19) characterized virus-specific CTLp that appeared in the epithelium 1 week after priming. Upon secondary *in vitro* restimulation, these CTLp gave rise to CTL that lysed reovirus-infected targets in an antigen-specific, MHC-restricted manner. Shortly after this paper was submitted for publication, Goodman and Lefrançois (20) and Bonneville et al. (21) reported that many murine IEL expressed γδ TCR. The hypothesis that the reovirus-specific CTLp were derived from γδ TCR bearing IEL was tested by examining both the CTLp and the CTL from reovirus-infected mice. It was found that the reovirus-reactive cells were conventional αβ TCR bearing T cells based on the findings that enteric infection in germ-free mice elicits a response that can be shown by flow cytometric analysis to be dominated by the appearance of αβ TCR[+] IEL (22); the CD8[+], Thy-1[+] CTL that appear following secondary *in vitro* culture are almost exclusively αβ TCR[+]; and CTL activity is blocked by anti-TCR complex antibodies. Furthermore, a large proportion of αβ TCR[+] IEL can be obtained from reovirus-infected severe combined immunodeficient mice (scid) that were reconstituted with immunocompetent Peyer's patch lymphocytes prior to infection (23, 24). Thus, enteric reovirus infection in mice provided a system to study the generation of CTL in gut-associated lymphoid tissue, including IEL, following an infection with an enteric virus. Additional studies describing the capacity of these cells to protect a host against infection are described below.

A similar system to study cellular mucosal immunity using enteric infection of mice with a simian strain of rotavirus, RRV strain 2, has been developed by Offit et al. (25). Unlike reovirus, rotavirus infection is a common cause of diarrhea in children worldwide. Rotaviruses are members of the *Reoviridae* family and share several structural and biologic features with the orthoreovirus used in our studies. Perhaps the most significant difference between rotavirus and reovirus is that, while reovirus specifically binds to M cells, rotavirus expresses a tropism for mature epithelial cells on the tips of villi in susceptible hosts. The tropism may be age-related because children, but not adults, are typically affected by rotavirus infection. In the rotavirus system, adult mice that are enterically infected with simian rotavirus mount an immune response that is characterized by the generation of CTLp in local and distal sites, and the transient appearance of virus-specific CTL in the epithelium (25). The rotavirus-specific CTL in IEL are also αβ TCR[+] based on blocking experiments with TCR-specific antibodies. Although enteric reovirus infection results in the generation in the epithelium of CTLp that are functionally and phenotypically identical to the CTLp that appear in the Peyer's patches, rotavirus infection does not induce CTLp in the IEL (26). Although a trivial explanation, such as culture conditions, could explain this observation, it is likely that differences in tissue tropism of the two viruses result in the induction of distinctive immune responses.

ROLE OF IEL IN IMMUNITY

Although it is possible to demonstrate *in vitro* CTL activity of IEL against alloantigens and viral pathogens, the role of IEL in protecting the host against infection is somewhat harder to demonstrate. Using a model of chronic rotavirus infection in scid mice, Dharakul et al. (27) reported that passive transfer of CD8$^+$, Thy-1$^+$ IEL from rotavirus-primed syngeneic donors into rotavirus-infected scid neonates transiently reduced rotavirus shedding in recipient mice. The IEL, given by the intraperitoneal route, appeared to migrate to the epithelium of the recipient mice and mediate a transient reduction in viral shedding in the absence of specific antibody.

We have examined the capacity of IEL to transfer protection against lethal meningoencephalitis in neonatal mice caused by reovirus serotype 3 clone 9 (28). Oral inoculation of 1 to 2-day-old mice with the neurotropic strain of reovirus causes an often fatal meningoencephalitis in infected neonates. Intraperitoneal transfer of reovirus-immune IEL can passively protect infected neonates against the lethal effects of the disease and the development of pathologic changes in the central nervous system of infected animals. The protective cells are CD8$^+$ and Thy-1$^+$, indicating that CTL could be responsible for protection, but the mechanism of protection and the site of viral clearance remains to be elucidated. Taken together, these data indicate that in addition to inducing a specific CTL response in the IEL, the effector cell population in IEL can play a role in ameliorating the effects of enteric viral infection.

ENTERIC VIRUS INFECTION INDUCES OTHER CYTOTOXIC CELL ACTIVITY

We have focused our discussion thus far on CTL in the IEL compartment that are inducible and specific. In addition to the aforementioned studies, we should also consider the effects of virus infection of the gut on the activation of other less well-defined cytotoxic cell function of IEL. In addition to classical CTL activity, atypical CTL activity has been shown to develop in IEL from animals following enteric infection. For example, Carman et al. (29) reported that enteric infection of specific pathogen-free mice with murine coronavirus (MHV-Y) induced the activation of a population of cytotoxic IEL that preferentially lysed MHV-Y infected NCTC-1469 cells. The cytotoxic IEL were not MHC-restricted, but they were specific because the cytotoxic IEL did not preferentially kill targets that were infected with nonenterotropic Pichinde virus. Based on depletion experiments, the phenotype of the cytotoxic population appeared to be asialoGm-1$^+$, but Thy-1$^-$ and Lyt-2$^-$. More recently, a similar resonse of bovine IEL was observed by Godson et al. (30). These investigators found that IEL from calves that were acutely infected with bovine coronavirus (BCV) preferentially lysed BCV-infected Madin Darby bovine kidney cells. It is plausible that the population(s) of murine and bovine IEL that react against coronavirus-infected mice are developmentally related to the broadly cytotoxic IEL that developed following alloimmunization described by Klein et al. (12–15).

γδ TCR$^+$ IEL AS CTL

The IEL contain a significant proportion of γδ TCR$^+$ IEL. It has been shown that these γδ TCR$^+$ IEL are cytotoxic in redirected lysis assays. However, the specificity of these cells, as well as the role of the γδ TCR$^+$ IEL in protecting the host against infection, remains to be elucidated. Some progress has been made in identifying molecules that might be important in the function of γδ TCR$^+$ IEL as CTL. Bonneville et al. (31) produced a γδ TCR-expressing hybridoma from adult thymocytes, designated KN6, which specifically recognized a molecule encoded by the TL locus of the MHC. This report raised speculation that the γδ TCR$^+$ IEL might recognize TL antigens expressed on the gut epithelium. This speculation was supported by reports from Hershberg et al. (32) and Wu et al. (33) that intestinal epithelial cells expressed TL-encoded proteins in a tissue-specific manner. Furthermore, this expression was observed in strains of mice previously thought to be TL$^-$. In a TL$^-$ mouse strain (C57Bl/6), expression of the T1 gene T3 was not observed in tissues where other γδ TCR$^+$ cells are commonly found, such as the lung, uterus, and epidermis. However, Vidovic et al. (34) also described γδ TCR$^+$ hybridomas that recognized similar nonpolymorphic class I MHC molecules encoded by the class I Qa locus. Thus, it is possible that TL or Qa-encoded surface proteins could serve as ligands for γδ TCR$^+$ IEL. These ligands could present microbial antigens or endogenous antigens such as heat-shock proteins to the γδ TCR$^+$ IEL, which could then act as CTL. Although this is an attractive, nearly irresistible hypothesis, supportive experimental data have not yet been reported.

THYMUS-INDEPENDENT IEL AS CTL

The observation reported by Rocha et al. (35), that IEL contain a population of αβ TCR$^+$ lymphocytes that express a novel form of CD8 (CD8αα or CD8αβ) and were not subject to the same selection processes as conventional T cells, renewed interest in reconsidering the intestinal epithelium as a site of extrathymic differentiation. This concept was suggested as early as 1968 by Fichtelius (36). However, the advances made in understanding T cell biology, thymic differentiation, and IEL phenotype have made it possible to manipulate experimental systems to assess the development and function of extrathymically derived IEL. The recent findings that significant numbers of IEL can express potentially autoreactive TCR, yet remain nonreactive in terms of *in vitro* proliferation (37), have implications in the study of CTL. The important issue is to determine whether these cells differentiate into CTL that recognize antigen following priming in the gut. Because these IEL express TCR that are normally deleted in the periphery, it is reasonable to speculate that the $\alpha\beta$ TCR$^+$ IEL have a potential repertoire that is larger than that of the T cells in the periphery. This may be useful in providing protection against pathogens that express determinants that resemble self-peptides. It remains to be determined how such potentially autoreactive CTL could distinguish between self and non-self, or if class I MHC molecules encoded by the K, D, L, TL, or Qa loci act as restriction elements for such CTL.

SUMMARY

The literature suggests that the IEL contains a population of CD8$^+$ cells that can act as antigen-specific CTL or CTLp following enteric challenge with antigen. It is our belief that in some cases, these cells are derived in the Peyer's patches from precursors that migrate from the Peyer's patches to the epithelium, as suggested by Guy-Grand et al. (38). Precursor frequency analysis of reovirus-specific CTLp from the Peyer's patches and epithelium supports this hypothesis in enteric reovirus infection (23,24). Because of the phenotype, TCR expression, antigen-specificity, and MHC-restriction of these cells, we consider them to be thymus-dependent, conventional T cells. It is likely that these T cells could play an important role defending the host from microbial invasion through the gastrointestinal tract, particularly in response to viral pathogens.

A second population of more promiscuous cytotoxic cells also are present in the epithelium. They appear to be either cross-reactive against tumor targets or antigen-specific but MHC-nonrestricted. These cytotoxic cells have some characteristics that are related to classical CTL in that they are, in some cases, inducible and antigen-specific. This is particularly true in systems utilizing enteric coronavirus infection (29,30). The developmental relationship between the classical CTL and these other cytotoxic cells remains to be elucidated. However, because cells with this promiscuous cytotoxic activity are typically not found at high frequencies in the periphery, and because the IEL contain populations of CD$\alpha\alpha$, $\gamma\delta$ TCR$^+$ and CD8$\alpha\alpha$, $\alpha\beta$ TCR$^+$ IEL that are not commonly found in the periphery, it is reasonable to speculate that the atypical cytotoxic cells are unique to the intestinal epithelium. What is needed is a demonstration that CD8$\alpha\alpha$ IEL, either the $\gamma\delta$ TCR$^+$ or $\alpha\beta$ TCR$^+$ populations, can mediate CTL activity that is inducible and specific. The next step would be to demonstrate that these cells could play a part in protecting the host against infection.

Not to be forgotten is the observation that the IEL contain populations of CD4$^+$, $\alpha\beta$ TCR$^+$ IEL that may also develop extrathymically. It may be of interest to determine whether these cells express CTL function, particularly in light of the observations that epithelial cells express class II MHC molecules and can present antigen (39).

In conclusion, we and others have made progress in characterizing the functional potential of IEL with regard to antigen-specific CTL activity. These cells may provide an important first line of defense against invasion by enteric pathogens, containing dissemination of microbes out of the intestine, or eliminating transformed epithelial stem cells. The relationship between the antigen-specific CTL and populations of lymphocytes that are unique to the epithelium, such as CD8αα cells, remains unresolved. The availability of probes such as reovirus to study biologically relevant, antigen-specific pertubations in the function and physiology of IEL will contribute to our understanding of the biology of IEL.

ACKNOWLEDGMENTS

The author thanks Drs. Thomas J. Rogers, Donald H. Rubin, and John J. Cebra. The author also thanks Dr. John J. Cebra for critically reviewing this manuscript. This work was supported by U.S. Public Health Service grant AI-23970 and Institutional Research grant IRG-181B from the American Cancer Society.

REFERENCES

1. Sanchez-Madrid F, Krensky AM, Ware CF, et al. Three distinct antigens associated with human T-lymphocyte-mediated cytolysis: LFA-1α, LFA-2 and LFA-3. *Proc Natl Acad Sci USA* 1982;79:7489–7493.
2. Chen L, Ashe S, Brady WA, et al. Costimulation of antitumor immunity by the B7 counterreceptor for the T lymphocyte molecules CD28 and CTLA-4. *Cell* 1992;71:1093–1102.
3. Budd R, Cerottini J, MacDonald HR. Phenotypic identification of memory cytolytic T lymphocytes in a subset of Lyt-2 + cells. *J Immunol* 1987;138:1009–1013.
4. Lefrançois L, Bevan MJ. Functional modifications of cytotoxic T lymphocyte T200 glycoprotein recognized by monoclonal antibodies. *Nature* 1985;314:449–451.
5. London SD, Cebra-Thomas J, Rubin DH, Cebra JJ. CD8 lymphocyte subpopulations in Peyer's patches induced by reovirus serotype 1 infection. *J Immunol* 1990;144:3187–3194.
6. Eichelberger M, Allan W, Zijlstra M, Jaenisch R, Doherty PC. Clearance of influenza virus respiratory infection in mice lacking class I major histocompatibility complex-restricted CD8 + T-cells. *J Exp Med* 1991;174:875–880.
7. Hou S, Doherty P, Zijlstra M, Jaenisch R, Katz J. Delayed clearance of Sendai virus in mice lacking class I MHC-restriced CD8 + T-cells. *J Immunol* 1992;149:1319–1325.
8. Muller D, Killer BH, Whitton JL, Lepan KE, Brigman KK, Frelinger JA. LCMV-specific class II-restricted cytotoxic T-cells in β₂ microglobulin deficient mice. *Science* 1992;255:1576–1578.
9. Janeway CA, Jones B, Hayday A. Specificity and function of T-cells bearing γ/δ receptors. *Immunol Today* 1988;9:73–76.
10. Davies MDJ, Parrott DMV. The early appearance of specific cytotoxic T-cells in murine gut mucosa. *Clin Exp Immunol* 1980;42:273–279.
11. Parrott DMV, Tait C, MacKenzie S, Mowat A, Davies MDJ, Micklem, HS. Analysis of the effector functions of different populations of mucosal lymphocytes. *Ann N Y Acad Sci* 1983;409:307–319.
12. Klein J, Kagnoff M. Nonspecific recruitment of cytotoxic effector cells in the intestinal mucosa of antigen-primed mice. *J Exp Med* 1984;160:1931–1936.
13. Klein JR. Ontogeny of the Thy-1 ⁻, Lyt-2 ⁺ murine intestinal intraepithelial lymphocyte: characterization of a unique population of thymus-independent cytotoxic effector cells in the intestinal mucosa. *J Exp Med* 1986;164:309–314.

14. Klein J, Lefrançois L, Kagnoff M. A murine cytotoxic T lymphocyte clone from the intestinal mucosa that is antigen specific for proliferation and displays broadly reactive inducible cytotoxic activity. *J Immunol* 1985;135:3697–3702.

15. Klein JR, Kagnoff MF. Spontaneous *in vitro* evolution of lytic specificity of cytotoxic T lymphocyte clones isolated from murine intestinal epithelium. *J Immunol* 1987;138:58–62.

16. Ernst PB, Clark DA, Rosenthal KL, Befus AD, Bienenstock J. Detection and characterization of cytotoxic T lymphocyte precursors in the murine intestinal intraepithelial leukocyte population. *J Immunol* 1986;136:2121–2126.

17. Wolf JL, Rubin DH, Finberg R, Kauffman RS, Sharpe AS, Trier JS, Fields BN. Intestinal M cells: a pathway for entry of reovirus into the host. *Science* 1981;212:471–472.

18. London SD, Rubin DH, Cebra JJ. Gut mucosal immunization with reovirus serotype 1/L stimulates virus specific cytotoxic T-cell precursors as well as IgA memory cells in Peyer's patches. *J Exp Med* 1987;165:830–847.

19. London SD, Cebra JJ, Rubin DH. Intraepithelial lymphocytes contain virus-specific, MHC-restricted cytotoxic cell precursors after gut mucosal immunization with reovirus serotype 1/Lang. *Reg Immunol* 1989;2:98–102.

20. Goodman T, Lefrançois L. Expression of γ/δ T-cell receptor on intestinal CD8[+] intraepithelial lymphocytes. *Nature* 1988;333:855–858.

21. Bonneville M, Janeway CA, Ito K, Haser W, Nakanishi N, Tonegawa S. Intestinal intraepithelial lymphocytes are a distinct set of γ/δ T-cells. *Nature* 1988;336:479–481.

22. Cuff CF, Hooper DC, Kramer D, Rubin DH, Cebra JJ. Functional and phenotypic analyses of the mucosal immune response in mice: approaches to studying the immunogenicity of antigens applied by the enteric route. *Vaccine Res* 1992;1:175–182.

23. Cebra JJ, Cuff CF, Rubin DH. Relationship between alpha/beta T cell receptor/CD8+ precursors for cytotoxic T lymphocytes in the murine Peyer's patches and the intraepithelial compartment probed by oral infection with reovirus. *Immunol Res* 1991;10:321–323.

24. Cuff CF, Cebra CK, Rubin DH, Cebra JJ. Developmental relationship between cytotoxic α/β T-cell receptor+ intraepithelial lymphocytes and Peyer's patch lymphocytes. *Eur J Immunol* 1993;23:1333–1339.

25. Offit P, Dudzik K. Rotavirus-specific cytotoxic T-lymphocytes appear at the intestinal mucosal surface after rotavirus infection. *J Virol* 1989;63:3507–3509.

26. Offit PA, Cunningham SL, Dudzik KI. Memory and distribution of virus-specific cytotoxic T lymphocytes (CTL) and CTL precursors after rotavirus infection. *J Virol* 1991;65:1318–1324.

27. Dharakul T, Rott L, Greenberg HB. Recovery of chronic rotavirus infection in mice with severe combined immunodeficiency: virus clearance mediated by adoptive transfer of immune CD8[+] T lymphocytes. *J Virol* 1990;64:4375–4382.

28. Cuff CF, Cebra CK, Lavi E, Molowitz EH, Cebra JJ, Rubin DH. Protection of neonatal mice from fatal reovirus infection by immune serum and gut derived lymphocytes. *Adv Exp Med Biol* 1991;310:307–315.

29. Carman PS, Ernst PB, Rosenthal K, Clark DA, Befus AD, Bienenstock J. Intraepithelial leukocytes contain a unique subpopulation of NK-like cytotoxic cells active in the defense of gut epithelium to enteric murine coronavirus. *J Immunol* 1986;136:1548–1553.

30. Godson DL, Campos M, Babiuk L. Non-major histocompatibility complex-restricted cytotoxicity of bovine coronavirus-infected target cells mediated by bovine intestinal intraepithelial leukocytes. *J Gen Virol* 1991;72:2457–2465.

31. Bonneville M, Ito K, Krecko EG, et al. Recognition of a self major histocompatibility complex TL region product by γδ T-cell receptors. *Proc Natl Acad Sci USA* 1989;86:5928–5932.

32. Hershberg R, Eghtesady P, Sydora B, Brorson K, Cherourtre H, Modlin R, Kronenberg M. Expression of the thymus leukemia antigen in mouse intestinal epithelium. *Proc Natl Acad Sci USA* 1990;87:9727–9731.

33. Wu M, Kaer LV, Itohara S, Tonegawa S. Highly restricted expression of the thymus leukemia antigens on intestinal epithelial cells. *J Exp Med* 1991;174:213–218.

34. Vidovic D, Roglic M, McKune K, Guerder S, MacKay C, Dembic Z. Qa-1 restricted recognition of foreign antigen by a γ/δ T-cell hybridoma. *Nature* 1989;340:646–650.

35. Rocha B, Vassalli P, Guy-Grand D. The Vβ repertoire of mouse gut homodimeric α CD8+ intraepithelial T cell receptor α/β + lymphocytes reveals a major extrathymic pathway of T cell differentiation. *J Exp Med* 1991;173:483–486.

36. Fichtelius KE. The gut epithelium: a first level lymphoid organ? *Exp Cell Res* 1968;49:87–95.

37. Poussier P, Philippe E, Lee C, Binnie M, Julius M. Thymus-independent development and negative selection of T cells expressing T cell receptor α/β in the intestinal epithelium: evidence for distinct circulation patterns of gut- and thymus-derived T lymphocytes. *J Exp Med* 1992;176:187–199.
38. Guy-Grand D, Griscelli C, Vassalli P. The mouse T-lymphocyte, a novel type of T-cell: nature, origin, and traffic in mice in normal and graft-versus-host conditions. *J Exp Med* 1978;148:1661–1677.
39. Bland PW, Kambarage D. Antigen handling by the epithelium and lamina propria macrophages. In: McDermott RP, Elson CO, eds. *Gastroenterology Clinics of North America*. Philadelphia: WB Saunders Co; 1991;20:577–596.

Subject Index

A